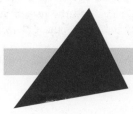

This text is dedicated to my wife Pat for her continuing patience and support during this and all of my professional endeavors.

Contents

CHAPTER 4

FLEXIBILITY   72

CHAPTER 5

DEVELOPING THE MUSCULAR COMPONENT   94

CHAPTER
6

DEVELOPING THE CARDIORESPIRATORY COMPONENT 130

CHAPTER
7

CARDIOVASCULAR DISEASES 148

**CHAPTER
8**

OTHER CHRONIC CONDITIONS 182

**CHAPTER
9**

THE BASICS OF NUTRITION   212

**CHAPTER
10**

THE REDUCTION EQUATION: EXERCISE + SENSIBLE EATING = FAT CONTROL   236

CHAPTER 11

THE CONSEQUENCES OF NEGATIVE CHOICES 270

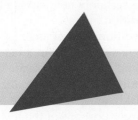

Preface

The aim of the third edition of this text is the same as the first—to establish through contemporary evidence the connection between physical fitness and wellness. The fact that this is a third edition attests to the unceasing interest in fitness and wellness by college and university instructors and their students. There has been an explosion of new information since the first edition appeared in 1986, and the proliferation of information has continued at a brisk pace since the second edition was published in 1990. The massive research effort in this exciting field is evident as a host of researchers submit the results of their work to medical, exercise science, and nutritional science journals for publication. The steady stream of new information clearly indicated that another revision was in order, and once again, several important challenges had to be addressed.

The first challenge was to solicit feedback from adopters of the book regarding the book's utility, level of difficulty, and research orientation. Most of the respondents to a marketing survey conducted by West Publishing Company, while applauding the up-to-date documentation, suggested the documentation be scaled down so as not to overwhelm the reader. This was a difficult but not insurmountable task that resulted in only the most important and representative references being cited in this edition. The references that were ultimately selected for inclusion in the text represent a fraction of those that were read in preparation for writing the manuscript.

A second challenge was deciding what and how much would be deleted from the second edition. These difficult decisions had to be made to keep the text within manageable proportions yet expansive enough to convey the nature of the relationship between physical fitness and wellness as it is scientifically observed at this writing. Every chapter in this new edition has been significantly improved by the addition of new information and the deletion of outdated material. As a result, this edition is a little larger than the second edition, which again attests to the ongoing explosion of information being generated in this field. On a number of occasions during the writing of the manuscript, concepts, principles, and standards that were once accepted as truths by the scientific community had to be changed, updated, or replaced with newer information. These changes were made to assure that the text would be as current as possible when it went to print.

Several goals were established for the third edition. The primary objective is to inform college-age students regarding the development of physical fitness and wellness. Carefully selected research is the foundation of the text and the method through which the primary objective of providing pertinent information is met. The second objective is to help students gain insight into their own physical fitness and health status by providing a variety of self-assessment instruments. A third objective is that the text would aid college and university instructors as they teach basic fitness and wellness courses, because the text pulls together current research data from exercise science, medicine, nutrition, and the allied health professions. To this end, this edition is amply referenced not only to validate the information that it contains but also to provide a convenient and handy source for those who are interested in pursuing information beyond the book's scope. This edition, like its predecessors, attempts to establish a sound base for lifetime participation in physical fitness activities and an active way of living. Although the "why" of exercise is emphasized, the "how" is certainly not neglected. In fact, this aspect has been somewhat expanded in this edition.

Many changes have occurred in the third edition that separate it from the first two editions. First and foremost, this edition has moved from a black-and-white format into a full-color text. The illustrations and photos have made the text more attractive. Second, more headings and subheadings have been strategically placed throughout the text so that the reader can quickly grasp the essence of the material that follows. The headings also break up larger portions of the text into smaller segments that are more easily digestible. To further facilitate comprehension of the material, some of the vocabulary and physiological terms have been simplified or deleted. Third, every chapter contains features entitled "Safety Tips" and "Facts, Fallacies, and Timely Tidbits" that enrich the text and add to the interest level. Boxed readings on selected current topics add flavor to the text.

Fourth, this edition features up-to-date statistics as well as new photos, illustrations, tables, charts, and figures. The summaries at the end of each chapter (Chapter Highlights) are in the form of individual statements rather than in narrative form, making it easier to identify important chapter concepts. (It might be helpful to read the Chapter Highlights before reading the chapter itself.)

Fifth, a total of 34 self-assessment instruments and tests are placed together in Appendix C at the back of the book. This procedure, which deviates from the format of previous editions, was chosen (1) so as not to bulk up each chapter, (2) so that the self-assessments would not interrupt the book's conceptual content, and (3) as a means to present them as a group. The tests are perforated for easy removal when they need to be handed in as part of a class assignment. The self-assessments may be administered and supervised by instructors, or they may be taken as outside assignments. Norms and standards are presented as a frame of reference for interpreting their results.

Sixth, adopters of the text will receive, upon request, an updated instructor's manual with chapter outlines and objectives, a test bank, and transparency masters. This convenient aid should help facilitate preparation for the delivery of instruction.

Seventh, items from previous editions that received favorable reviews such as "Points to Ponder," "Margin Notes," and "Miniglossary" were retained and expanded to reflect the new information being presented.

The third edition represents a substantial revision of its predecessor. The chapters not only have been significantly revised but also are presented in a different order. The rationale for changing the order was to present the material as much as possible in approximately the same order that an experienced exerciser would begin a workout or a novice would initiate an exercise program. For example, Chapter 1 lays a foundation for the attainment of wellness through physical fitness. It is important to understand the link between the two and that the fitness component is voluntary, important, and achievable within one's own potential.

Chapter 2 provides a variety of motivational techniques that have been successfully used by both beginners and seasoned exercisers to maintain interest in and enthusiasm for participating in their fitness activities. Chapter 3 issues exercise guidelines with which one must become familiar to maximize the likelihood of effectively and safely achieving one's fitness and wellness objectives. Chapter 4 presents a rationale for improving flexibility through appropriate stretching exercises that should be practiced during every exercise warmup and cooldown period. Chapters 5 and 6 introduce the principles of exercise and their application to the development of musculoskeletal and cardiorespiratory strength and endurance.

Chapters 7 through 11 are primarily informational in nature. It is necessary to understand selected diseases and disorders that can be delayed or prevented through a sound exercise program. Chapters 7 and 8 provide this information. Chapters 9 and 10 cover the basics of nutrition and provide the principles for successfully losing weight in a healthful manner. It seemed important to add Chapter

11, which deals with drugs and sexually transmitted diseases, since the target audience for this text is substantially affected by both.

A textbook is usually not the work of one person, and this effort is no exception. The ideas of many people are represented here. The contributions begin with the data generated by all of the researchers whose works provide the cognitive base for this text. They extend from there to the reviewers whose ideas and suggestions helped to refine the finished product, to the models who contributed to the aesthetics of the text, and to the professional staff of West Publishing Company. Jerry Westby, Manager, College Editorial, directed this project with assistance from Dean De Chambeau, Development Editor, whose cut-and-paste analyses of the reviewers critiques made my job easier; Christine Hurney, Production Editor, who made sure that I met deadlines; and Deborah Cady, Copyeditor, who fine-tuned the language and clarified the ideas.

Many thanks to my good friend Sheri Seiser, who took the photographs that have substantially enhanced the written word. Thanks also to the people who were willing to serve as models for this edition: Wayne Gutch, Renee Moss, Mimi Nguyn, Rob Pearse, Angela Redden, and Duane Sanders. I wish to extend my gratitude to the managers of Q the Sports Club for allowing us to take photos at their premises of our models performing exercises on the club's state-of-the-art equipment. The managers were very patient in allowing us to disrupt their very busy schedules.

Special thanks to Angie Newton who expeditiously transcribed my handwritten scrawl onto a computer disk.

Acknowledgements

As previously mentioned, the reviewers for this text deserve both praise and appreciation for the timely and knowledgeable comments. These individuals are:

Nikki Assman
Ball State University

James W. Jones
Henderson State University

Ralph Barclay
Wayne State College

Timothy Kirby
Ohio State University

Frederick C. Beyer
County College of Morris

Jerry Krause
Eastern Washington University

Sandy Bonneau
Golden West College

Richard W. Latin
University of Nebraska—Omaha

Kay Carter
University of Wisconsin—Stout

Mark Loftin
University of New Orleans

R.L. Case
Sam Houston State University

Joseph J. Lopour
Southern Utah University

Lonnie J. Davis
Eastern Kentucky University

James R. Marett
Northern Illinois University

Brian M. Don
Boston University

Wayne F. Major
University of Georgia

Sandra Flood
Northern Illinois University

Elizabeth Ready
University of Manitoba

Susan Hunter
Memphis State University

Forrest C. Tyson
Springfield College

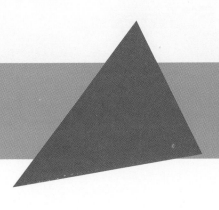

Fitness for Wellness
The Physical Connection

Third Edition

CHAPTER 1

Introduction to Wellness Through Physical Fitness

CHAPTER OUTLINE

INTRODUCTION

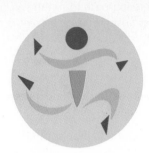

High-level wellness is within reach of most students who read this text. Required first is the basic knowledge of what constitutes a wellness lifestyle along with those behaviors that promote optimal health and well-being. Such a lifestyle can delay or prevent the onset of the chronic diseases (heart attack, stroke, cancer, diabetes, atherosclerosis, and chronic obstructive lung disease) that are disabling and killing the majority of Americans. A second requirement involves the motivation necessary to make the effort to act upon that knowledge. In other words, appropriate behavioral patterns consistent with and based upon the best evidence available today will pay substantial health benefits. This text identifies these behaviors and provides discussions regarding their impact on the quality and quantity of life.

A mountain of contemporary data clearly differentiates positive from negative behaviors and the effect that each has upon wellness or illness. After reading this text, you will understand why the behaviors impact health the way they do.

The text emphasizes the attainment of wellness through physical activity and a physically active lifestyle. The connection between the two will become very evident. If you follow the suggestions made here, you can expect many or all of the following physical fitness and wellness benefits to occur:

1. Improved physical appearance (more muscle, less fat, improved posture).
2. Increased level of energy.
3. Improved self-concept and self-esteem.
4. Greater ability to relax and handle stress, anxiety, and tension.
5. Enhanced mental and emotional well-being.
6. Greater resistance to such chronic diseases as heart disease, strokes, cancer, diabetes, osteoporosis, low-back problems, and other musculoskeletal disorders.

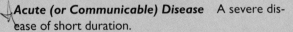

Acute (or Communicable) Disease   A severe disease of short duration.

Agility   The ability to rapidly change direction while maintaining dynamic balance.

Balance   Involves the maintenance of a desired body position either statically or dynamically. Also referred to as equilibrium.

Body Composition   The amount of lean versus fat tissue.

Cardiovascular Disease   A complex of diseases of the heart and circulatory system.

Cardiorespiratory Endurance   The ability to take in, deliver, and extract oxygen for physical work.

Chronic Disease   A long-lasting and/or frequently occurring disease.

Chronological Age   An individual's calendar age.

Coordination   The integration of body parts resulting in smooth, fluid motion.

Flexibility   Range of motion around a specific joint.

Health Age   An individual's biological age.

Health-Related Fitness   A type of fitness that enhances one's health status by modifying many of the risks associated with lifestyle diseases.

Muscular Endurance   The capacity to exert repetitive muscular force.

Continued

—Continued

Muscular Strength   The maximum amount of force that a muscle can exert in a single contraction.

Performance-Related Fitness   A type of fitness that allows one to perform physical skills with a high degree of proficiency.

Power   A function of work divided by the time that it takes to perform the work.

Psychoneuroimmunology   Branch of medical science that studies how the mind affects the endocrine and immune systems.

Reaction Time   The elapsed time between the presentation of a stimulus and the stimulus's response. Also called response latency.

Risk Factor   Genetic tendencies and learned behaviors that increase the probability of premature illness and death.

Speed   Performance of a movement in the shortest amount of time. Also known as velocity.

Wellness   A dynamic approach to health enhancement that emphasizes positive health behaviors and preventive practices.

---

7. Reduction in risk factors for disease, such as high blood pressure, blood serum cholesterol and triglyceride levels, obesity, and stress.

Two Self-Assessment activities appear in Appendix C that apply directly to the contents of this chapter:

1.1 Health/Wellness Inventory

1.2 Your Fitness Attitudes

WELLNESS DEFINED

Wellness is a generic concept characterized by the lifelong pursuit of optimal well-being. High-level wellness is a dynamic approach to health enhancement that emphasizes positive health behaviors and preventive practices. It is a process of growth that evolves and changes. It is not achieved suddenly at a specific time, such as a college degree. Rather, it is an ongoing process—indeed a way of life—through which one encourages the development of every aspect of the body, mind, and emotions.[1] One does not have to live like a monk to achieve high-level wellness. Consistent application of the principles presented in this text will result in health enhancement and a satisfying sense of accomplishment that should motivate one to continue the quest.

Wellness involves optimal development of the physical self, the constructive use and management of stress energy, effectiveness in communicating and dealing with emotions, positive use of the mind, environmental sensitivity, and the development of productive relations with other people. From this description, it is quite clear that the quality of one's health and the quest for total well-being are primarily the responsibility of each individual and not the responsibility of physicians or the conventional medical care and delivery system, government, or society. It is not our intention to denigrate this country's medical care system, which is currently the best in the world. Medical training focuses upon treating diseases rather than preventing them, and there will always be a critical need for these skills. Even if medicine shifted its priorities toward prevention (and this entails considerable resources), the fact remains that we are to a large extent the masters of our own destinies. We ultimately make the choices that influence our health.

Wellness is composed of several interrelated dimensions: social, spiritual, physical, intellectual, and emotional. Each contributes to the overall quality of one's life, but none operates in isolation. Taking care of the physical body has ramifications for the mind and the spirit. After all, the human body is a marvelously integrated amalgam of many systems working together in harmony to

We must stop trying to buy health with our dollars and start earning it with our behaviors.
— Don Ardell *Planning for Wellness*

maintain the life force. Exercising the body for the attainment of total fitness—a reasonable and desirable goal—impacts virtually every facet of wellness. In addition to providing the obvious physical effects on the body, exercise improves self-concept, self-esteem, body image, and emotional well-being, and for some, it provides a sense of spiritual focus. It also provides greater energy for work, study, and meeting intellectual challenges. This is important at every stage of life, but certainly critical during the college years.

Intellectual performance in the classroom affects total well-being. Academic difficulties may negatively permeate other phases of one's life, such as disturbed sleep and emotional stress. They may lead to destructive behaviors such as substance abuse or produce overeating, weight gain, and possibly depression.

The mind and body are interrelated—what affects one will affect the other. Beliefs have the potential to become reality. Programming the mind that it can, in fact, influence the body creates the physiological climate that could fortify the immune system. This proposition, supported by case studies of people who have overcome illness by methods other than medical or clinical, is known as **psychoneuroimmunology.** This area of scientific research focuses on the interactions between the mind and the nervous, endocrine, and immune systems. The immune system is the body's most effective defense against disease, but when weakened, it leads to increased vulnerability to disease. It is now well established that psychological and emotional stress are debilitating to the immune system.

The power of the mind to influence physical health, either positively or negatively, is being vigorously investigated. Medical researchers have developed sophisticated techniques and equipment to study the changes that occur in the immune system as a function of different mental states. For example, such disparate groups as grieving widowers, medical students prior to exams, and depressed people, all of whom were experiencing stress from different sources, exhibited similar responses in their immune systems. The life changes indicated that their immune systems had been weakened. The emotions these people experienced produced chemical changes in the nervous and endocrine systems that resulted in corresponding cellular changes in the immune system. It is only in the past few years that science has been able to identify and document these cellular modifications and to connect them to the mental and emotional conditions that appear to have caused them.

If the immune system is weakened by negative mental and emotional states, how would it react to positive influences? Although enhancement of the immune system from a positive frame of mind is not as well documented, the available evidence does support the notion that the immune system is strengthened by positive influences.

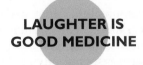

LAUGHTER IS GOOD MEDICINE

A few years ago, Norman Cousins (magazine editor, author, and university professor) claimed that laughter helped speed up his recovery from a serious disease. The study of humor and its effects on the human body has a name: gelotology. In a recent article for the *Journal of the American Medical Association,* Dr. William Fry of Stanford University, a well-known gelotologist, noted that besides increasing heart rate and hormone production, laughter also improves muscle tone and circulation. Indeed, a good laugh is a kind of workout, he says, It's not exactly a major calorie burner—you can laugh yourself silly, but not thin—yet it does help move nutrients and oxygen along to the body's tissues. That might be one reason why a fit of mirth makes people feel better. But don't throw away your running shoes, since aerobic guffawing is hard to do.

If you really want to get serious about laughing, there are at least two groups to contact. The American Association for Therapeutic Humor, at 1163 Shermer Road, Northbrook, Illinois 60062 (telephone 708-291-0211), can supply you with bibliographies on various aspects of humor-as-therapy, as well as a newsletter, *Laugh It Up.* The Humor Project, at 110 Spring Street, Saratoga Springs, New

Continued

—Continued

York 12866 (telephone 518-587-8770), provides workshops, courses, and seminars for people who wish to use humor as a positive force in their work; it also supplies a free information packet on the positive power of humor (send a 9-by-12-inch, self-addressed envelope with 75 cents postage) as well as a magazine called *Laughing Matter*.

Adapted from "Divine Comedy," *University of California at Berkeley Wellness Letter* 8, no. 11 (August 1992): 3.

Spirituality as a dimension of wellness deals with feelings and experiences whereby individuals perceive that they are connected to some spiritual force or higher power that adds significance to their lives. For some, this occurs as a result of membership in an organized religion, for others it comes from science and nature, and for still others it comes from personal and philosophical ethics. Regardless of the mode, in its truest sense, having spirituality confers feelings of inner peace and harmony. Spiritual awareness enables one to lead a healthier life characterized by resiliency in coping with its unrelenting peaks and valleys. These ups and downs are part of life. Learning to handle them with equanimity brings peace, acceptance of oneself, and tolerance of others. True spirituality leads to *joie de vivre*, or joy of living.

HEALTH: A MATTER OF CHOICE

We make choices, both positive and negative, about smoking cigarettes, wearing seat belts, exercise, weight control, nutrition, alcohol intake, frequency of medical examinations, and so on. These choices and the ensuing behavior patterns profoundly affect the state of our health.

Some people make seemingly inappropriate choices and live to a ripe old age, but they are the exception rather than the rule. They have beaten the odds and make headlines as a result. Winston Churchill was an example of one who defied the principles of good health and lived more than 80 years. But one must wonder how much longer he might have lived had he been less indulgent when it came to the harmful excesses in his life. Genetically, he was probably well-endowed for longevity, but his lifestyle practices seemed to detract from his biological potential. The majority of those who follow similar lifestyles die early and become mere statistics in some esoteric piece of research. These people do not make headlines, because their fate is the norm: it is expected, and it is not newsworthy. By featuring these exceptions, the media inadvertently promotes a cavalier attitude toward good health practices.

Figure 1.1 emphasizes the importance of self-responsibility in a wellness lifestyle by assigning to it a central position in the constellation of factors. Living in accordance with this model fosters an attitude of responsibility for our actions and removes the compulsion to blame others or to make excuses for our predicament.

During the past 20 years, many Americans have positively altered their daily habits and accepted responsibility for their own health. Unfortunately, these people still represent a minority of the population. Although the notion that good health is represented by the absence of disease and the avoidance of disability has outlived its usefulness, it continues to persist. Consequently, high-level wellness escapes most Americans, since many continue to rely upon the annual or semi-annual medical exam in the hope that they will receive a "clean bill of health." If they do, the old lifestyle is reinforced, regardless of the healthy or unhealthy practices that characterize it. If the old lifestyle includes cigarette smoking, a diet high in fat and cholesterol, sedentary habits, and an inability to effectively cope with stress, it is virtually certain to lead to premature disease. In fact, the **chronic diseases** (cardiovascular diseases, cancer, diabetes, etc.) that

You the individual can do more for your own health and well-being than any doctor, any hospital, any drug, any exotic medical device.

— Joseph Califano

FIGURE 1.1

A Constellation of Selected Wellness Factors

Adapted from D. Ardell, *Planning for Wellness*, Dubuque, Iowa: Kendall/Hunt, 1982.

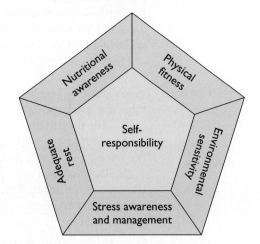

To a greater extent than most of us are willing to accept, today's disorders of overweight, heart disease, cancer, blood pressure, and diabetes are by-and-large preventable. In this light, true health insurance is not what one carries on a plastic card, but what one does for oneself.

— Lawrence Power, M.D.

"Americans annually lose 15 million years of living from preventable causes."

— Surgeon's General Report

TABLE 1.1

Leading Causes of Death Among the U.S. Population

1. Heart disease
2. Cancer
3. Injuries
4. Stroke
5. Chronic lung disease
6. Pneumonia/influenza
7. Suicide
8. Diabetes
9. Liver Disease
10. Atherosclerosis

Source: *Healthy People 2000*, DHHS Publication No. (PHS) 91–50212, Washington, D.C.: U.S. Government Printing Office, 1990.

have replaced the **acute** or **communicable diseases** as the leading causes of death in the past four to five decades are the result of such a lifestyle (see Table 1.1). The chronic diseases are not transmitted from person to person through contact; rather, they are voluntary or self-inflicted. The tendency for developing a few of the chronic diseases appears to run in some families. Whether or when these diseases manifest themselves is influenced substantially by the living habits of those involved. The chronic diseases are not prevented by inoculation, nor can they be cured with antibiotics. They are the calamitous results of the choices people make and the behaviors they practice. Consider the following:

1. Seven of the ten leading causes of death can be substantially reduced by controlling blood pressure, quitting the cigarette habit, eating more wisely, getting regular exercise, and reducing alcohol consumption.
2. The heart attack risk is doubled in men who are cigarette smokers.
3. Ten percent of all deaths in the United States are alcohol related.
4. Occupational hazards are responsible for approximately 20 percent of cancer mortality.
5. Highway accidents are responsible for nearly 50,000 deaths annually. A significant number of them can be prevented with seat belts, shoulder harnesses, and sobriety. According to the National Highway Traffic Administration, 40 percent of all Americans will be involved in an alcohol-related crash during their lives.
6. High blood pressure, a precursor of 500,000 strokes and 1.5 million heart attacks per year, afflicts approximately 17 percent of Americans.
7. Suicide is steadily rising as a leading cause of death among teenagers and young adults.
8. Eighty million Americans are overweight; 70 million have arthritis.
9. Premature employee deaths account for the loss of $20 billion per year.

The difference in the health status of any two Americans is primarily determined by factors beyond a physician's control. By following reasonable rules for healthful living, we can reduce the rate of premature morbidity and mortality. This has become imperative as the cost of disease care rises to a staggering and disproportionate amount of the gross domestic product (GDP). The United States spends a greater share of its GDP on health care than any of the other industrialized nations. In 1979, the nation's total health care bill was $212.2 billion, and it has risen precipitously every year since.[2] By 1992, health care costs reached an astounding $817 billion.[3] Unless the government enacts major health care reform, costs are predicted to escalate to $1 trillion by 1995 and $1.9 trillion by the year

2000. This will represent approximately 16 percent of the GDP and will be the largest single expenditure for Americans. Nearly 12 percent, or $4,296 of the average family income, was spent for health care in 1992.[4] By the year 2000, the cost will exceed 16 percent of the average family income.

Highly sophisticated technology developed to aid physicians in the diagnosis and treatment of disease has added materially to the cost of health care. Table 1.2 gives some examples of the cost of selected medical procedures. Although the table indicates the economic toll, it does not illustrate the human suffering associated with the treatment and rehabilitation associated with these diseases. The earnest pursuit of high-level wellness and the prevention of disease is certainly the wisest and most prudent course of action.

Wellness embodies a characteristic lifestyle—a mindset that personifies a positive approach to health. It is the antithesis of our present health care system, which many have more accurately labeled a "disease care" system. The following article, written by John Grossman, was published in 1981, but its message is as appropriate now as it was then. Not much has changed in the intervening years.

HEALTH CARE OR DISEASE CARE?

Wellness goes beyond prevention in that it initiates a whole new way to conceive of health: not simply as the absence of disease, as most of us have been led to believe, but as a continual process of attaining greater and greater personal well-being. Wellness does not describe dos and don'ts; it's much more than that.

Health promotion is the fiber of wellness. These two words may have a familiar ring to them, since they have indeed been part of our vocabulary for years. In fact, they have long been drowned out by organized medicine's traditional orientation not toward health, but toward illness.

To understand this orientation, it may help to call to mind a legendary Cornish test of sanity. Imagine a running faucet, beneath which sits a bucket rapidly filling with water. Handed a ladle, you are instructed to empty the bucket. As Cornish legend has it, if you fail to shut off the water before you start ladling, you may find yourself declared insane.

So it goes, say many critics, with our current health-care system, a system that ladles frantically—removing cancerous lungs, bypassing blocked coronary arteries, prescribing all manner of pills—with hardly a glance at the still-running faucet. In name, we speak of our health-care system. In truth, we have built a multi-billion dollar disease care system, which according to many estimates, allocates up to 96 percent of these dollars for treatment and only 4 percent or less for prevention and education. Ergo, we ladle with 96 percent of our resources and expend only 4 percent of our efforts trying to slow the flow from the faucet. The wellness movement seeks to bring these numbers considerably closer together.

It does so in the belief that significant society-wide gains in health can no longer be expected from fancier hospitals, more sophisticated surgical procedures and more potent drugs.

John Grossman, "Inside the Wellness Movement," *Health*, Family Media, Inc., November/December, 1981. Reprinted by permission.

 ## CONTRIBUTING TO THE SOLUTION

Commenting on the cost of health care, George Sheehan, a cardiologist who recommends running, says, "The rules of health require less monetary outlay when you abide by them than when you break them."[5] The solution is obvious when you think about it, but at the behavioral level, developing good health habits is very difficult for many people. A lack of knowledge is responsible for some peo-

TABLE 1.2 **Cost of Treatment for Selected Conditions That Are Potentially Preventable**

CONDITION OR DISEASE	INTERVENTION	COST PER PATIENT
Heart Disease	Coronary bypass surgery	$ 30,000
Lung Cancer	Treatment	$ 29,000
Cervical cancer	Treatment	$ 28,000
Stroke	Hemiplagia treatment and rehabilitation	$ 22,000
Hip fracture	Surgery and rehabilitation	$ 40,000
HIV infection	AIDS treatment	$ 75,000 (lifetime)
Liver transplant	Surgery and rehabilitation	$250,000
Drug abuse	Treatment of cocaine-exposed baby	$ 66,000 (5 years)

Source: Adapted from *Healthy People 2000*, DHHS Publication No. (PHS) 91–50212, Washington, D.C.: U.S. Government Printing Office, 1990.

Health has become one of America's biggest businesses. It is the nation's second largest employer, after education, and third largest industry in consumer spending, behind only food and housing.

— Joseph Califano

ple's poor health practices, while other people know what to do but find it too easy to slip back into bad habits.

Self-Assessment 1.1 in Appendix C provides you with an opportunity to evaluate your health/wellness behaviors. Read the directions, answer each of the 60 items honestly, and read how to interpret your scores. We have all given good advice to our friends and family regarding *their* health behavior: Dad needs to lose weight, Mom needs to quit smoking, friends need to eat more wisely, others need to use seat belts, and so on. This inventory will help you to define your own behaviors. The test is: Can we take our own advice?

The importance of living a healthy life was demonstrated and quantified in several studies produced in California.[6] More than 6,000 residents of Alameda County were randomly selected and followed for five years. A definite relationship was observed between selected health practices and longevity. The following positively influenced length of life:

1. Eat breakfast regularly.
2. Eat moderately, with no snacking between meals.
3. Maintain normal body weight.
4. Never smoke cigarettes.
5. Drink no alcohol, or drink only moderately.
6. Exercise regularly.
7. Sleep 7 to 8 hours per night.

The data indicated that people who lived in accordance with these health principles lived longer than those who did not. For example, 45-year-old men who followed six of these practices lived, on the average, 11 years longer than 45-year-old men who followed three or fewer. The data for 45-year-old women who followed similar health patterns as the males in this study were less dramatic but still highly significant. The healthful-living group showed a seven-year advantage in longevity. These convincing data prompted the researchers to conclude that "the daily health habits of people have a great deal more to do with what makes them sick and when they die than all the influences of medicine."[7] This is a powerful statement, but one that seems to be consistent with research and authoritative opinion. The importance of our behaviors is illustrated in a statement by that well-known think tank, the Rand Corporation, which has developed a theoretical model that projects that each mile that a sedentary person walks or jogs will add 21 minutes to her or his life and save society 24 cents in medical and other costs.

A nine-year followup of the Alameda County study showed that five of the seven health habits (the maintenance of normal weight, having never smoked cigarettes, use of alcohol in moderation, regular exercise, and sleeping 7 to 8 hours)

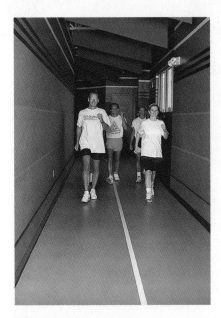

Fitness walking is an excellent physcial activity for all age groups.

were associated with lower mortality from all causes.[8] Eating breakfast regularly and not snacking between meals were not related to lower mortality. This very sophisticated study essentially reconfirmed the results of the original study. The evidence continues to accumulate, confirming what knowledgeable people already knew: we are the chief determiners of our own health. We are not hapless victims of disease; instead, we set our course and chart our destiny. We are victims only in the sense that we have been victimized by our lifestyle choices. As George Sheehan remarks, "We have come to an era in which aberrant life-style can no longer be ignored."[9]

Where difficult decisions are concerned—about surgery, risky procedures, or medicines with side effects—people often ask physicians, "What would you do if you were in my place, doctor?" Perhaps we should also ask about the decisions our physicians make on a daily basis about matters that are long-term and not crisis oriented but yet critical to their own health. Ten years ago, a survey of the Harvard Medical School clinical faculty did just that by asking the faculty members about their personal health practices. Five hundred and ninety-five faculty members responded. The survey was repeated in 1991.[10] Six hundred and seventy-two responses were obtained, and comparisons were made between the two sets of data. The first administration of the survey revealed that many of the physicians were practicing what they were preaching but that there was room for improvement. The second survey revealed that further behavior changes occurred during the intervening years. Some of the more relevant comparisons appear in Table 1.3.

Fourteen percent of the Harvard physicians consumed fish more than three times per week; 71 percent included fish in the diet one to three times per week. Vitamins, minerals, and other supplements were not favored in 1981 and continued to remain so in 1991. For the few who took supplements, the two most popular were calcium and beta carotene.

Ten years ago, 29 percent of the physicians were concerned with losing 10 pounds. In 1991, this figure rose to 39 percent. Either the faculty has become fatter, or they have become more worried about their weight. The researchers suggest the latter because of the evidence indicating that even small amounts of excess fat stored inappropriately are a risk for cardiovascular disease and diabetes.

Approximately 78 percent of the physicians avoided sunbathing, and more than 75 percent said they used sunscreens when they could not avoid exposure. Their behavior is reflective of the evidence linking exposure to the sun and skin cancer.

The Harvard physicians reported relatively low alcohol consumption: 70 percent took fewer than four alcoholic drinks per week, 12 percent abstained from alcohol, and 11 percent had as many as one or two drinks per day.

TABLE 1.3   Health Habits: What Do the Doctors Do?

BEHAVIORS	1981	1991
Seat-belt usage	73%	86%
Cigarette smoking	8% smokers	3% smokers
Diet		
Red meat consumption	44% restrict red meat	90% restrict red meat
Egg consumption	79% eat 3 or fewer per week	95% eat 3 or fewer per week
Margarine or butter usage	69% use margarine	78% use margarine
High-fiber diet	41% eat high fiber	59% eat high fiber
Aspirin usage to prevent heart attacks	7%	25%
Exercise habits—20 minutes a day at least 3 times a week.	49%	53%

Source: "What Doctors Do—Ten Years Later," *Harvard Health Letter*, Special Supplement, January 1992, p. 9.

Seventy-four percent of the physicians regularly drank caffeinated coffee, and 71 percent consumed other caffeine-containing beverages. (The current evidence indicates that moderate consumption of caffeine is not harmful to health. The key is *moderate* consumption. Since caffeine dehydrates the body, if you drink coffee or cola, you need to make sure you consume other beverages as well.)

It appears that the health behaviors of the Harvard physicians are essentially in concert with the best evidence available from research. The physicians have integrated their knowledge and behaviors into a balanced approach that avoids excesses and extremes in the pursuit of optimal wellness. We can all learn from their example.

AMERICA'S HEALTH REPORT CARD

Prevention magazine initiated a national health report card in 1984 called the "Prevention Index." An annual survey has been conducted by the Louis Harris pollsters for *Prevention* magazine. The survey consists of 21 health promotion questions, each of which is associated with behaviors that can be controlled by each individual. The nation scored highest on the 1992 index—66.5 points. This was a five-point improvement over the first survey in 1984 but still far short of the 100 points possible on the index. A score of 100 would indicate that every American was engaging in all 21 healthy behaviors.

The following are a few of the survey's most important findings:

1. Americans are feeling more stress today than 10 years ago. The percentage reporting "a great deal of stress" at least once a week has risen from 55% to 62%. More women than men—37% to 27%—report experiencing great stress more than once a week.

2. The percentage of Americans who smoke has fallen from 43% to 25% since 1973, but the decline has slowed to less than one-half percent per year during the past several years.

3. More Americans are watching their fat and cholesterol intake, but fewer are limiting their intake of salt and sugar.

4. In spite of all the media coverage regarding weight control, the percentage of American adults whose weight falls in the recommended range has decreased from 23% to 19% since 1983.

While the nation's health index has creeped up since 1984, its score indicates a grade of D+, or just barely passing.

Source: "News Briefs—America's Health Report Card," *ARAPCS Newsletter* 9, no. 2 (Winter 1993): 16.

 POINTS TO PONDER

1. How would you define and describe wellness?
2. What is the role of the individual in developing and maintaining optimal wellness?
3. What are the components of a wellness lifestyle?
4. Why are the chronic diseases the leading causes of death at the present time?
5. What is important about the Harvard Medical School survey of the school's teaching faculty?
6. Why has the cost of medical care increased disproportionately in the past 15 years?

HEALTHY PEOPLE 2000

In September 1990, Dr. Louis Sullivan, Secretary of the U.S. Department of Health and Human Services, released a monumental document entitled *Healthy People*

1. In 1990, Americans spent
   a. $16.7 billion on milk
   b. $47.3 billion on soft drinks
   c. $86.7 billion on alcohol
2. There are approximately 20.7 million junior and senior high school students in the U.S.
   a. 8 million drink alcoholic beverages weekly.
   b. In 1990, this group consumed 1.1 billion cans of beer.
3. In 1990, only 22 medical schools required a course in nutrition. Another 100 offered nutrition as an elective course, but only 5% of the medical students elected it.
4. The number of American adults who have had their cholesterol checked rose from 35% in 1983 to 65% in 1990.
5. The average American consumed the equivalent of 556 cans of soft drinks in 1990. If these were regular soft drinks, the sugar that they contained would be equal to 83,400 calories. This is the number of calories in 23.8 lbs.
6. A Harris survey in 1990 of 10 industrialized nations found that Americans were least satisfied with their health care system and that Canadians were most satisfied with theirs.
7. Forty-four states have enacted laws prohibiting the sale of cigarettes to minors but do not prohibit smoking by minors. An estimated one billion cigarettes are sold each year to underage Americans.
8. People who live in Montana and Colorado are the least sedentary of all Americans. The most sedentary state is Kentucky, where 42% of the people report that they do not participate in any leisure physical activity.
9. The most popular fruit in the U.S. is bananas, followed by apples. The most popular vegetable is potatoes, followed by iceberg lettuce, one of the least nutritious of foods.
10. There are nearly 300 alcohol-related deaths every day in the U.S.
11. About 21 million Americans regularly use smokeless tobacco products.
12. The myth that long-distance running is harmful to women continues to persist. The truth is that women benefit from exercise in much the same way as men. The two major concerns are that the uterus will become displaced and the ligaments supporting the breasts will stretch. The uterus has the best shock-absorbing system in the human body. There has not been a documented case of uterine prolapse caused by running. A good running bra should alleviate worries about structures that support the breasts.
13. Myth: As we age, we need to slow down. Inactivity is one of the major reasons that obesity and the chronic diseases are so prevalent in America. Age is not a deterrent to exercise and a physically active way of life. Exercise is important during every phase of the life cycle, including older age.
14. In 1990, deaths from gun injuries in Texas surpassed traffic fatalities (3,443 vs. 3,309) for the first time. (This was the first time that this has occurred for *any* state in the U.S.)

Far from being simply the absence of disease, health is a dynamic and harmonious equilibrium of all the elements and forces making up and surrounding a human being.

— Andrew Weil, M.D.

2000—*National Health Promotion and Disease Prevention Objectives,*[11] the product of more than two years of intensive effort involving approximately 10,000 health professionals representing varied disciplines. The purpose of the document is to provide objectives for enhancing the health of the nation during a 10-year time frame. The document includes more than 300 specific health objectives that are attainable targets by the year 2000.

The objectives are categorized into 22 categories, one of which relates to physical activity and physical fitness. This category contains 12 of the 300 objectives, synopsized in Table 1.4.

PHYSICAL FITNESS OBJECTIVES

For centuries, humans have been intrigued with the concept and applications of physical fitness. Many cultures, both past and present, have been concerned with the development of fit people for the utilitarian purposes of war and conquest. During the Golden Age of Greece, fitness was elevated from the level of necessity to a lofty goal, along with the development of the mind, as individuals attempted to achieve their full potential. The Greeks were truly ahead of their time. Twenty-

TABLE 1.4 Physical Activity and Fitness Objectives

1. Reduce the mortality rate from coronary heart disease.
2. Reduce the incidence of overweight among adolescents and adults.
3. Increase the number of people of all ages who on a regular basis participate in light to moderate physical activity.
4. Increase the number of people of all ages who participate in vigorous physical activity at least three times per week for a minimum of 20 minutes per workout.
5. Increase the number of people of all ages who regularly participate in exercises that build muscular strength, muscular endurance, and flexibility.
6. Increase the number of people of all ages who combine regular exercise with sound nutritional practices.
7. Reduce the number of people of all ages who engage in no leisure physical activity.
8. Increase the number of schools that provide daily physical education in grades 1–12.
9. Increase physical education class offerings to include more lifetime physical activities.
10. Increase the number of employer-sponsored worksite physical fitness programs and facilities.
11. Increase community availability and accessibility to physical activities and fitness facilities.
12. Increase the number of physicians who are trained to counsel their patients regarding (1) the need for exercise and (2) how to develop a sound program of exercise.

Source: *Healthy People 2000*, DHHS Publication No. (PHS) 91–50212, Washington D.C.: U.S. Government Printing Office, 1990.

five centuries later, we have finally come full circle by resurrecting this worthy concept.

The objectives that people expect to accomplish through exercise provide the basis for the type of fitness that is most appropriate for them. For instance, some people exercise for health, some for performance, and some for physical fitness. These are not necessarily mutually exclusive; in fact, they often overlap in the same fitness program. Sometimes the primary focus is all that differentiates exercise programs.

Exercise for Health

The primary purpose of health-related exercise is to attain well-being and prevent disease. Health-related exercise is characterized by regular participation in mild to moderately vigorous exercise for the purpose of reducing body weight, serum cholesterol, hypertension, and stress. To achieve these benefits, it is not necessary to achieve a demonstrable increase in physical fitness from the exercise program.

It is important for people to understand that the attainment of **health-related fitness** does not depend upon athletic ability or physical activities that are highly performance related. Health-related fitness can be achieved with minimal psychomotor ability. Almost anyone, including those with varying degrees of physical disability, can participate in such natural activities as walking and jogging. Other activities, such as biking (including use of a stationary bike), hiking, backpacking, orienteering, swimming, and rope jumping, require minimal cognitive and psychomotor abilities when one participates for physical fitness purposes rather than for skill development. Health-related fitness training differs from competitive training because the objectives of each program differ. The adage that most of us grew up with, "No pain, no gain," while probably necessary for competitive athletes, is inappropriate for the purpose of health-related fitness.

Most authorities agree that fitness for health consists of the development of cardiorespiratory endurance, muscular strength, muscular endurance, flexibility, and a lean body composition. **Cardiorespiratory endurance** refers to the ability of the body to take in, deliver, and extract oxygen for physical work. It is the best physiological index of total body endurance. **Muscular strength** is the maximum amount of force that a muscle can exert in a single contraction. **Muscular endurance** is the capacity to exert repetitive muscular force. **Flexibility** refers to the range of motion around specific joints. **Body composition** refers to the amount of lean versus fat tissue.

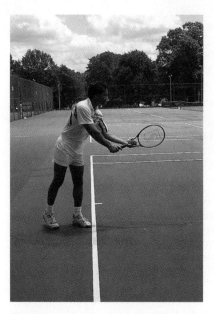

Tennis is one of the more popular sports for fun and fitness.

The relative contribution of each component to health and wellness is one of degree. Although cardiorespiratory endurance is the most important component, recent evidence has shown that the means through which muscular strength and muscular endurance are developed also contribute substantially to wellness. This is fully explored later, along with a rationale for the other components.

● Exercise for Performance

Performance-related fitness, though not essential for health, is necessary for the execution of sports skills. Speed, power, balance, coordination, agility, and reaction time are the components of performance-related fitness. **Speed** refers to velocity, or the performance of a movement in the shortest amount of time. **Power** refers to work divided by the time it takes to perform the work; the faster the completion of work, the greater the power. **Balance,** or equilibrium, refers to the ability to maintain a desired body position either statically or dynamically. **Coordination** is the integration of the body parts to produce smooth, fluid motion. **Agility** is the ability to rapidly change direction while maintaining dynamic balance. **Reaction time** represents the time that it takes to respond physically to a given stimulus. It is usually measured in fractions of a second.

Highly skilled athletes possess these abilities in a highly refined state. The sports in which they participate may also require one or more of the health-related components, because mutual exclusivity does not exist between the two types of fitness. The primary objective for noncompetitors may be health-related fitness, but the activities such people use to achieve this goal may also require some or all of the performance-related components. In fact, some people prefer the challenge of developing skill and fitness concurrently. These people are usually athletic and enjoy athletic competition. Their principal mode of developing and maintaining fitness is through athletic games. Literally millions of people participate in racquetball, handball, tennis, and other games that combine both types of fitness.

● Exercise for Physical Fitness

Exercise for physical fitness requires individuals to work vigorously enough to improve cardiorespiratory endurance, muscular strength, and muscular endurance. People who exercise to develop physical fitness do so to increase their energy level, to feel better, to look better, and to derive an inner satisfaction of accomplishment. Competition is usually not a major factor for these exercisers. Such people normally do not compete in races and other events, and if they do, winning is relatively unimportant. Rather, these people view the event as an opportunity to participate in a different environment and to visit with friends and old acquaintances.

 HOW FITNESS FITS

Physical fitness is an integral part of a multifaceted wellness lifestyle. It can be developed and maintained only through persistent and progressively increasing effort, but the payoff includes an impressive array of predictable physiological, emotional, social and health benefits. Participation in a vigorous physical fitness program, one that attempts to develop all the components of health-related fitness, has far-reaching effects upon the quality and quantity of life. Practitioners of a wellness lifestyle present physical profiles that are synonymous with vibrant and robust health. Significant differences exist in health status between them and sedentary people matched for age and sex. In general, active people are leaner, have lower levels of blood fats and lower blood pressure, handle stress more effectively, and smoke less.

Comparisons made between active and inactive groups using health risk appraisal analyses indicate that the **health age** (or biological age) of the active group is generally lower than the **chronological age.** That is, an active 52-year-old is likely to be the equivalent of a 45-year-old with regard to health. We often see the converse when people enter our Fitness and Wellness Center. The health age of our entry-level clients is likely to be higher than the chronological age. This is undesirable, but some positives are associated with it; for example, it acts as a powerful motivator for change. We usually see favorable changes when people participate in our programs for several months.

Health risk appraisals are questionnaires used to assess lifestyle habits. Respondents react to questions about such behaviors as tobacco and alcohol usage, exercise habits, dietary habits, use of seat belts, frequency of self-exams and medical evaluations, and monitoring of blood pressure and blood lipid values. These appraisals also project, on the basis of heredity and lifestyle habits, an individual's likely age at death. Of course, the prediction is only as good as the data base upon which it is conceived, the respondent's honesty, and the built-in error associated with laws of probability. None of these appraisals predict infallibly, but they do graphically identify negative and positive health behaviors while providing suggestions for improving health status and longevity. Regardless of their shortcomings, the predictions for active people are generally more favorable than for sedentary people.

The attainment of physical fitness seems to act as a catalyst for change in other facets of our life. The evidence in this regard is anecdotal, but literally thousands of people have capitalized upon fitness as a springboard for successfully changing their nutritional, smoking, alcohol, and rest habits. In effect, they are maximizing the health benefits they initially acquired through regular exercise. Exercise as a change agent certainly requires more investigation, but it is considered to be one of the vehicles for altering some unhealthy behaviors.

IS FITNESS A FAD?

Since the inception of the fitness movement in the 1960s, skeptics have proclaimed the movement a passing fancy—a fad akin to streaking and the hula hoop. Thus far, the movement has survived, and it continues to attract new participants.

A national survey in 1986 revealed some interesting characteristics about the fitness movement during that time.[12] Seven out of ten respondents reported that they had participated in sports or fitness activities during the previous 12-month period. On the surface, this was indeed impressive, but closer inspection of the data indicated that the respondents participated an average of only 53 times per year, or about once a week. Only one out of ten respondents reported participating four or more times per week, and 27 percent of all respondents indicated that they never participate in sports or physical fitness activities.

The same survey was repeated in 1990. The only significant change between it and the original poll—and it is an encouraging sign—was that the frequency of exercise had risen from 53 to 74 times per years.[13] Seventy-three percent of Americans claim to exercise at least one and one-half days per week. If they can be convinced to double the frequency of exercise, approximately 75 percent of Americans will be exercising frequently enough to enhance their health. The most popular activities among those surveyed were swimming (45 percent), cycling (34 percent), fishing (33 percent), exercise machines (33 percent), bowling (26 percent), and calisthenics/aerobics (24 percent).

A survey conducted by the National Sporting Goods Association revealed that the number of Americans who exercised at least twice a week increased from 30.8 million in 1987 to 32.2 million in 1989.[14] However, that still leaves about 80 percent of the adult population (age 25 or older) who do not exercise or who exercise less than twice a week.

The Gallup Poll completed a survey for IDEA (International Dance and Exercise Association).[15] It surveyed only people who exercised regularly and not

Nations have passed away and left no traces, and history gives the naked cause of it. One single, simple reason in all cases—they fell because their people were not fit.
— Rudyard Kipling

the entire population. It found that of all of the age groups that exercise regularly, the younger groups have the greatest number of participants, but the older participants who do exercise, do it more frequently. The survey reconfirmed what was previously known about the exercise movement; that is, its primary participants are young, well-educated, and of middle and upper socioeconomic class. Twenty-five percent of the regular exercisers were in the 18-to-24-year-old group, even though this group constitutes only 11 percent of the U.S. population. Eighteen percent of the population is over 65, but only 8 percent of this group exercises regularly.

The three primary reasons that people in this survey exercised were (1) to lose weight (21 percent), (2) to relieve stress (17 percent), and (3) to improve physical appearance (13 percent). Ninety million Americans exercise fewer than 25 days a year because of (1) not enough time, (2) not enough self-discipline, (3) inability to find an interesting activity, (4) inability to find a partner, and (5) inability to afford equipment.[16]

Over 10 percent of the nonexercisers would participate if their physicians would allow it, 34.6 percent would exercise if they were convinced that they could benefit from it, and 38.1 percent said they would exercise if they could find an easy activity.[17] Obviously, many Americans are not convinced of the benefits of exercise, nor do they understand how hard or how often to exercise to achieve their objectives. Many would be surprised to learn how little time and effort are required if health enhancement is the goal.

 ## THE FITNESS LEVEL OF AMERICAN YOUTH

For several decades, data regarding the physical fitness level of American youth have been accumulating. The perception is that the youth fitness level has declined and youth are less fit today than their age group in previous generations.[18] Evidence also appears to support the notion that today's youth are fatter than youth in the past.[19] In 1984, 62 percent of high school students (grades 9–12) reported exercising vigorously for at least 20 minutes a day three days per week. In 1990, only 37 percent of the high school students exercised at that level.[20] The least active of the students were twelfth-grade females. Only 17 percent of this group exercised three or more times per week.

This study corroborated the work of previous studies on the inverse relationship between time spent viewing television and exercising. The more one watches the tube, the less one exercises. Television seems to be making a substantial contribution to an inactive lifestyle.

Some authorities agree that while some physical fitness components have slipped among today's youth, others have not.[21, 22] These authorities point to the fact that some of the standards as well as the instruments for measuring physical fitness have been inappropriate and therefore lead to inaccurate results. This issue is far from being resolved. At this time, the conclusion about the state of youth fitness that best fits the research evidence is that most American youngsters are not as poorly fit than previously thought but that a substantial number continue to be below that which is expected for this age group.

A study of 10,000 youngsters (ages 10 to 18) has produced some insights into the reasons for sports participation (reported in Table 1.5). The study also explored the reasons that youngsters stop participating (see Table 1.6).[23]

It appears that fun is the most important motivator of young people. When physical activity ceased to be fun or if it did not contain a fun element, it was discontinued or avoided. Therefore, it is quite clear that marketing efforts designed to stimulate participation by this age group in physical activities should stress the fun aspect.

TABLE 1.5

Most Important Reasons for School Sports Participation

- To have fun
- To improve skills
- To stay in shape
- To do something I'm good at
- For the excitement of competition
- To get exercise
- To play as part of a team
- For the challenge of competition
- To learn new skills
- To win

TABLE 1.6

Most Important Reasons for Discontinuing Sports Participation

- Lost interest
- Was not having fun
- Took too much time
- Coach was a poor teacher
- Too much pressure (worry)
- Wanted nonsport activity
- Was tired of it
- Needed more study time
- Coach played favorites
- Sport was boring
- Overemphasis on winning

TABLE 1.7

Percentage Increase in Sports/Recreational Activities 1987–1990

ACTIVITY	INCREASE
Stair climbing	500
Treadmill exercise	300
Mountain biking	250
Ice hockey	75
Low-impact aerobics	66.7
Fitness walking	43.7
Home gym exercise	35.3
Free-weight exercise	25.8
Resistance machines	18.8
Basketball	18.5

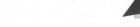

ACTIVITIES THAT ARE GROWING IN POPULARITY

The percentage of adults who exercise has been quite stable over the past few years. Fitness devotees participate in a variety of activities. From 1987 through 1990, the greatest increase in frequency of participation occurred in activities that emphasize the development and maintenance of physical fitness.[24] These activities are listed in Table 1.7.

U.S. exports of sports equipment and athletic footwear to other countries exceeded $1 billion in 1991, the third consecutive year that exports have exceeded this amount.[25] The sale of roller skates rose significantly, representing the largest increase in export items.

On the homefront, the interest in physical fitness has also been reflected in the increasing amount of literature devoted to promoting health/wellness and physical fitness. Books featuring exercise of all types for fitness purposes have regularly appeared on the best-seller list. Every month popular magazines feature articles on some aspect of exercise and health. Exercise videos have become very popular regardless of the credentials and expertise of the producers of these items.

Pulse meters of different types and degrees of sophistication have been developed to monitor the intensity of exercise. Pedometers measure distance to tell us how far we have traveled, and skinfold calipers measure the thickness of skin, telling us how much fat we have lost.

Sports drinks touted to replace the exercising body's lost nutrients are heavily advertised. It is not uncommon to see athletic teams consuming such beverages during television coverage of their games. Certain foods are hawked as energy foods, and vitamin and mineral supplements are sold in large quantities with the promise of enhancing performance.

Some advertising agencies have gone to the extreme in affiliating with the fitness movement. Products that have nothing to do with fitness are advertised using a fitness motif. This is an eloquent commentary by those advertisers who recognize the importance of associating their products, however marginally, with the public's generally positive attitude toward fitness. The object, of course, is to transfer that positive attitude from fitness to the product being promoted. Whole new industries have developed around the fitness movement, while others have been revitalized. Membership in health clubs, spas, YMCAs, and so on, have increased or at least remained steady over the past decade.

FITNESS IN BUSINESS AND INDUSTRY

In an effort to cut escalating health care costs, many businesses and corporations have turned to fitness and wellness programs. According to the Association for Worksite Health Promotion, American businesses paid out more than $70 billion in health care costs in 1986, and 500 million workdays were lost to illness and disability.[26] To the average person, these numbers are so large that they are incomprehensible.

To better understand the scope of these costs, we may need to look at them from the following perspective: "Ten percent of a company's payroll goes to health insurance, and the health-related expenses of a typical Fortune 500 corporation are equal to 24 percent of its profits."[27] These are significant expenditures that are in need of reduction.

The Ford Motor Company reported paying more than $600 in employee health care costs for each vehicle it produced in 1989.[28] These costs accounted for 16 percent of Ford's payroll expenses—a 150 percent increase over payroll expenses for health care in 1970.

Many companies have instituted fitness and wellness programs in an effort to lower health care costs, and the early data are indeed encouraging. Containing the

WELLNESS

One should apply the principles of a wellness lifestyle on a consistent basis for a lifetime. The following is a selection of some of the important principles:

1. Drink alcohol sparingly or not at all.
2. Do not drink and drive.
3. Take drugs only as prescribed by a physician for a specific ailment.
4. Do not use tobacco products in any form.
5. Exercise consistently—four to five times a week for at least 20 minutes per exercise session. Be sure to include both cardiorespiratory and musculoskeletal activities in your program.
6. Cut fat consumption to less than 30% of total calories.
7. Eat three to five servings of vegetables and two to four servings of fruit every day.
8. Reduce consumption of sugar, salt, and cholesterol.
9. Carry less than 18% of your total weight as fat if you are a male and less than 25% of your total weight as fat if you are a female.
10. Perform self-examinations (breast, testicles, etc.) on a regular basis.
11. Have preventive medical exams as suggested for your sex and age by various medical agencies.
12. Since stress cannot be avoided in today's world, learn to manage it to avoid suffering its consequences.
13. Get adequate rest, which is essential to a wellness lifestyle.
14. Always use seat belts and shoulder restraints.
15. Put your emphasis on preventing disease rather than on having to treat it after the fact.

spiraling cost of health care seems to be worth the effort and the initial expense of developing and implementing the program.

The effects of wellness programs, of which physical fitness constitutes but one component, cannot be measured overnight. It takes time, effort, and an educational emphasis to change such long-standing behavior patterns as cigarette smoking, overeating, eating a high-fat diet, and following a sedentary lifestyle. However, corporations that have implemented wellness programs have found that health care costs have been reduced and there is less worker absenteeism, greater productivity, less worker turnover, and fewer on-the-job accidents.[29] Having a wellness program with fitness facilities is often used as a perk by corporations to recruit and keep key personnel.

The initial capital outlay for a comprehensive wellness program usually can be recovered in two to three years. From that point on, the potential company savings may be in the range of $2 to $6 in reduced medical costs, reduced absenteeism, increased productivity, and decreased turnover for every dollar the company invested in a wellness program.[30] Estimates are that more than 50 percent of the firms with 50 or more employees have health care programs.[31]

The medical profession has become aware of the importance of regular exercise and the development and maintenance of physical fitness. A growing number of medical schools are offering courses in the physiology of exercise, and a number of physicians have expressed the opinion that physicians should be able to prescribe exercise with as much skill as they prescribe medicine.

The attitude of the American public toward exercise is generally positive. Most people feel that exercise is good for them, although many are not quite sure why or how. This is probably one of the reasons that only 10 percent to 20 percent of the exercisers are working hard enough and often enough to become physically fit. Although the exercise surveys indicate that increasing number of people are exercising—and this is a positive trend—a large segment of our society does not participate, and a larger segment exercise at a level below that which is required to promote health and fitness. We need to continue to educate people regarding the importance of an active lifestyle and regular exercise.

In an effort to educate the American public regarding the need for a physically active way of life, The American College of Sports Medicine (ACSM) has established the ACSM Fit Society,[32] a membership association geared to and open to the general public. The Fit Society is designed to deliver current health/fitness information to the consumer. For a 20-dollar annual fee, a member receives a quarterly newsletter plus discounts on ACSM consumer literature. ACSM is the most influential and most recognized professional organization for exercise science and sports medicine. The literature this organization generates is of the highest quality.

THE MECHANIZATION OF AMERICA

The health of nations is more important than the wealth of nations.
— Will Durant

The fitness movement was largely a reaction to developments in science and technology and their relationship to the changing disease and death patterns in the nation. The communicable diseases (tuberculosis, pneumonia, typhoid fever, smallpox, scarlet fever, etc.) were the leading causes of death during the early years of this century. Advances in medical science have virtually eradicated these maladies and threats to life, but they have been replaced by such chronic and degenerative diseases as heart disease, stroke, cancer, and diabetes. This group of diseases is largely lifestyle induced and has reached epidemic proportions. Cardiovascular disease (diseases of the heart and circulatory system) accounts for approximately 44 percent of all deaths in the United States.[33] Atherosclerosis, a progressive degenerative disease resulting in narrowed blood vessels, is responsible for most of the deaths from heart attack and stroke.

The risk factors that lead to heart disease and stroke were identified by the ongoing landmark Framingham Study, which began in 1949.[34] As these risk factors were identified, the realization evolved that these diseases were not the inevitable consequences of aging but are acquired and are therefore potentially preventable. Risk factors are genetic tendencies and learned behaviors that increase the probability of premature illness and death. Cigarette smoking, high blood pressure, elevated levels of blood fats, diabetes, overweight, stress, lack of exercise, and a family history of heart disease are some of the risk factors for heart attack and stroke.

Most risk factors can be modified or controlled by adopting appropriate lifestyle behaviors. During the past 40 years, millions of Americans have made healthy lifestyle changes. It was no coincidence that during this time the death rate for cardiovascular disease decreased by a formidable 51 percent.[35] Other factors were involved in this favorable trend, but modifications in lifestyle behaviors have made a significant contribution.

Our lives today are considerably different from life in the early years of this century. Scientific and technological advances have made us functionally mechanized. Labor-saving devices proliferate all phases of life—our occupations, home life, and leisure pursuits—always with the promise of more and better to come. Each new invention helped foster a receptive attitude toward a life of ease, and we have become accustomed to the easy way of doing things. The mechanized way is generally the most expedient way, and in our time-oriented society, this became another stimulus for us to indulge in the sedentary life.

Today, exercise for fitness is contrived; it is programmed into our lives as an entity separate from our other functions. On the other hand, the energy expenditures of our forefathers were integrated into their work, play, and home life. Physical fitness was a necessary commodity, and fit people were the rule rather than the exception. Tilling the soil, digging ditches, and working in factories were physically demanding jobs. Lumberjack contests and square dances were vigorous leisure pursuits. Being a wife and mother and taking care of home and family required long hours at arduous tasks. In the early years of this century, much of the energy for operating our factories came from muscle power. By 1970, this figure dropped to less than one percent and is reflective of the declining energy demand of our jobs.

The turn of the century found 70 percent of the population working long, hard hours in the production of food. Children of that era walked several miles to school and did chores after they returned home. Today, only 3 percent of the population, using highly mechanized equipment, are involved in the production of food. Children ride to school, and adults drive to the store, circle the parking lot to get as close as possible to the entrance, and ride elevators and escalators while there. People mow the lawn with a riding mower, play golf in a cart, wash dishes and clothes in appropriate appliances, change television channels with a remote control, open garage doors in the same manner, and so on.

These are simply observations of life in America and are not intended to imply that the fruits of science and technology be repudiated, but rather that their results along with their impact on us be viewed in perspective and acted on accordingly. Mechanization has reached our leisure time, and it is in this sphere that we must commit some time to vigorous activity, because such activity has been effectively removed from other areas of life.

Programming exercise into one's leisure time is getting tougher, since both the white-collar and the blue-collar workweek have been increasing over the past few years.[36] Actually, the length of the factory workweek is the longest it has been since the mid 1950s. Americans had 26.2 hours per week for leisure in 1973. In 1989, this dropped to 16.6 hours per week.[37] The average workweek in 1976 was 40.6 hours, but by 1989, it had increased to 46.8 hours. Effective management of time takes on greater importance as we attempt to fit work, leisure activities, and sleep into 24 hours. To commit the time and effort required to participate in regular exercise, one must understand its relevance to a healthy life.

TIPS FOR MANAGING YOUR TIME

Good time managers are very effective in identifying and setting goals. Your goals should establish what you ultimately wish to accomplish. Following are some guidelines for developing your goals. First, the goals that you identify should be yours. (While this may seem obvious, it really isn't, because the goals that important people in your life have for you sometimes conflict with your own.) Second, your goals should be listed in order of importance. Third, your goals should be as specific as possible so that you can evaluate your progress toward their accomplishment. Fourth, your goals should be realistic and attainable, but not without effort. Fifth, your goals should be accompanied by a timeline for their accomplishment.

After establishing your goals, devise a weekly or monthly calendar or schedule of events. Post it in a prominent place so that you will come into contact with it several times during the day. This calendar should contain the fixed items that occur every week, such as classes, work, meals, and meetings, plus the important non-fixed items, such as tests, due dates for written assignments, and vacations. One of the important insights to be attained from such a calendar is the amount of time left over during the day that is available for physical activity, study, and other pursuits.

Another helpful time management tool is keeping a list of things to do. Write what you need to do each day on a 3 × 5 card or in a pocketsize notebook and keep the list with you. Cross off the items as you complete each one during the day.

For more information, read *Personal Time Management* by Marion E. Haynes, Los Angeles: Crisp Publishing, 1987; or *Manage Your Time, Manage Your Work, Manage Yourself* by Melville and Donna Douglas, New York: American Management Association, 1980.

Man has inhabited the earth for many centuries, but only the past 75 years have generated such drastic changes in lifestyle. Our basic need for physical activity has not changed. Our bodies were constructed for and thrive on physical work, but we find ourselves thrust into the automobile, television, and sofa age, and we simply have not had enough time to adapt to this new sedentary way of living. Perhaps 100,000 years from now, the sedentary life will be the healthy life. However, at this stage of our development, the law of use and disuse continues to work, and that which is used becomes stronger and that which is not becomes weaker. For simple verification of this physiological principle, just witness the results of a leg in a cast for eight weeks and note the atrophy that has occurred to the limb during that time.

It is the belief of many people, this author included, that our new ways of living are precipitating—or at least significantly contributing to—the diseases that are affecting modern affluent man. These diseases are unique to the highly industrialized nations. By contrast, the underdeveloped nations, with their different lifestyles, do not experience this phenomenon to the same extent.

FITNESS: BOOM OR BUST?

The American College of Sports Medicine has established criteria that should be met if exercise is to produce desirable physiologic and health-related goals.[38] The following criteria apply to aerobic exercise (walking, jogging, cycling, swimming, and other continuous low to moderate physical activities): the intensity or vigorousness of exercise should correspond to 60 percent to 90 percent of the maximum heart rate, the appropriate intensity should be maintained for 20 to 60 minutes, and exercise should be engaged in 3 to 5 times per week. The following guidelines apply to weight training: a minimum of 8 to 10 exercises performed two times per week; and a minimum of one set of 8 to 12 repetitions to near fatigue.

The ACSM suggests that beginners select from activities that allow the participant to control the pace or the resistance. Self-paced activities are those that are individual in nature and do not require competition, such as walking, jogging, cycling, swimming, and backpacking. After a period of conditioning, for variety, these activities can be supplemented with games and sports that are not self-paced. The intensity of these activities is dependent upon the skill level and motivation of the competitors.

When gauged by these criteria, the results of the national surveys appear to be far from satisfying. The surveys also indicate that the fitness movement has not pervaded all segments of society. Most of the participants are young, affluent, and well educated. Also, the activities selected by many proclaimed exercisers are questionable with respect to meeting the ACSM exercise guidelines. However, many Americans are exercising today, and many more are becoming aware of the importance of regular exercise. Many people are beginning to understand that even light exercise performed at least three times per week will confer some health benefits.

The American Heart Association has finally accepted—and has begun to publicize the fact—that physical inactivity is a major risk for heart disease. This change in policy will probably appear in its 1993 literature. The American Heart Association's endorsement of exercise should function as a motivator for some Americans. Other prestigious organizations have increased their efforts to make the general public aware of the need to exercise, including the President's Council on Physical Fitness and Sports; the American Alliance for Health, Physical Education, Recreation, and Dance; the Association for Worksite Health Promotion; and various medical organizations. Many of these groups are urging the public schools to reinstitute daily physical education programs for grades K through 12 to improve the fitness level of youth and increase the knowledge and need for physical activity throughout their lives.

At this point, the evidence in support of a physically active life is irrefutable and mounting. Will the fitness movement bog down and eventually run out of steam? The answer can be found in the evidence, and it is a resounding no.

POINTS TO PONDER

1. Explain the importance and the influence that *Healthy People 2000* may have on the American Public.
2. Discuss the objectives and the differences among the concepts of exercise for health, exercise for performance, and exercise for fitness.
3. Is fitness a fad? Defend your answer.
4. Why do American youth participate in sports?
5. Why should business and industry invest in a wellness program?
6. Will the fitness movement survive? Defend your answer.

CHAPTER HIGHLIGHTS

- Wellness is a dynamic approach to health enhancement that emphasizes positive health behaviors and preventive practices.
- Wellness is composed of five dimensions: social, spiritual, physical, intellectual, and emotional.
- Our state of mind has a profound effect on our immune system.
- Self-responsibility is the core of a wellness lifestyle.
- The chronic diseases have replaced the communicable diseases as the leading causes of death in the U.S.
- The U.S. spends a greater share of its GDP on health care than any of the other industrialized nations.
- Highly sophisticated technology developed to aid physicians in the diagnosis and treatment of disease has added considerably to the cost of disease care.
- The majority of the physicians on the faculty of Harvard Medical School diligently practice health behaviors intended to result in optimal well-being.
- *Healthy People 2000* is a joint effort of the federal government and thousands of health professionals who have set health care goals for the U.S. to attain by the year 2000.
- Health-related fitness includes the development of cardiorespiratory endurance, muscular strength and endurance, flexibility, and body composition.
- Performance-related fitness is composed of speed, power, balance, coordination, agility, and reaction time.
- National polls and surveys indicate that the majority of Americans either do not exercise or exercise infrequently.
- American youngsters are not as poorly fit as previously thought, but a substantial number of them are below that which is expected for their age group.
- Stair climbing has attracted more participants in the past four years than any other fitness activity.
- Business and industry have determined that fitness and wellness programs for employees are cost effective and that the initial monetary outlay can be recovered in the first few years of operation.
- Since the average workweek in the U.S. has been increasing during the past two decades, it is more difficult to schedule exercise during dwindling leisure time.

REFERENCES

1. G. Edlin and E. Golanty, *Health and Wellness—A Holistic Approach,* Boston: Jones and Bartlett, 1992.
2. "U.S. Health Care Bill $943 Per Person in 1979." *President's Council on Physical Fitness and Sports Newsletter,* December 1980, p. 8.
3. "Your Stake in Reform," *AARP Bulletin* 33, no. 6 (June 1992): 8.
4. "Health Woes of the Future," *U.S. News and World Report,* December 23, 1991, p. 12.
5. G. Sheehan, "Living with Style," *The Physician and Sportsmedicine* 11, (1983): 65.
6. L. Breslow, "A Quantitative Approach to the World Health Organization Definition of Health: Physical, Mental, and Social Well-Being," *International Journal of Epidemiology* 1 (1972): 347; L. Breslow, "A Policy Assessment of Preventive Health Practice," *Preventive Medicine* 6 (1977): 242.
7. Ibid.
8. D. L. Wingard et al., "A Multivariate Analysis of Health-Related Practices: A Nine-Year Mortality Follow-up of the Alameda County Study," *American Journal of Epidemiology* 116 (1982): 765.
9. Sheehan, "Living with Style," 1983, p. 65.
10. "What Doctors Do—Ten Years Later," *Harvard Health Letter, Special Supplement* (January 1992): 9.
11. *Healthy People 2000,* DHHS Publication No (PHS) 91–50212, Washington, D.C.: U.S. Government Printing Office, 1990.
12. *Sports Illustrated,* "Sports Poll '86," Time, Inc., 1986.
13. "Sports Illustrated on Sports," *ARAPCA Newsletter,* XIII, no. 2 (Winter 1992): 12.
14. "Exercise Boom Continues," *ARAPCA Newsletter,* XII, no. 2, (Winter 1991): 8.
15. "IDEA Fitness Participant Survey," *ARAPCA Newsletter,* XII, no. 2 (Winter 1991): 8.
16. "Couch Potatoes Speak," *The Walking Magazine* 6, no. 2, (March/April 1991): 12.
17. "My Dog Ate My Running Shoes," *The Physician and Sportsmedicine* 19, no. 5 (May 1991): 7.
18. Updike, W. F., "In Search of Relevant and Credible Physical Fitness Standards for Children," *Research Quarterly for Exercise and Sport* 63, no. 2 (June 1992): 112.
19. C. T. Kuntzleman and G. G. Reiff, "The Decline in American Children's Fitness Levels," *Research Quarterly for Exercise and Sport* 63, no. 2 (June 1992): 107.
20. "Workouts Wanting Among High School Students," *Harvard Heart Letter* 2, no. 9 (May 1992): 8.

21. C. B. Corbin and R. P. Pangrazi, "Are American Children and Youth Fit?" *Research Quarterly for Exercise and Sport* 63, no. 2 (June 1992): 96.
22. S. N. Blair, "Are American Children and Youth Fit? The Need for Better Data," *Research Quarterly for Exercise and Sport* 63, no. 2 (June 1992): 120.
23. M. E. Ewing and V. Seefeldt, *American Youth and Sports Participation,* North Palm Beach, Fla.: Athletic Footwear Association, 1990.
24. "News Briefs," *President's Council on Physical Fitness and Sports Newsletter* 91, no. 4 (July/August 1991): 8.
25. "News Briefs," *President's Council on Physical Fitness and Sports Newsletter* 92, no. 3 (May/June 1992): 8.
26. P. Gambaccini, "The Bottom Line on Fitness," *Runner's World* 66 (July 1987).
27. Ibid.
28. "Fascinating Facts," *University of California at Berkeley Wellness Letter* 7, no. 7 (April 1991): 1.
29. R. Bertera, "The Effects of Workplace Health Promotion on Absenteeism and Employment Costs in a Large Industrial Population," *The American Journal of Public Health,* July 1, 1991, p. 68.
30. N. Feineman, "From Boardroom to Locker Room: A Look at the 10-year Metamorphosis of Corporate Fitness Plans," *Health* 22, no. 8 (September 1990): 49.
31. Bertera, "Effects of Workplace Health," July 1, 1991, p. 68.
32. "Fit Society Is New ACSM Outreach, *Fitness Management* 8, no. 8 (July 1992): 11.
33. American Heart Association, *1992 Heart and Stroke Facts,* Dallas, Tex.: American Heart Association, 1991.
34. W. B. Kannell and others, "Epidemiology of Acute Myocardial Infarction: The Framingham Study," *Medicine Today* 2 (1968): 50.
35. American Heart Association, *1992 Facts.*
36. J. Liscio, "America Is Going Back to Work Again," *U.S. News and World Report,* May 11, 1992, p. 55.
37. D. Hales, *Your Health,* Redwood City, Calif.: Benjamin Cummings, 1991.
38. American College of Sports Medicine, "The Recommended Quantity and Quality of Exercise for Developing and Maintaining Cardiorespiratory and Muscular Fitness in Healthy Adults," *Medicine in Science and Sport* 22, no. 2 (April 1990): 265.

CHAPTER 2

Motivation for a Physically Active Life

CHAPTER OUTLINE

INTRODUCTION

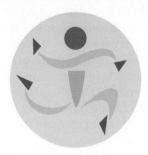

Chapter 1 established the importance of self-responsibility as the cornerstone of a wellness lifestyle. Adherence to a regular program of exercise is one of the program's vital elements. This chapter addresses the challenge of motivating people for involvement in those lifetime activities that lead to high-level wellness as well as the development and maintenance of physical fitness.

Initiating and complying with an exercise program are dependent upon education (which includes explaining why and how people should exercise) and motivation.[1] Both are important because many sedentary people plunge into exercise with unrealistic impressions of what constitutes effective yet safe training practices. The importance of education was attested to by the results achieved with the publication of Kenneth Cooper's first book, *Aerobics*. Cooper provided the whys and hows in that text, which literally motivated millions of people to exercise. The publication of this book was timely because Americans were ready to do something positive for themselves, but they needed a plan, and Cooper's book seemed to provide that plan. The print and broadcast media also got into the act, and the public soon began to learn about the value of exercise.

People must have sufficient motivation to sustain an exercise program during the first six months, because 40 percent to 50 percent of those who start exercising drop out during this time,[2] with the largest percentage dropping out during the first three months.[3] Exercise programs lasting a year or longer experience less than 50 percent **adherence** (continuation in the program), and the situation worsens as time goes by. The first six months of the exercise program have been called the critical period. These estimates apply to exercise programs in supervised settings. It is quite possible that more moderate forms of exercise performed individually have better adherence rates.[4]

Miniglossary

Adherence Long-term participation.

Blood Lactate A metabolite that produces fatigue and results from incomplete breakdown of sugar.

Burnout A loss of energy, creativity, and direction.

Extrinsic (External) Reward Any positive reinforcement emanating from an outside source—e.g., friends, coaches—that increases the strength of a response.

Goal Something toward which effort or movement is directed; an end or objective to be achieved.

Intrinsic (Internal) Reward Reinforcement coming from within; the degree of satisfaction derived from participation in the absence of some visible reward.

Motivation The internal mechanisms and external stimuli that arouse and direct behavior.

Positive Reinforcement A reward; positive reinforcement increases the strength of a response or responses.

Self-Concept The set of people's beliefs about and evaluations of themselves as persons.

Stimulus Any energy impinging upon an organism that results in a response.

Three self-assessment activities appear in Appendix C that apply directly to the content of this chapter:

2.1 Exercise Adherence Scale
2.2 The Physical Activity Questionnaire
2.3 Personal Fitness Contract

EXERCISE DROPOUTS AND ADHERERS

Recent research has suggested that exercise and physical activities consist of behaviors that are more complex than other health-related behaviors. Exercise shares some common dimensions with other health behaviors, but it has inherent uniqueness (effort, exertion, sweat, etc.) that separates it from the other behaviors. As a result of exercise's uniqueness, researchers are currently attempting to develop a model of behavior applicable to exercise that will enable them to identify potential dropouts and adherers. The advantages of such a model are obvious. If the potential dropouts can be identified early, they can be targeted for appropriate intervention by program staff to increase the probability of adherence.

Studies of this type are complex and difficult because (1) terminology has not yet been standardized and (2) participants change their behaviors. For instance, many people who enroll in supervised exercise programs drop out but continue to exercise on their own, while others drop out and do not continue exercising on their own. This confounds the adherence statistics unless viable followup of dropouts occurs to determine their exercise status.

The reasons most often offered by exercise dropouts include lack of time, inconvenient or inaccessible exercise site, work conflicts, and poor spousal support.[5] Dropouts frequently cite situational factors, such as the travel requirements of their jobs, as impediments to regular participation.

From a purely biological perspective, dropouts may be at an initial disadvantage because of higher than normal levels of body fat. Exercise intensities that are appropriate for the development of physical fitness may be too demanding for dropouts, thus causing them to discontinue the effort. Lack of self-regulatory and time management skills also contributes to the drop-out rate.

It is difficult to determine whether these barriers to exercise are actual or perceived. Evidence indicates that adherers often live farther away from the exercise facility and have no more leisure time than do dropouts. Spousal support repeatedly has been shown to be a predictor of adherence, but some adherers have indicated that it is less important than other factors. Perhaps one of the differences between those who continue to exercise and those who don't is that impediments to exercise are perceived as real barriers by dropouts. These same barriers are perceived by adherers as mere inconveniences that are easily surmounted. Turning dropouts into adherers may be accomplished by changing the dropouts' perceptions. Providing instruction in time management and flexible exercise hours and developing home exercise programs for such people might be a productive approach.

Wood has advanced several additional reasons for dropping out.[6] One reason is a poor attitude toward exercise. Wood states, "Our schools have produced two or three generations of adults who, generally speaking, are philosophically opposed to exercise."[7] A second reason involves poor choice of exercise. Since exercise comes in many forms, people have ample opportunity to select activities that are fun, enjoyable, and appropriate for their needs. Third, people drop out because of injuries. Wood claims that many of these injuries are preexisting—that is, they were sustained early in life primarily through participation in school contact sports. The majority of such injuries involve knee problems resulting from

The acquisition of habits of increased physical activity is viewed as a process with three stages: (a) the decision to start exercising, (b) the early states of behavior change, and (c) maintenance of the new behavior.
— Dorothy Knapp

Although numerous variables affect participant exercise compliance, perhaps the most important is the exercise leader.
— Barry Franklin

Exercise programs should be designed not only to develop optimal fitness but also to enhance long-term adherence to training.
— Michael Pollack

cartilage damage. These injuries are aggravated rather than developed by vigorous exercise of the wrong type later in life. The advent of an injury during a program is generalized to all exercises and not merely the program in which the injury occurred. Actually, people with preexisting injuries should be evaluated and guided into activities that will not aggravate those injuries. For instance, severe lower limb injuries might not be aggravated by nonweight-bearing activities such as swimming and cycling.

Some generalizations regarding exercise adherence may be advanced that tend to endure regardless of subjects, methods, time frames, and programs.[8] They include the following:

1. Blue-collar workers, smokers, and the obese are less likely to begin and sustain exercise in either a supervised or an individual program.

2. People who are highly self-motivated are more likely to continue nonsupervised exercise.

3. Perception of lack of time and inconvenience lead to dropping out, but some exercisers continue despite the same barriers.

4. Health enhancement encourages adopting an exercise program, but reinforcement from health and exercise professionals, support from significant others, feelings of well-being, and the attainment of one's goals seem to be more important for continuation.

WHO IS EXERCISING?

The fitness and wellness movement has created the opportunity for the development of new industries while providing for the development of new product lines for established businesses. The market for such products has expanded to such an extent that the money spent in the pursuit of fitness and wellness exceeds the gross domestic products of most third world countries.[9]

Having the money to spend on fitness apparel, equipment, and membership in fitness and health clubs is positively related to participation in fitness and wellness endeavors. Although a healthy lifestyle is theoretically within reach of nearly everyone, the typical practitioner is the relatively wealthy, educated, white American. Tables 2.1 and 2.2 present the results of a national survey of upper management regarding their attitudes about health and physical fitness. Sixty-four percent of these executives exercise regularly, only 10 percent smoke, and the executives' average blood pressure is an excellent 124/79. Even though they devote an average of 54 hours per week to their jobs, these executives take time to exercise. The following are some of their tips:

EXERCISE TIPS FOR BUSY PEOPLE

> Schedule exercise as a regular business appointment, to minimize the likelihood that the day's demands will intrude; park a mile or two away from the office (or communting point) and "walk-in;" never stay in a hotel that doesn't have a pool, fitness center or exercise path (nearby if not on the premises); and finally, don't treat travel as an excuse to interrupt your routine. Your running or walking shoes can be a reminder and incentive. Never leave home without 'em![10]

While the wealthy were discarding bad health habits, the poor were not.[11] Cardiovascular disease has decreased among those with higher socioeconomic status, but the poor continue to suffer more than their share.[12] Some researchers have concluded that the high prevalence of chronic disease among blacks and other minorities is evidence that the fitness movement has passed them by.[14] LaPorte (researcher in the area of health and exercise) has stated, "The exercise boom has been a result of efforts to target the sedentary white-collar executives

TABLE 2.1	Attitudes of 3,000 Executives Regarding Health and Exercise*		
	VERY IMPORTANT (%)	IMPORTANT (%)	NOT IMPORTANT (%)
Healthy Habits			
Don't smoke	87	8	5
Exercise regularly	76	19	5
Eat less sugar, salt, fat	73	21	6
Get adequate sleep	56	33	11
Control stress	55	35	10
Limit alcohol intake	51	39	10
Exercise Motivation			
Overall health benefits	87	10	3
Improved sense of well-being	74	20	6
Weight control	71	19	10
Reduced stress	56	26	18
Better productivity	53	31	16

*Figures represent percentage of respondents.

Source: Adapted from K. M. Cahill, "The 3-Martini Lunch Is Long Gone," *The Walking Magazine* (March/April 1989): 33.

who have money. But those excluded from the fitness boom are the ones who need it the most. If researchers want to use activity to reduce the prevalence of chronic disease, they have to go where the chronic diseases are—among the lower socioeconomic groups."[14] Efforts aimed at this segment of society are under way in California, Arizona, and Georgia, and each program has achieved success in changing health and exercise behaviors. Health professionals administering these programs are convinced that it is fruitless to bring Jane Fonda and Richard Simmons to the ghetto, and it is much more productive to develop fitness programs that respect cultural values.[15] A sound fitness program developed for middle-class America will not work in non-middle class settings, but a sound program adapted for local consumption will.

MOTIVATION: SOME BASICS

Motivation is a label invented by people to describe a characteristic type of behavior. Since it cannot be measured directly, it is inferred through observations of behaviors and actions. Such imprecision often results in inaccurate perceptions about presumed levels of motivation. The matter is confused further because motivation, as with other aspects of human behavior, lacks a uniformly acceptable definition. For this text, we will adopt Sage's (researcher in the area of motor behavior) definition that **motivation** is "the internal mechanisms and external stimuli that arouse and direct behavior."[16] According to this definition, motivation is affected by both internal and external forces. External forces, represented by **extrinsic** (external) **rewards,** often are a necessary stimulus for people to continue in an exercise program during those critical early months. For instance, membership in an exercise group provides a setting where compliments and positive strokes from one's peers furnish the external reinforcement for adherence during this time.

The rewards provided to the novice exerciser can be (1) symbolic (a badge, pin, T-shirt), (2) material (money, prizes, payment of fitness club dues), or (3) psychological (attention, recognition, encouragement).[17] Such rewards are important, particularly during the early stages of exercise, since at this point many facets of

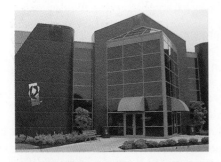

Q, The Sports Club in Memphis, Tennessee. This is an example of a prototype fitness and wellness center featuring qualified instructors. This is an excellent place for people to pursue their fitness goals.

TABLE 2.2	Physical Fitness Participation of 3,000 Executives*		
FAVORITE ACTIVITIES	**PEOPLE WHO PARTICIPATE (%)**	**PEOPLE WHO PARTICIPATE 3 TIMES A WEEK OR MORE (%)**	
Jogging/running	35	72	
Tennis	35	7	
Golf	32	2	
Fitness walking	31	66	
Stationary cycling	22	64	
Weight training	27	56	
Calisthenics	18	94	
Racquetball	12	26	
Outdoor cycling	10	10	

*Figures represent percentage of respondents.

Source: Adapted from K. M. Cahill, "The 3-Martini Lunch Is Long Gone," *The Walking Magazine* (March/April 1989): 33.

the program—cost of exercise apparel, equipment, investment of time, pain, discouragement, failure to realize goals, fatigue, and possible alienation of family—may be perceived as deterrents to continuing. However, excessive dispensation of extrinsic rewards or the use of rewards as bribes rather than as indicators of accomplishment can be counterproductive in the long term. An event of considerable import in exercise motivation occurs when the individual transcends dependence on external rewards and begins to internalize the feelings of well-being as prime motivators of exercise.

Franklin (researcher in the field of exercise and wellness) stated, "The benefits derived from extrinsic rewards, while initially important, are also short-lived. Ultimately, the motivation to continue an exercise program must be intrinsic rather than extrinsic in nature. The individual must develop an attitude toward exercise which reinforces adherence."[18] Each individual is his or her own best motivator, for greatest motivational energy comes from within.[19] **Intrinsic** (internal) **rewards** are rewards that come from the degree of satisfaction derived from participation.

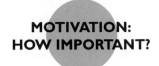

MOTIVATION: HOW IMPORTANT?

There are those who argue that motivation is the most-valued human commodity. It separates the successes from the failures, the winners from the losers, and the spectacular from the mundane. What does motivation look like? Take a good look inside yourself. You'll find it.

P.W. Buffington, "Getting Going," *Sky* 112 (April 1985).

There is some question regarding the staying power produced solely by external rewards, and there is speculation regarding such rewards' possible depressant effect upon intrinsic motivation. For instance, two researchers showed that "play could be turned into work,"[20] and two others declared that "token rewards may lead to token learning."[21] The epitome of the adverse effect of external rewards upon intrinsic motivation is represented by the following fable:

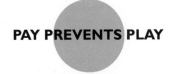

PAY PREVENTS PLAY

Once upon a time, there was an old man who was bothered by the noise made by a group of young boys who would play in an area near his house. As the story is told, the old man, desperately trying to come up with a way to rid himself of the disturbances, decided to pay the boys. He offered them 25 cents apiece to return the next day and play by his house. Naturally, the boys thought they had found a good thing and returned to play the next day, at which time the old man offered them 20 cents if they would repeat their performance on the morrow.

Continued

The drive producing long-term adherence in any endeavor, exercise included, must be intrinsically motivated. But more recent research indicates that external rewards do not necessarily subvert internal motivation. In fact, prudently selected external rewards that are contingent upon quality of performance do not impair (and may even augment) intrinsic motivation.

Human behavior is purposeful—that is, it is goal-directed. The objective of motivated behavior is the achievement of our goals. **Positive reinforcements** (intrinsic supplemented with extrinsic) motivate us to persist in the attainment of these goals. A workable plan for achieving **goals** involves knowing what we want to accomplish in the long run. In other words, we should be able to identify our long-range goals. Then we should set realistic short-term goals that we may reach within a realistic time. The achievement of each short-term goal acts as both a reinforcer and a stimulus motivating us to strive for the next goal, while each accomplishment brings us closer to realizing our long-term goal. The key is realism: setting goals that are difficult enough to provide a challenge but that we have a reasonable chance of achieving. This is a functional plan for achieving objectives, and physical fitness should be approached in this manner.

Some psychologists have determined that a moderate level of motivation is optimal.[22] Too little is likely to result in early failure, and too much may result in injury and burnout (see Figure 2.1). In either case, motivation is adversely affected, adherence wanes, and the program, with all of its good intentions and potential benefits, is terminated. To avert this all too familiar scenario, we must cultivate the philosophy that our fitness goals should be approached slowly and patiently, albeit progressively. We must learn to contain our enthusiasm so as not to attempt too much too soon during the early phases of the program. Remember, physical fitness is not achieved with two weeks of training. The development and maintenance of physical fitness should be a lifelong affair. This requires a sizable commitment of time and knowledgeable effort, but the results are eminently worthwhile. You supply the time and the effort, and this text will provide you with the necessary knowledge. The appropriate application of these ingredients will increase your likelihood of success.

FIGURE 2.1

The Inverted U Hypothesis
Moderate levels of motivation produce the best results. Motivation levels that are too high or too low tend to result in poor adherence and failure.

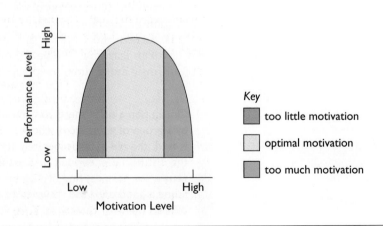

1. It is a fallacy that motivation must be present for learning to occur. Oftentimes, some degree of learning must occur for motivation to develop. For instance, parents may pay for music lessons for a child who is not motivated to learn. But after a few sessions, the child finds some satisfaction in the progress she has made, and her motivation to learn begins to grow. Or a college student is required to take a square dancing course as part of his physical education requirement. He puts it off until the last semester because he is sure he will not like it. Square dancing doesn't fit his image. But after a few classes, he begins to realize how much fun square dancing can be, so his motivation to learn begins to increase. In these two examples, learning precedes motivation.

2. Self-efficacy involves one's perception of how successful one might be in any given situation. People with low self-efficacy often quit or give up when faced with a difficult problem or task; people with high self-efficacy tend to persist to overcome the challenge. People with high self-efficacy tend to "stick with the program," and this would include an exercise program. Self-efficacy can be enhanced by direct action—experiencing an exercise program based on sound principles. Self-efficacy can also be enhanced by observing others who are similar to yourself who successfully continue their exercise programs. You will realize that if they can do it, so can you. Also, through verbal persuasion—logical arguments regarding your ability to succeed—you will increase your self-efficacy.

3. How do people come to enjoy activities that at first are frightening? Why do people skydive or rock climb or hang glide or run Iron Man triathalons? First-time skydivers are usually terrified. However, repeated jumps lessen the fear and increase the thrill. After the first jump, the skydiver experiences a brief but exhilarating sense of relief, whereas veteran skydivers experience a sense of euphoria for several hours after each jump. The sequence of emotions for a first jump is anxiety before, terror during, and relief after the jump. The emotional sequence for a veteran jumper is eagerness before, a thrill during, and exhilaration after the jump. This sequence powerfully reinforces skydiving activity.

 ## WHY PEOPLE EXERCISE

People participate in physical activities for a variety of reasons. Knowledgeable people in the fitness business can list many reasons that people in general are attracted to exercise. Although we know, in general, why people participate, we need to learn more about which **stimulus** or combination of stimuli will motivate a given individual to exercise.

The evidence is quite clear that the majority of middle-aged and older adults exercise primarily for health enhancement. Several investigations of college students also indicated that health was the major reason for engaging in exercise.[23] A recent study of this population suggested, however, that previous studies may have misinterpreted student motives by not including questions related to aesthetics. As a result, student interest in exercise and weight control was interpreted as reflective of students' desire to enhance their health status. Koslow's (physical educator) study indicated, however, that student interest in exercise and weight control were motivated primarily by students' desire to develop a pleasing physical appearance.[24] Exercise for health was rated highly by this group, but second to aesthetics. The appeal of exercise for this group should stress both, but greater effort should be devoted to the potential of exercise to effect desirable changes in physical appearance. College students are *young* and essentially in good health. They don't relate to the threats of heart disease, stroke, cancer, etc. at this age. These are diseases that occur as one ages. College students further perceive that physical appearance is of paramount importance, particularly with regard to relations with the opposite sex.

According to a Harris Poll, some people exercised because their jobs had become more demanding, and a sizable segment of this group exercised to combat on-the-job burnout.[25] **Burnout,** a relatively vague term, implies a loss of energy, creativity, and direction. Forty-three percent of the Harris respondents who exercised a minimum of five hours per week reported more creative energy as well as more total energy devoted to their jobs. Becoming and remaining fit may do as much for occupational health as it does for personal health.

The enhancement of body image and self-concept are the prime motivators of exercise for some people. **Self-concept** refers to our perceptions about ourselves and is molded from how we see ourselves and how we think others see us. It involves the personal self, physical self, moral and ethical self, and family self. Body image, which represents the physical self, is an important constituent of self-concept.

A national panel of experts was convened by the National Institute of Mental Health to produce a state-of-the-art summary regarding the effect of exercise on mental health.[26] The experts concluded that long-term participation in exercise leads to a significant increase in self-esteem and significantly enhances one's estimation of the physical self. Body image improves as fitness level improves.

Loss of excess weight, development of muscle tissue, and desirable changes in body composition all contribute to a better physical appearance and thus to a better body image. The research indeed suggests that the enhancement of physical fitness is pervasive. It leads to an improvement of body image that enhances the entire self-concept.

Most exercisers who participate regularly derive important mental and emotional benefits, including mood elevation, relief from tension, and improved self-image.[27] Scientists at the National Center for Health Statistics in Maryland have been studying the relationships between exercise and mental health. After analyzing data from surveys that collectively involved more than 75,000 adults representing a broad spectrum of individuals in the United States and Canada, they concluded that a positive association exists between exercise and mental health.[28] Initially, exercise may seem stressful, but those who continue begin to feel better about themselves.[29] The gains in self-esteem, coupled with decreased feelings of tension, become powerful positive reinforcers. These desirable changes, which are subtle at first, do not become evident until the tenth or twelfth week of exercise. Unfortunately, many would-be exercisers drop out before this time, having never fully experienced these benefits. Psychologist Robert Brown indicated that his files are packed with cases that support the notion that many people exercise primarily to control their moods and because of the way they feel about themselves.[30]

An interesting aspect of the effects of physical fitness upon self-concept relates to one's perceptions of one's level of fitness. Several studies reported that subjects' perceptions of their improved level of fitness, even in the absence of an actual improvement, beneficially affected their self-concept.[31] This suggests that merely participating in an exercise program has the potential to positively impact the self-concept.

The importance of developing a positive self-concept, or the degree of satisfaction that we derive from who and what we are, was most appropriately advanced by Dr. Norman Vincent Peale, who stated that "you have to spend every minute of your life in your own company. If you don't enjoy it, you're going to be miserable." By comparison, a few minutes spent in fitness activities three to five times a week may help us enjoy living with ourselves. Fitness is not a panacea, but the evidence indicates that it improves the self-concept.

As previously stated, it takes some time and effort—a small price to pay for such a profound payoff. A poor self-concept often leads to feelings of inferiority. Eleanor Roosevelt once said, "No one can make you feel inferior without your consent." You do not have to accept your lot in life: you can make a change. Do something positive for yourself: make exercise a part of your life.

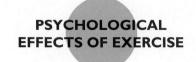

PSYCHOLOGICAL EFFECTS OF EXERCISE

Most regular exercisers not only feel healthier, but they also think exercise helps them feel good about themselves. In a recent study most seasoned runners said that their good feelings about running stem from psychological rather than physical satisfaction. For example, vigorous exercise may act as a release

Continued

—Continued

for anxiety and tension, and it has been favorably compared with tranquilizing drugs, meditation, and various relaxation techniques as a means of reducing muscle tension.

Good self-esteem is another strong deterrent to psychological problems. Feelings about the body and especially about appearance are intimately related to self-concept, so improved fitness usually results in improved self-esteem.

A. Weltman, and B. Stamford, *The Physician and Sportsmedicine* 11, no. 1 (January 1983).

Some people enjoy the social interactions with others while they exercise. They jog with a partner or group, participate in aerobic dance, compete in sporting activities, enjoy backpacking, and so on, partially to satisfy a need to do things with others but also to receive the benefits of exercise. This is carried to the extreme by those individuals who exercise because it is the "in thing" to do. This may not be the best of reasons, but from our perspective, the motive that initiates the program is irrelevant as long as the program endures. If the program is continued, the superficial motives that spurred the individual to exercise will probably yield to more substantial ones.

The risks inherent in some activities are the major lure for some people. Rock climbing, rappelling, mountain climbing, white-water canoeing, kayaking, hang gliding, skydiving, and, currently, bungee jumping are some activities that basically satisfy the need for people to challenge themselves. Participants involved in these activities are often after the ultimate physical and psychological experience and are willing to assume the risks necessary to achieve their goal. The exhiliration of looking danger in the face and prevailing is a powerful reinforcer for future risk-taking behavior.

Some people are influenced by the aesthetic appeal or beauty of graceful and proficient physical movement, while others are attracted by the potential that movement has to improve physical appearance. Favorable changes in body composition—loss of fat and gain of muscle—enhance physical appearance and, at least by Western standards, create a more pleasing silhouette.

Others are drawn to exercise for catharsis, that is, to reduce the twentieth-century malady known as chronic stress. Regular exercise is a powerful relaxer. It is an excellent vehicle for taking out one's frustrations; it acts as a safety valve for pent-up emotions; it removes the by-products of chronic stress (adrenaline

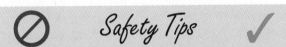

⊘ *Safety Tips* ✔

STARTING AN EXERCISE PROGRAM

1. Be patient with your exercise program. Beginners tend to exercise beyond their ability, which results in pain and injury. Do not do too much too soon.
2. Older people need to be a bit more cautious about starting an exercise program.
3. Medical clearance for exercise is in order for people of any age if they have two or more major coronary factors or if they have symptoms of cardiopulmonary or metabolic disease.
4. Overweight people should probably engage in non-weight bearing activities, such as water aerobics, stationary cycling, and rowing, in the beginning stages of their exer-

cise program. They can progress to weight-bearing activities as they lose weight and become more fit. Walking would be the best weight-bearing activity until weight is lost and fitness is gained. The obese should avoid high-impact activities (jogging, sports such as racquetball and basketball, or high-impact aerobic classes) until they lose weight.

5. Exercise no more than four to five days a week for 20 to 30 minutes each workout at a relatively low intensity level (50% to 60% of max heart rate). More than this amount, when just beginning the exercise program, can lead to injury and loss of motivation.

and noradrenaline) from the blood stream; and it dilates blood vessels, resulting in more effective blood flow.

A small number of people exercise for ascetic reasons. The discipline associated with the rigors of training is appealing to this group. The reasons that people exercise are many and varied. Factors that motivate one person may not have the same effect on another because of differences in experience, values, interests, objectives, intelligence, and so on. The selection of the exact factor or factors that might motivate a given individual to participate is conjectural at best.

There is general agreement that adherence on a regular basis for a long period of time is greatly enhanced if the activity selected is fun and enjoyable.[32] You can readily see how a given activity (for example, jogging) may be fun for some and drudgery for others. Therefore, we must try to match activities with people on the basis of what gives them enjoyment while meeting their physiological, psychological, and other needs, interests, and objectives. This is not always easy to do. This task would be much more manageable if we had highly qualified physical education teachers in the elementary schools. During these formative years, children who are exposed to top-notch programs that teach the need for and the physiology of fitness as well as the motor skills to attain it may retain the interest, knowledge, and skill bases for later participation. We cannot prove this, but it seems to be a logical place to begin establishing lifelong exercise habits.

In the absence of such programs, we must continue to carry the message to youngsters and adults about the value of exercise. Millions of Americans quit smoking cigarettes as a result of the antismoking messages on television during the early 1980s. Other media messages over the years regarding the devastating effects of tobacco usage have also contributed to the quit rate. However, not all cigarette smokers who have been exposed to the messages have quit. Likewise, millions of Americans have changed their lives for the better by exercising regularly, but in spite of positive media messages, the majority of Americans either do not exercise at all or don't exercise enough. These is still much work to be done.

 POINTS TO PONDER

1. Describe the characteristics of those who exercise and those who don't.
2. What are the primary reasons given by those who do not exercise?
3. Identify the reasons that adults and college students exercise. Is the major motivator different for each group?
4. What are the psychological and emotional effects of exercise?

 MOTIVATIONAL STRATEGIES

With regard to exercise, educational/promotional approaches are based on two premises: (1) that individuals are motivated for self-enhancement and (2) that knowing the how and why of exercise is indispensible for motivating people to commit to an active way of life. The rationale for this approach is that people usually don't change their behaviors unless they know why they should change and how to change. Knowledge alone works for some but certainly not all people. As previously mentioned, Kenneth Cooper's book motivated many to exercise, and the antismoking campaign on television was so effective in advertising the downside of cigarette smoking that many people responded by quitting. But facts alone are not enough incentive for many people to change their behaviors. This text is providing you with the facts about exercise and the necessity of an active lifestyle. For some of you, this won't be enough. Therefore, the remainder of the chapter presents a number of proven motivational strategies in the hope that you will try them. You may be pleasantly surprised at how effective they can be.

> Exercise to eat. Working out offers one of the few remaining excuses to eat more, to indulge occasionally without guilt.
>
> — James Rippe

Define Your Goals

Because exercise is multifaceted and can be programmed in numerous ways, it can meet many different objectives. The selection of appropriate types of activities and the proper application of exercise principles can help the overweight to lose and the underweight to gain, but first it must be determined what is to be accomplished through the exercise program. The more specific your goals the better. Do you wish to gain or lose weight, increase your energy level, reduce your risk for chronic disease, or improve your physical appearance? Would you like to participate competitively in swimming, cycling, running, or court games? Your reasons for participation will determine which types of activity are best as well as how hard and how often they should be performed. If you have several goals, rank them in order of importance and work on them one at a time. Often, more than one goal may be pursued concurrently. For instance, weight loss and an increase in energy level can be accomplished together, and an increase in both muscle tissue and strength may be accomplished at the same time.

Knowing your objectives and goals is a very important first step if an appropriate exercise program is to be developed. Without objectives, the exercise program becomes a hit-or-miss proposition that might be analogous to sightseeing in Chicago with a map of Philadelphia. You might reach your destination, but the odds are against it. The Physical Activity Questionnaire (Self-Assessment 2.2 in Appendix C) will help you to clarify your present exercise status, your reasons for exercising, and your attitude regarding regular participation in exercise.

Set Realistic Goals

The commonly used phrase "do your best" does not result in as great a performance improvement as does a specific goal.

— Richard MaGill

Set realistic, attainable, and behavioral goals. The more specific the goal, the better. An example of a nonspecific goal is reflected in the commonly heard statement: "I have finally had it; I'm going to lose weight." Contrast that statement with, "I'm going to lose 30 pounds, and I'm going to do it by losing one pound a week for 30 weeks." This statement is specific and provides a timetable or a plan of attack. A nonbehavioral goal is "I'm going to reduce my resting heart rate to 56 beats per minute," which can be made behavioral by adding "by jogging 30 minutes a day, four days a week." Realistic goals expressed specifically and behaviorally are more helpful because they provide information and guidance for their attainment.

Don't expect too much too soon. Be patient, because fitness takes time. At the same time, don't become excessively goal oriented. Remain flexible and change your goals and activities if and when the need arises. Do not go beyond your exercise capacity by raising the intensity too abruptly. This can lead to discomfort and possibly injury. In either case, you will probably terminate the program. The injury rate rises when you exercise more than five times per week for more than 45 minutes per session.[33] Beginners would do well to exercise every other day and limit the duration of each workout to 20 to 30 minutes exclusive of warmup and cooldown.

Exercise recommendations for the average participant would be to decrease the intensity while increasing the frequency and duration. High-intensity exercise is not appropriate, enjoyable, or well tolerated by those who participate for reasons other than competition.[34] Nor is it appropriate for the overweight, the sedentary, older people, and people who have cardiovascular disease. Studies have shown that increasing the frequency and/or duration of exercise is an effective way to equalize the caloric expenditure of higher intensity exercise. The increase in aerobic capacity is similar for both training schedules. The intensity of exercise should be sufficient to meet the exerciser's objectives but not so high as to be a deterrent.

People differ genetically in their potential for aerobic activity. Not everyone can achieve the same level of performance, but everyone can improve his or her level of fitness. Consistency is the key: you must exercise regularly to achieve your objectives. Set short-term goals that you can achieve in a few weeks. This will give

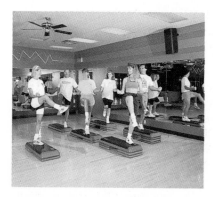

Aerobic Exercise with a Group

you the feeling of success and provide a boost for you to achieve the next goal, because success breeds success and motivates you to work harder. If the ultimate goal is to lose 30 pounds, it can be approached in stages, with each stage covering a loss of six to eight pounds. If the task is not broken down into a series of small steps, it may appear to be insurmountable. Reward yourself upon the successful completion of each stage. The closer you get to the ultimate goal, the more reinforcement you will get from other people who notice the positive changes in your physical appearance.

You may occasionally experience a setback or two on the way to your goals, but don't let them deter you. You may not be progressing as rapidly as you would like, or a minor injury or illness might keep you out of action temporarily. Since these and similar delays occur to almost everyone who exercises, expect occasional problems, handle them philosophically, and don't get discouraged. If an injury means that you cannot engage in your favorite physical activity, find a substitute. A knee injury might prevent you from playing tennis or racquetball or jogging, but swimming might be an acceptable alternative. It may not be your favorite form of exercise, but concentrate on the results rather than the means of attaining the results. Above all, don't become impatient with temporary setbacks. A classic example of maintaining motivation in spite of a string of setbacks was displayed by a nineteenth-century politician. The man lost his business, was defeated running for the legislature, failed in business once again, suffered an emotional breakdown, twice lost an election for the U.S. Congress and twice for the U.S. Senate, and was defeated running for vice president of the United States. In 1860, he was elected president. In the face of adversity, Abraham Lincoln never lost his motivation to succeed.[35]

● Exercise with a Group

Two investigators compared Kenneth Cooper's individualized aerobics program to the group approach and found that after 28 weeks, only 47 percent of those in the individualized program continued to participate, compared to 82 percent in the group system.[36] An attractive feature of group participation is the possibility of developing social relationships with other participants. The group provides reinforcement, camaraderie, and an element of competition as well as a spirit of cooperation. In the early days of exercise, allegiance to a group enhances compliance; one's commitment to the group is not as easily dissolved as a commitment to oneself.[37]

When the individual becomes committed to regular participation in exercise, the need for group support will probably decrease, and the program can be continued without such support. However, a recent one-year study using middle-aged men and women who were more representative of the general population than were people in previous studies—this study included the overweight and smokers as subjects—showed that a home-based exercise program was more effective than a group program in maintaining exercise adherence.[38] The reason given for this unexpected result was that the group program became too inconvenient over the one-year period for the participants to justify the benefits. Convenience and accessibility of the exercise facility are extremely important considerations when one is in the process of selecting a group exercise program. If you cannot satisfactorily meet these two conditions, you would be better off exercising at home.

● Enlist the Aid of Significant Others

Spouses, other family members, friends, and coworkers—those with whom the individual frequently interacts and whom the prospective exerciser considers to be special—can be a primary source of support. Social support from such people (particularly one's spouse) includes a favorable attitude and encouragement toward the individual's exercise endeavors. Spousal support has been a source of

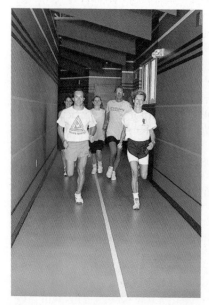

Jogging with a Group

positive motivation in a number of studies.[39] A better scenario exists when spouses or other family members are regular exercisers. Such people can be role models who can draw on their experiences and knowledge to provide information, counsel, and advice. They may act as reinforcers of exercise by working out with the novice exerciser.

Exercise with a Buddy

The effectiveness of the buddy support system was examined in two independent investigations,[40] which indicated that this model might provide the necessary support for sustaining an exercise program. Two people with similar training routines and compatible levels of fitness can reinforce each other. Knowing that your training buddy will be waiting for you at a designated time and place makes it difficult to skip the workout even when you would rather do something else.

Having someone to share your training problems with is another benefit of the buddy system. It is very helpful to get objective advice from someone whose judgment you trust.

Associate with Other Exercisers

Associate with people who motivate you in a positive manner and avoid those who are negative and pessimistic. Seek out others who exercise and discuss with them training, nutrition, weight loss, the reasons that they began exercising, what they have already accomplished, and what you hope to do and learn from each other. Catch their enthusiasm and give them some of yours. Enthusiasm is prevalent and contagious when people who exercise get together. As a result of such interaction, you will eagerly approach your next workout.

Build on Successful Experiences

Stress the importance of regular participation in exercise rather than superior exercise performance. Skill level and physical fitness improvement should be approached slowly and patiently. Expect gradual changes and focus on the results that you are achieving.

Keep a Progress Chart

Maintaining a daily record (self-monitoring) (see Table 2.3) of your exercise can be motivating, particularly if the record sheet is posted where you can regularly observe it.[41] A daily record provides objective data that show the actual rate and amount of progress achieved. Exercisers who keep records substantially increase their level of exercise.

Looking back at the record and observing the gains made can be a source of motivation when one becomes discouraged. The chart should reflect changes in body weight, type and amount of exercise, duration, and the exercise and resting heart rates. There should also be room for a short accompanying statement on how the participant felt during and after the workout.

Weighing yourself before and after the workout is important, particularly in hot weather when fluid loss can become a major problem. Since most of the weight lost during the workout is liquid, the difference between pre- and post-exercise weight is an approximation of the amount of fluid loss. This figure should not exceed 4 percent to 5 percent of your body's weight. This process of determining and/or approximating fluid loss is one of the functional aspects of the progress chart. Over the long term, a trend for weight loss or gain, type and amount of exercise, distance covered or time spent, and heart rates (exercise and resting) will become discernible, and you will have a record of improvement.

Exercise to Music

Music provides a sense of rhythm, and it tends to take the mind off the effort. A researcher at Ohio State University tested experienced runners with and without

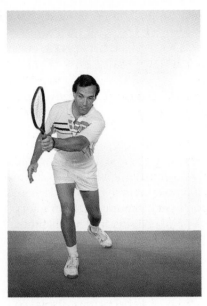

Exercise with a Buddy

TABLE 2.3 Progress Chart

DATE	BODY WEIGHT		EXERCISE		INTENSITY**			COMMENTS
	Pre-Exercise	Post-Exercise	Type	Duration*	RHR	THR	PE	

*Time, distance, etc.

**RHR = resting heart rate; THR = training heart rate; PE = perceived exertion.

upbeat music.[42] The runners stated that music made the bout of exercise seem easier. They ran two trials—one with and one without music—both at the same workload. Measures of working heart rates and **blood lactate** indicated that the runners were working equally hard on both trials; only their perception of the difficulty of the workload was changed. Music can be easily provided indoors, and portable radio headsets are gaining in popularity for outdoor exercise.

● Set a Definite Time and Place for Exercise

It is best to set a definite time and a convenient place in the initial stages of the program. Resolve to exercise at least three times a week and schedule your workout as you would any other important activity.

Cardiologist James Rippe suggests that the day and time of each workout should be written on one's daily calendar so that it will be scheduled in the same way as appointments and other important activities.[43] Resist the temptation to replace your workout with some other pursuit that might be more appealing. Skipping workouts becomes habit forming: like any habit, the more you do it, the easier it becomes. But once you become hooked on exercise, the time and place may be varied to meet the vagaries of weather, job responsibilities, and aesthetic sensibilities.

If lack of time is causing you to skip workouts, you might try exercising less frequently but more intensely at each session. While this is not optimal, it is much better than dropping the exercise program completely. High-intensity exercise performed two times a week will not increase your level of fitness, but it will attentuate or postpone the effects of detraining. Then, if and when your schedule allows for a return to a normal pattern of exercise, your fitness level will not have deteriorated, and you won't be starting from scratch again.

● Participate in a Variety of Activites

Varying the activities is one of the ways to maintain enthusiasm and combat boredom. Select activities that are enjoyable and randomly rotate them. You may also wish to participate in more than one activity on any given day. If you are not participating competitively in a particular activity, you have great flexibility of choice.

The selection of activities for inclusion in your physical fitness program will probably be based on past experience plus some trial-and-error experimentation. Don't exclude an activity because of lack of experience with it. The same applies to exercise equipment. You won't know whether you enjoy using a stationary cycle or rower, a stair stepper, or any other device unless you have had an opportunity to experience it.

Members of fitness clubs have access to many exercise devices and can choose those that meet their needs. The opportunity to experiment with different types of exercise equipment is limited for those who exercise on their own. An alternative for such people is to borrow or rent the equipment for a few weeks, which is usually enough time to decide whether the equipment is needed and will be enjoyed.

The same advice applies to the selection of the activities that the exercise program will comprise. Try a number of different activities to determine which ones will produce what you want. It is quite possible that you will shift from one activity to another several times during your lifetime as your needs, interests and abilities change.

● Dwell on the Positive

People tend to notice the negatives associated with the workout, such as the sore muscles, the effort required, and the feelings of fatigue. Instead, concentrate on the positives—as the song states, "Accentuate the positive and eliminate the negative." Pay attention to the sense of accomplishment and the feeling of relaxation after exercise. Notice that your mind roams freely during exercise. Let it go where it may. You may work out the solution to a nagging problem while you jog or bike, or you may organize in your mind that paper that is due next week, or you may simply daydream. Also, as the weeks pass, you will notice a difference in energy level and a feeling of general well-being. Concentrate on these factors, and they will keep you in the right frame of mind about exercise.

● Don't Become Obsessive About Exercise

You should relax and enjoy exercise, which should be recreative, not obstructive. Don't become so obsessive that you feel and act miserable because you missed a day of exercise. Sometimes unplanned circumstances make it difficult to exercise on a particular day. Develop the mature philosophy that tomorrow is another day, and you will get your chance then. If you become ill, don't exercise. Resume your program when you feel better. The major point is that missing an occasional day of exercise will not detract from the fitness benefits that you have achieved. Later on in this text you will find that a couple of days off from exercise in a week's time is important. The second point is that one need not feel guilty because occasionally a day slips by without a workout. If you rest two days a week, you can use one of the days to make up the missing workout.

● Know That There Are No Failures

Physical fitness may be attained without competing against others or the clock. McGlynn;[44] has summarized this concept very nicely in this manner, "There are no complex skills to learn, no condescending instructors, no embarrassing situations, no last-place finishes, no critical peers, no intimidation." In other words, just go out and do your thing.

PERSONALIZE YOUR EXERCISE PROGRAM

Personalizing your fitness program involves those suggestions in this chapter that are relevant for you. It means that you take ownership and responsibility for the program. Personalizing the program includes the objectives that you wish to achieve, the activities employed to attain those objectives, whether you will exercise alone or with others, whether you will join a health or fitness center, whether you will take a fitness-oriented physical education course, how hard and how often you will exercise, and how physically fit you ultimately wish to become.

One of the tools that you can use to personalize your program is to develop and sign a contractual document with yourself or some significant other person. Complying with the terms of the contract is highly motivating for some—it may be for you. An example of a personal contract appears in Self-Assessment 2.3 in Appendix C. Completing this contract will answer some of the questions needed to personalize your program.

POINTS TO PONDER

Identify and discuss the various motivational strategies that one may employ to enhance starting and/or continuing an exercise program.

Give some examples of specific and behavioral fitness objectives.

How would you respond to someone who says that he or she doesn't exercise because of lack of time?

Define extrinsic and intrinsic reinforcement.

How would you go about the process of personalizing an exercise program?

Why would you keep a progress chart or daily record of exercise? What items would you include in the progress chart?

 CHAPTER HIGHLIGHTS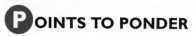

- Education and motivation are necessary minimums for the establishment and maintenance of a personal physical fitness program.
- About 50% of the people who begin exercise programs drop out during the first six months.
- Lack of time, inconvenient exercise site, work conflicts, and poor spousal support are the reasons most offered by people who quit exercising.
- Blue-collar workers, smokers, and the obese are less likely to begin and continue to exercise.

- Intrinsic motivation will sustain an exercise program; extrinsic motivation is important but supplementary.
- Moderate levels of motivation are optimal for continuing an exercise program.
- Adults exercise for health enhancement; college age people exercise to improve their physical appearance.
- There are many motivational strategies for improving exercise adherence. This chapter discusses many of them. Try them all and find out which one you are comfortable with.

REFERENCES

1. J. H. Wilmore, "Individual Exercise Prescription," *American Journal of Cardiology* 33 (1974): 757.

2. R. K. Dishman, "Exercise Compliance: A New View for Public Health," *The Physician and Sportsmedicine* 14 (1986): 127; R. J. Sonstroem, "Psychological Models" in R. K. Dishman (Ed.) *Exercise Adherence,* Champaign, Ill.: Human Kinetics, 1988.

3. M. L. Pollock, "Prescribing Exercise for Fitness and Adherence," in R. K. Dishman (Ed.), *Exercise Adherence,* Champaign, Ill.: Human Kinetics, 1988.

4. S. Biddle and R. A. Smith, "Motivating Adults for Physical Activity: Towards a Healthier Present," *Journal of Physical Education, Recreation, and Dance* 62, no. 7 (September 1991): 39.

5. R. K. Dishman, "Exercise Compliance," 1986, p. 132.

6. J. M. Rippe (Moderator), "The Health Benefits of Exercise (Part 2 of 2)," *The Physician and Sportsmedicine* 15 (1987): 120.

7. Ibid., p. 124.

8. R. K. Dishman, "Exercise Compliance," 1986, p. 141.

9. S. G. Aldana and W. J. Stone, "Changing Physical Activity Preferences of American Adults," *Journal of Physical Education, Recreation, and Dance* 62, no. 4 (April 1991): 67.

10. B. Ketchum, "Fit for the Fast Lane," *The Walking Magazine* (March/April, 1989): 4.

11. Louis Harris and Associates, Inc. *The Prevention Index: A Report Card on National Health,* Emmaus, Pa.: Rodale Press, 1988.

12. "Report of the Secretary's Task Force on Black and Minority Health," U.S. Dept. of Health and Human Services, Publication No. 0/N/174/N/719, Washington, D.C. U.S. Government Printing Office, August 1985.

13. D. Giel, "Fitness and Exercise Issues for Black Americans," *The Physician and Sportsmedicine* 16 (1988): 162.

14. T. Monahan, "Is Fitness Reaching Only the Wealthy?" *The Physician and Sportsmedicine* 17 (1989): 200.

15. D. Giel, "Fitness and Exercise Issues," 1988, p. 168.

16. G. Sage, *Motor Learning and Control: A Neuropsychological Approach*, Dubuque, Iowa: William C. Brown, 1984.

17. R. J. Shepard, "Motivation: The Key to Compliance," *The Physician and Sportsmedicine* 13 (1987): 88.

18. B. A. Franklin, "Motivating and Educating Adults to Exercise," *Journal of Physical Education and Recreation* 49 (1978): 6.

19. J. H. Buffington, "Getting Going," *Sky* 112 (1985): 113.

20. D. Greene and M. R. Lepper, "How to Turn Play into Work," *Psychology Today* 8 (1974): 49.

21. F. Levine and G. Fasnacht, "Token Rewards May Lead to Token Learning," *American Psychologist* 29 (1974): 816.

22. P. Klavora, "Customary Arousal for Peak Athletic Performance," in P. Klavora and J. V. Daniel (Eds.), *Coach, Athlete and Sport Psychologist,* Champaign, Ill.: Human Kinetics, 1979.

23. S. Blair, "Values of Physical Activity as Expressed by Physical Education Majors," *The Physical Educator* 41 (1984): 186; T. R. Trimble and L. D. Hensley, "The General Instruction Program in Physical Education at Four-Year Colleges and Universities, 1982, " *Journal of Physical Education, Recreation, and Dance* 59 (1988): 28.

24. R. E. Koslow, "College Fitness Courses—What Determines Student Interest?" *Journal of Physical Education, Recreation, and Dance* 59 (1988): 28.

25. T. G. Harris and J. Kagan, "The Fitness Advantage," *American Health* 4, (1985): 12.

26. W. P. Morgan and S. E. Goldston (Eds.), *Exercise and Mental Health,* Washington, D.C.: Hemisphere Publishing, 1987.

27. K. E. Callen, "Mental and Emotional Aspects of Long-Distance Running," *Psychosomatics* 24 (1983): 145.

28. T. Monahan, "Exercise and Depression: Swapping Sweat for Serenity?" *The Physician and Sportsmedicine* 14 (1986): 192.

29. J. M. Rippe, "The Health Benefits of Exercise," 1987, p. 122.

30. T. Monahan, "Exercise and Depression," 1986, p. 193.

31. R. A. Hayes, "Relating Physical and Psychological Fitness: A Psychological Point of View," *Journal of Sports Medicine and Physical Fitness* 18 (1978): 399; G. R. Leonardson, "Relationships Between Self-Concept and Perceived Physical Fitness," *Perceptual and Motor Skills* 44 (1977): 62; G. R. Leonardson and R. M. Garguilo, "Self-Perception and Physical Fitness," *Perceptual Motor Skills* 46 (1978): 338.

32. J. M. Rippe, "The Health Benefits of Exercise," 1987, p. 122; B. A. Franklin, "Program Factors That Influence Exercise Adherence: Practical Adherence Skills for the Clinical Staff," in R. K. Dishman (Ed.), *Exercise Adherence,* Champaign, Ill.: Human Kinetics, 1988.

33. M. L. Pollock et al., "Effects of Frequency and Duration of Training on Attrition and Incidence of Injury," *Medicine and Science in Sports* 9 (1977): 31.

34. M. L. Pollock, "Prescribing Exercise," 1988, p. 222.

35. D. Greene and M. R. Lepper, "How to Turn Play into Work," 1974, p. 49.

36. J. F. Massie and R. J. Shepard, "Physiological and Psychological Effects of Training—A Comparison of Individual and Gymnasium Programs, with a Characterization of

Exercise Drop-Out," *Medicine and Science in Sports* 3 (1971): 110.

37. D. N. Knapp, "Behavioral Management Techniques and Exercise Promotion," in R. K. Dishman (Ed.), *Exercise Adherence,* Champaign, Ill.: Human Kinetics, 1988.

38. A. C. King et al. "Group- vs. Home-Based Exercise Training in Healthy Older Men and Women: A Community Based Clinical Trial," *Journal of the American Medical Association* 266, no. 11 (1991): 1535.

39. G. M. Andrew et al., "Reasons for Dropout from Exercise Programs in Post-Coronary Patients," *Medicine and Science in Sports and Exercise* 13 (1981): 164; D. Knapp et al., "Exercise Adherence Among Coronary Artery Bypass Surgery (CABS) Patients," *Medicine and Science in Sports and Exercise* 15 (1983): 120.

40. A. C. King and L. W. Frederiksen, "Low-cost Strategies for Increasing Exercise Behavior: Relapse Preparation Training and Social Support," *Behavior Modification* 8 (1984): 3; J. E. Martin et al., "Behavioral Control of Exercise in Sedentary Adults: Studies 1 Through 6," *Journal of Consulting and Clinical Psychology* 52 (1984): 795.

41. R. O. Nelson et al., "Self-Reinforcement: Appealing Misnomer or Effective Mechanism?" *Behavior Research and Therapy* 21 (1983): 557.

42. R. J. Trotter, "Maybe It's the Music," *Psychology Today* 8 (1984): 19.

43. J. M. Rippe, "29 Tips for Staying With It," *Annual Edition—Health 89/90,* Guilford, Conn: The Dushkin Publishing Group, 1989.

44. G. McGlynn, *Dynamics of Fitness: A Practical Approach,* Dubuque, Iowa: William C. Brown, 1987.

Guidelines for Exercise

CHAPTER OUTLINE

INTRODUCTION

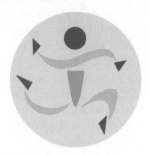

This chapter presents exercise guidelines developed by the American College of Sports Medicine (ACSM) for the achievement of physical fitness and wellness. For safe and effective exercise, it is important for you to understand and apply these guidelines. The chapter presents warming-up and cooling-down procedures. It identifies and discusses the principles of conditioning from the perspective of applying them to your personal needs. The chapter gives suggestions for manipulating the exercise principles to accommodate your objectives and the environment in which you exercise. It also presents suggestions regarding the effects of exercise on prepubescent children and pregnant women and their fetuses.

Two Self-Assessment activities appear in Appendix C that apply directly to the contents of this chapter:

3.1 The Karvonen Formula

3.2 Your Personal Exercise Program

Miniglossary

Active Warm-Up Dynamic movements for the purpose of readying the body for physical activity.

Adenosine Diphosphate (ADP) A complex, high-energy compound from which ATP is resynthesized.

Adenosine Triphosphate (ATP) A complex, high-energy compound stored in the cells from which the body derives its energy.

Aerobic Literally means "with oxygen."

Anaerobic Literally means "without oxygen."

Anaerobic Threshold That point at which exercise cannot be totally sustained by the aerobic processes. Anaerobic processes contribute to the production of ATP and lactic acid begins to accumulate in the blood.

Conduction Transference of heat from one object to another by physical contact.

Convection Transfer of heat from the body to a moving gas or liquid.

Creatine Phosphate (CP) A chemical that donates its phosphate to ADP for the resynthesis of ATP.

Cross-training Selection and participation in more than one physical activity on a consistent basis.

Dehydration Excessive loss of body fluids.

Electrolyte Any solution that conducts an electrical current through its ions.

Evaporation The loss of heat by changing a liquid to a vapor.

Glycogen The stored form of sugar.

Heat Exhaustion A condition characterized by a buildup of body heat. Symptoms include dizziness, fainting, rapid pulse, and cool skin.

Heat Stroke The most dangerous of the heat-stress illnesses. Symptoms include a temperature of 106° F and above, absence of sweating, dry skin, and often delirium, convulsions, and loss of consciousness.

Hemoglobin Iron pigment of the red cells that combines with oxygen.

Hyperthermia Overheating; abnormally high body temperature.

Hypothermia Abnormally low body temperature.

Lactic Acid A fatiguing metabolite resulting from the incomplete breakdown of sugar.

Passive Warm-Up Inactive means of preparing for physical activity; may include massage and dry and wet heat.

Radiation Transfer of heat from the body to the atmosphere by electromagnetic waves.

The energy for muscular contraction comes from the foods that we eat, but our muscles cannot directly use carbohydrates, fats, and proteins for fuel. Protein liberates only a very small portion of its energy to generate human movement. Its primary function centers on building and repairing bodily tissues as well as synthesizing hormones and enzymes. No other food source can perform these functions. Protein becomes a substantial energy source under two conditions: (1) during starvation, when the body is consuming its own muscles, and (2) during prolonged exercise, such as marathons, ultra-marathons, or other long-distance continuous events.

Carbohydrates and fats are our major energy sources. Both substances are metabolized enzymatically in a series of complex chemical stages to provide the fuel for movement. The chemical processes by which this is accomplished are very complex and beyond the scope and purpose of this text, but we will cover the anaerobic and aerobic operations associated with metabolic processes to emphasize the major differences between aerobic and anaerobic exercise.

Carbohydrates are broken down to water and carbon dioxide, which releases the energy needed to form **adenosine triphosphate (ATP).** The energy for muscular contraction occurs when ATP splits into **adenosine diphosphate (ADP)** and phosphate (P). A small quantity of ATP is stored in the muscles, along with **creatine phosphate (CP),** to provide an instant source of energy for muscular contraction. The splitting of CP to creatine and inorganic phosphate provides the energy to resynthesize ATP from ADP, thus restoring ATP levels in the muscles.

Fats are also oxidized to yield energy to form ATP. The type of fuel—carbohydrate or fat—used to manufacture ATP depends upon the intensity or the amount of effort required to perform an exercise or activity. Exercise and physical activity—indeed, all movement—may be categorized as being predominantly, if not exclusively, anaerobic or aerobic. **Anaerobic** literally means "without oxygen." Anaerobic activities, then, are high-intensity movements that can be continued for only a matter of seconds. Sprinting 100 yards, lifting a heavy weight, shot-putting, and running up two flights of stairs are some examples of anaerobic activities. The oxygen demand of these activities is higher than that which can be supplied by the body during their performance. As a result, these events rely on the short-term fuel supplies of ATP or CP stored in the muscles that can be mobilized rapidly in the absence of adequate oxygen. Sugar in the form of **glycogen** (the stored form of glucose) is broken down to pyruvic acid, which is temporarily shunted to **lactic acid** (a fatiguing metabolite that results from the incomplete breakdown of sugar) when oxygen cannot be supplied rapidly enough for processing by the muscle cells (see Figure 3.1). This process produces a very small quantity of ATP and a large quantity of lactic acid. Since the cells cannot tolerate

---

FIGURE 3.1

Simplified Schematic of the Anaerobic Pathway Without sufficient O$_2$, pyruvic acid is converted to lactic acid, and only 2 ATP are formed from each molecule of glycogen. Carbohydrates are the fuel source for this type of high-intensity work. No oxygen is required for glycogen to break down to pyruvic acid.

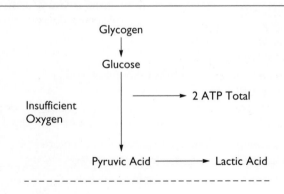

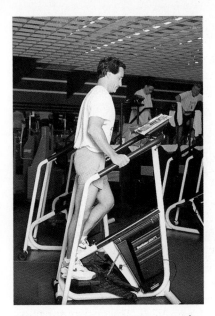

Stair-step exercise is becoming one of the most popular of the aerobic exercise alternatives.

high levels of lactic acid, performance must cease until the lactic acid is removed. In the anaerobic cycle, one molecule of glucose yields only two molecules of ATP.

Fat is not utilized as a fuel source during high-intensity anaerobic activity, because lactic acid blocks the action of epinephrine, a fat-mobilizing hormone. Epinephrine makes fat available from its storage depots for use as a fuel during low-intensity exercise because lactic acid production is inconsequential. Anaerobic activities are fueled entirely by carbohydrate metabolism (see Figure 3.2). The limited production and storage capacity of ATP in this process dictates that high-intensity exercises can be sustained for only a matter of seconds.

Carbohydrates are the preferred source of fuel during very vigorous exercise because they are our most efficient source of fuel. Carbohydrates produce about 5 percent more energy per liter of oxygen consumed than fat. This is important for performing anaerobic or high-intensity exercise because we need to extract as much energy as possible from each unit of oxygen that we are capable of consuming.

Aerobic means "with oxygen." Aerobic activities depend on a continuous and sufficient supply of oxygen to burn fats and carbohydrates to support endurance or sustained activity. For exercise to be aerobic, the level of intensity is such that the oxygen needs of the activity can be adequately supplied by the body during the activity. In other words, the participant achieves a balance or "steady state" between oxygen supply and demand. This is a "pay as you go" system (see Figure 3.3).

Walking, jogging, biking, swimming, stair-skipping, and aerobic dancing are some of the more popular forms of aerobic exercise. Carbohydrates and fat supply large quantities of ATP aerobically to fuel these activities. Walking, slow jogging, and prolonged exercises that are performed at less than 55 percent of one's oxygen utilization capacity rely primarily on fat for ATP production. Those activities that are sustained above 80 percent of one's capacity depend upon carbohydrates as the predominant source of ATP production.

When sufficient oxygen is available, carbohydrates are broken down to pyruvic acid, which in turn is converted to carbon dioxide and water through a series of intermediate stages without the production of lactic acid. This process is accompanied by the systematic production of large quantities of ATP—19 times the amount produced anaerobically (see Figure 3.4). Fats make their contribution to ATP production by entering the cycle below the level of pyruvic acid.

In terms of ATP production, it is readily apparent why aerobic exercise can be prolonged and anaerobic activities cannot. B. J. Sharkey summarizes this way: "Aerobic pathways must be used if we are to delay fatigue. They are more efficient and the fuels are more abundant. As exercise intensifies from a walk to a jog we switch from fat as the predominate source of energy to a fat-carbohydrate

---

FIGURE 3.2

Lactic Acid Effect on Fat Metabolism   Lactic Acid blocks the action of epinephrine so that fat cannot be removed from storage in adipose cells during high-intensity exercise. This action inhibits the use of fat as a fuel during vigorous exercise.

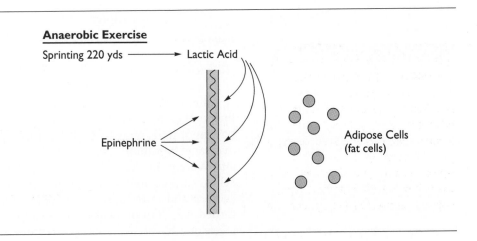

Anaerobic Exercise

Sprinting 220 yds ⟶ Lactic Acid

Epinephrine

Adipose Cells (fat cells)

FIGURE 3.3

Oxygen Demand This is a typical curve representing the achievement of a steady state between the oxygen demand of exercise and the exerciser's ability to meet it.

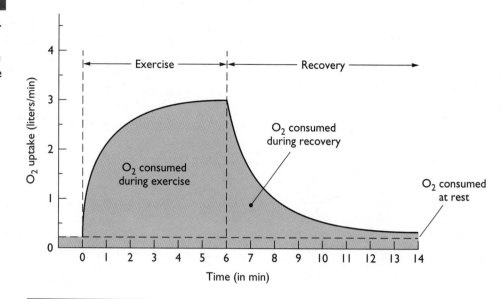

(glycogen) mixture. Switch from a jog to a run, and glycogen becomes the main source of energy. Sprint and glycogen is the sole source of energy."[1]

Aerobic activities, which are dependent upon a constant supply of oxygen, stress the cardiovascular and respiratory systems. In this manner, they increase aerobic capacity and produce the training effect that enables people to improve their performance in endurance activities while concomitantly attaining the health-related benefits. On the other hand, anaerobic activities apply their stress for periods of time that are too short to enhance the aerobic system unless they are employed in circuit or interval training (discussed in Chapter 5).

PRINCIPLES FOR EXERCISE

This chapter attempts to provide the type of information beginners need to intelligently assess their fitness needs and develop a sound program to meet those needs. A sound program will avert many of the pitfalls that have beset and curtailed thousands of fitness programs. Start right and give yourself every chance to succeed. Optimal benefits accrue by regular participation beginning early in life and continuing without the years of interruption that commonly occur between graduation from school and middle age.

> Choose what is best; habit will soon render it agreeable and easy.
> —Pythagoras

Starting Out Right

Exercise must become habitual if it is to make an optimal contribution to physical fitness and health. Regular and consistent participation for three to six months will yield a variety of physiological and psychological benefits that may ultimately provide the stimulus for lifetime continuation.

An important lesson that prospective fitness devotees must learn is to contain their enthusiasm in the initial stages of the exercise program. Ten years of inactivity cannot be expunged with ten furious days of activity. Impatient beginners, overeager to rapidly attain fitness, tend to exercise beyond their capacity. Such efforts are predictably doomed to fail because the usual results are a profusion of aches, strains, and pains and no enjoyment of exercise. As exercise becomes a chore, enthusiasm subsides and the program, with all of its good intentions, is discarded. Recall from the inverted U hypothesis covered in Chapter 2 that moderate levels of motivation are best for perseverance at a task.

The Medical Exam

The ACSM, in conjunction with the American Medical Association (AMA), has established guidelines for medical screening before starting an exercise program.[2] People under the age of 45 who are apparently healthy can begin exercising without medical screening. However, they need to start at a level compatible with their degree of physical fitness, and they should progress slowly. All people regardless of age should have a medical screening prior to exercise if they are at high risk, that is, if they they have two or more risk factors for cardiovascular disease or if they have previously diagnosed cardiovascular disease, diabetes, or any other chronic disease.

Warming Up for Exercise

Warming up, or getting the body ready for exercise, is one of the often slighted and sometimes neglected phases of a workout. Warm-up may be passive, active, or a combination of the two. A **passive warm-up** includes massage, steam or sauna, hot towels, hot showers, and whirlpool baths. These activities might alleviate the stiffness and soreness that can carry over from the previous workout. A passive warm-up might be an adjunct to, but not a replacement for, an active warm-up prior to exercise. Passive warm-up may be counterproductive because it increases surface temperature by dilating the blood vessels in the skin, resulting in the diversion of blood to the skin rather than to the muscles that will be involved in the activity.

An **active warm-up** usually includes a general and a specific component. The general component consists of stretching and large-muscle activities designed to slowly raise the heart rate while increasing muscle temperature. The specific component of warming up involves participation in the activity to be performed or a related activity. For example, subsequent to the completion of the general phase of warm-up, joggers might run in place or jog the first half mile of the workout at a leisurely pace, slowly increasing to the desired speed. In this way, the body is allowed to selectively and gradually adapt to the specific stress to be imposed upon it. The concepts of general and specific warm-up apply to most activities—including swimming, biking, rope jumping, racquetball, and tennis.

The primary reason for warming up before exercise is to gradually increase the heart rate and thus the circulation of blood. This smooths the transition from inactivity to activity with minimum oxygen deprivation to the tissues and organs. In the absence of warming up, the heart rate rapidly increases from the resting to the

---

FIGURE 3.4

Simplified Schematic of the Aerobic Pathway   When sufficient oxygen is present, pyruvic acid is broken down to its end products of carbon dioxide and water, and in the process, large quantities of ATP are produced. Fats are a primary energy source during low-intensity work.

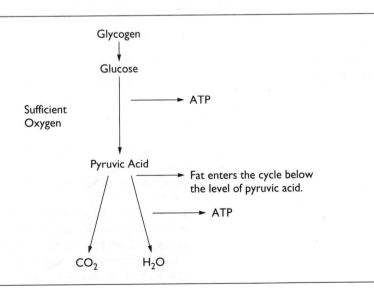

exercise state, and the body is forced to employ anaerobic processes to generate fuel, resulting in an undesirable and unnecessary accumulation of lactic acid. Circulation does not increase proportionately to heart rate, causing a brief interval when the heart is not fully supplied with oxygen. This delay can be hazardous for people whose circulation is compromised. Although the healthy, well-conditioned heart can usually endure such treatment, even a sound organ may be at risk. One study indicated that 44 healthy male subjects ages 21 to 52 had normal electrocardiographic (EKG) responses to exercise that followed a warm-up consisting of two minutes of easy jogging.[3] But 70 percent of the group developed abnormal EKG responses to the same exercise when it was not preceded by a warm-up. You have probably warmed-up sufficiently when you begin to sweat because this signifies that the core temperature is slightly elevated.

● Intensity

Intensity refers to the degree of vigor associated with each bout of exercise. The ACSM recommends an exercise intensity level of 60 percent to 90 percent of the maximum heart rate for aerobic exercise.[4] The intensity level as recommended by most authorities for weight training is approximately 70 percent to 80 percent of a maximal lift.[5] The ACSM suggests doing 8 to 12 repetitions to near maximal fatigue for each exercise.[6] These guidelines reflect the fact that the training effect for the cardiorespiratory and muscular systems occur at a level of exercise below maximum capacity. This rather nicely dispels the myth that exercise must be very vigorous, and therefore painful, to be beneficial. Exercising individuals who cannot talk without gasping for breath between each word are performing at a pace too vigorous for their fitness level. Although this is a good subjective check that lessens the probability of overexertion, it doesn't indicate whether the participant is exercising at the level needed to achieve optimal results.

A more precise test utilizes the heart rate for calculating the upper and lower limits for exercise. The calculating procedure for target heart rate (training heart rate) is quite simple. Follow these steps:

1. Estimate maximal heart rate by subtracting your age from the constant 220.

2. Multiply the result by the percent of your capacity at which you which to train.

3. The following example is for a 20-year-old.

> 220 (constant)
> −20 (age)
> 200 (predicted maximal heart rate in beats per minute—bpm)
> × .70 (percent of maximum heart rate that you wish to exercise at)
> 140 (target exercise heart rate in bpm)

The target heart rate for exercise is a ballpark figure based on an estimated maximum heart rate. The error of estimation can be as high as 12 beats per minute for some people. The average 20-year-old will have a maximum heart rate of 200 bpm. The maximum heart rate (MHR) is affected by age—the older the person, the lower the MHR, so that the average 40-year-old has an MHR of 180 beats per minute.

The Karvonen formula is also a popular and functional method for determining exercise heart rate (pulse rate). This method was developed in 1957 and validated in 1975.[7] The resting heart rate must be known to use this formula. Since many factors (caffeine, nicotine, environmental temperature, anxiety, eating a meal, etc.) affect the resting heart rate, it is important to establish this parameter under standard conditions. The best way to determine the resting heart rate is in the sitting position after waking up in the morning.[8] You may need to empty your bladder first, then sit down and stay calm for a few minutes before taking the pulse. Repeat this for four to five consecutive days and average the readings. This method should produce a good representation of the normal resting heart rate.

There are two advantages to using the Karvonen formula. First, the individual's resting heart rate (RHR) is used in the calculation of the exercise heart rate. The RHR yields an estimate of one's fitness level. Generally speaking, the lower the RHR, the more fit the individual. The second advantage is that the formula uses the individual's cardiac reserve, which is the difference between the maximum heart rate (MHR) and the resting heart rate (RHR), in the calculation of the target heart rate (THR). The more fit the person, the greater the cardiac reserve because of a lower RHR. Conversely, the less fit the person, the lower the cardiac reserve because of a higher RHR.

Table 3.1 gives an example of how to use the Karvonen formula. The example is based on a 22-year-old exerciser with an RHR of 72 bpm who is in average physical condition and will train at an intensity level of 70 percent. Table 3.2 presents guidelines that should help you select the proper training intensity to use in calculating the Karvonen formula based upon your level of fitness.

Learning to take the heart rate by palpating the pulse is a skill that you must develop to determine the RHR and to monitor the intensity of exercise. The pulse can be felt at several sites in the body. The two most practical are the radial pulse, located in the wrist at the base of the thumb while the hand is held palm up, and the carotid pulse, which can be felt in the large arteries at either side of the neck (see Figure 3.5). Use the middle three fingers of the preferred hand to count the pulse. To locate the carotid pulse, slide your fingers down from the angle of the jaw below the earlobe to your neck. Remember to start counting the pulse as soon as possible after exercise to get an accurate indication of the exercise heart rate, because the rate declines rapidly when activity ceases. It takes some practice to quickly locate the pulse, begin the count, and count accurately.

The carotid pulse may not be the most appropriate site for estimating exercise heart rate, because the arteries in the neck are pressure sensitive. Pressure applied to the carotid arteries stretches their walls, which in turn signals the brain to slow the heart rate. This will result in an inaccurate, underestimated exercise heart rate. To minimize or possibly circumvent this effect, the pressure applied to the carotid should not exceed that required to feel the beat.

To calculate exercise heart rate, the participant should periodically stop exercising, immediately count the pulse rate for ten seconds, and multiply this figure by six to obtain heart rate per minute.

Monitoring exercise by heart rate is generally an effective method, but it is not without flaws. First, stopping to take pulse rates become tedious and tends to interrupt the workout. Second, unless the maximum heart rate is assessed by an exercise tolerance test, the possibility of substantial error exists. Third, such monitoring might encourage slavish dependence upon heart rate to the exclusion of

TABLE 3.1 **Calculating Target Heart Rate for Exercise by the Karvonen Formula**

1. Calculate MHR (maximum heart rate)	220 (constant)
	− 22 (age)
	198 (MHR)
2. The Karvonen formula is	
THR	= cardiac reserve × TI% + RHR
Where	
THR	= target or training heart rate
Cardiac reserve	= MHR − RHR
TI%	= training intensity as a percentage
RHR	= resting heart rate
Therefore	
THR	= (MHR − RHR) × TI% + RHR
	= (198 − 72) × .70 + 72
	= 126 × .70 + 72
	= 88.2 + 72
THR	= 160 bpm

TABLE 3.2

Guidelines for Selecting Exercise Intensity Level

FITNESS LEVEL	INTENSITY LEVEL (%)
Low	60
Fair	65
Average	70
Good	75
Excellent	80–90

A perceived exertion rating of 12 to 13 corresponds to approximately 60% of the heart rate range. A rating of 16 corresponds to approximately 90% of heart rate range.

—ACSM

perceived exertion or one's subjective impression regarding how difficult the workout feels. It is important that you tune into your body and that you learn to recognize and pay attention to the signals it gives. Some of the notable signals that form our perception of exertion during exercise include rate and depth of breathing, heart beat, body temperature, musculoskeletal stress and pain, and overall discomfort. Gunnar Borg had developed a rating scale that rather accurately predicts actual exercise heart rate.[9] (See Figure 3.6).

Note that the scale ranges from 6 to 20, with 6 being very, very light and 20 corresponding to very, very hard. When multiplied by a factor of 10, the numbers on the scale represent heart rates. A rating of 6 is translated as a heart rate of 60, and a rating of 20 is translated as a heart rate of 200. Published data indicate that the rating of perceived exertion not only correlates quite well with actual exertion as exhibited by exercise heart rate but also is oftentimes a better criterion measure, since it considers more than just the exercise heart rate.[10] It encompasses sensory input from all of the systems associated with the generation of energy for movement.

Perceived exertion is an excellent technique for monitoring exercise, particularly when maximum heart rate is estimated. If the heart rate maximum is overestimated, so too will the exercise target rate. Perceived exertion may be used to compensate for the error, thus averting overwork and its consequences. Also, we all experience days when exercise is more difficult, where the hills seem steeper and the track seems longer. Much like a sputtering auto engine, our body is trying to tell us something. When we experience such feelings, we should adjust the intensity downward and shorten the duration of the workout instead of pressing on as usual. Tomorrow will probably be a better day. The point is that we should not neglect what our body is attempting to communicate, and we should capitalize upon this source of feedback to make adjustments when needed.

A perceived exertion rating of 12 to 13 is equivalent to approximately 60 percent of the maximum heart rate.[11] A rating of 16 corresponds to approximately 85 percent of the maximum heart rate. Most people should exercise within this range of scores, since it reflects the ACSM recommendations for exercise.

To avoid confusion and repetition, the training principles in this chapter will apply primarily to cardiorespiratory or aerobic endurance. The principles that apply to the development of muscular strength, muscular endurance, and flexibility are discussed specifically in each of the chapters dealing with these topics.

FIGURE 3.5

Common Sites for Taking Pulse Rates   Locating the Pulse at the carotid artery (a) and at the wrist (b).

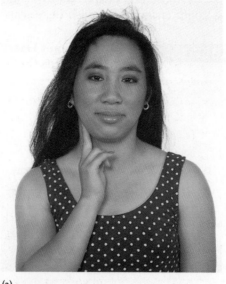
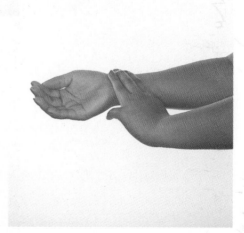

(a)   (b)

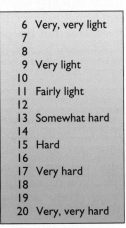

6	Very, very light
7	
8	
9	Very light
10	
11	Fairly light
12	
13	Somewhat hard
14	
15	Hard
16	
17	Very hard
18	
19	
20	Very, very hard

RECOGNIZING THE SIGNS OF OVERTRAINING

● Frequency

The ACSM recommends that exercise be pursued three to five times per week.[12] Fewer than three times a week is not enough of a stimulus to develop physical fitness, and more than five times a week increases the likelihood of injury.[13]

The frequency of exercise should vary according to the objectives you are attempting to achieve. Those of you who are interested in weight loss and altering body composition would do well to exercise five or possibly six times a week at a lower intensity, whereas three to four days of higher intensity exercise would suffice for those who are lean and whose major concern is the development of more energy or endurance. The intensity and duration of exercise should have some bearing upon frequency. Low-intensity exercise of moderate duration (20 to 40 minutes), such as walking, could be pursued every day without producing physiological or orthopedic problems, but high-intensity, longer-duration exercises such as jogging, biking, and aerobic dancing need to be performed only three to five times a week.

A study at Stanford University indicated that exercise can be split into several shorter sessions in a day and still produce adequate health and fitness benefits.[14] Two groups of men exercised for 30 minutes three times a week at 65 percent to 75 percent of their maximum heart rate. One of the groups achieved their workout with one bout of 30 continuous minutes of exercise, while the other group split the 30-minute workout into three separate 10-minute bouts. At the end of the eight weeks, both groups had improved their cardiorespiratory endurance, but the one-bout-of-exercise-per-day group showed more improvement. However, both groups lost the same amount of weight—4 pounds—during the eight weeks. The researchers concluded that people on tight work and/or academic schedules can squeeze shorter sessions of exercise between other responsibilities and attain significant health and fitness benefits. Shorter bouts of exercise spaced throughout the day represent a realistic option for busy people.

Days of rest are an important part of the training programs of people who exercise for health-related reasons—even world-class competitive athletes need to take an occasional day off to recharge the physiological and psychological batteries. Rest days should be spaced rather than taken consecutively. Periodic rest days also make sense with regard to lowering the likelihood of incurring an injury and combating the possibility of becoming "stale."

A fine line exists between the amount of exercise that produces maximum gains and the amount that results in the negative effects (staleness) associated with overtraining.[15] Overtraining occurs when exercisers do too much too often. The following are signs of this phenomenon:

- A feeling of chronic fatigue and listlessness.
- Inability to make further fitness gains (or there may be a loss of fitness).
- A sudden loss of weight.
- An increase of five beats or more in the resting pulse rate taken in the morning prior to getting out of bed.
- Loss of enthusiasm for working out (the exerciser no longer looks forward to the workout).
- Susceptibility to injury and illness.
- Feelings of anger and depression.

Staleness can be both psychological (lack of variety in the program or boredom after years of training) and physiological. It is probably a combination of both, but the treatment is the same: either stop training for a few days to a few weeks (depends upon the severity of staleness) or cut back substantially. In either case, rebuild and regain fitness gradually. Prevention is the best treatment. Recognize the signs and adjust accordingly before staleness becomes a problem.

Duration

Duration and intensity are inversely related: the more intense the exercise, the shorter its duration, and vice versa. Intensity is always an important consideration, but for people who exercise for health enhancement, it is best to sacrifice some degree of intensity for duration. The ACSM recommends that the length of each bout of exercise be 20 to 60 minutes of continuous or noncontinuous aerobic exercise.[16]

Epidemiological data have indicated that burning 1,000 to 2,000 calories per week in physical activity resulted in fewer heart attacks and longer life.[17] Achieving this level of energy expenditure is not as difficult as it may sound (see Table 3.3 for an example). Of course, you can use different activities from those in the example, and you can spread the activities over fewer days, but the point is that almost any level of energy expenditure above the sedentary level will produce health benefits.

Overload and Progression

Overload involves subjecting the various systems of the body to gradual and unaccustomed stresses. It is only through overload that the body adapts and improvements occur in strength, cardiovascular endurance, and flexibility. Without overload, no adaptation or improvement occurs. The principle of progression actually functions as the schedule for the application of overload. All physical fitness programs have three phases of progression: (1) the initial phase, (2) the improvement phase, and (3) the maintenance phase.

The initial phase features low-level intensity exercises performed three days a week. An entry program such as this should produce minimum muscle soreness and a decreased likelihood of physical injury. Pay attention to exercise heart rate and perceived exertion during this phase, adjusting them to suit your fitness level. The duration of the exercise session during the initial phase should be about 30 minutes, including the time spent warming up and cooling down. The initial phase should last four to six weeks, depending upon your fitness level at the entry point. During this phase, you are adapting to the exercise program.

The improvement phase lasts a minimum of four months to several years. During this time, the frequency and duration of exercise are increased slowly and

TABLE 3.3 Caloric Expenditure for a 150-lb. Person*

DAY	ACTIVITY	CALORIES EXPENDED
Monday	Brisk walking (30 min)	160
	Stair climbing (5 min)	35
Tuesday	Swimming (20 min)	180
	Jogging (10 min)	95
Wednesday	Stationary cycling (15 min, 10 mph)	105
	Stationary rowing (10 min)	65
	Stair climbing (10 min. fast)	85
Thursday	Mow lawn (20 min)	150
	Rake grass and yard work (20 min)	135
	Housecleaning (20 min)	80
Friday	Brisk walking (30 min)	160
	Stationary cycling (20 min)	135
Saturday	Brisk walking (30 min)	160
	Wash car (20 min)	65
	Gardening (20 min)	135
Sunday	REST	
		Total 1,745 calories

*If you weigh less than 150 lb., you will burn fewer calories; if you weigh more than 150 lbs., you will burn more calories. The figures in this example are not exact but are representative estimates.

progressively. When you are able to exercise continuously for 30 minutes exclusive of warmup and cooldown, you are ready to increase exercise intensity. The key to overloading the body is to apply stress slowly and progressively, only when it is warranted, and not before.

Overload is applied by increasing the frequency, duration, and intensity of exercise. Beginners should stress increasing frequency and duration, and when fitness improves, they can begin to increase intensity. Three observations might be noted regarding the application of overload:

1. Patience is necessary.
2. Improvements occur in small increments, but the greatest amounts occur during the first six to eight weeks of the exercise program.
3. Overload should be applied only when certain criteria are met that indicate that the individual is ready to accept a newer challenge.

When people attain a level of fitness that meets their needs and further improvement is no longer desired, the program switches from the development of fitness to the maintenance of fitness. The maintenance phase may be initiated after the first six months of training. This represents a point where many exercisers are no longer willing to increase the workload. However, some competitors are willing to work harder to achieve the small gains that are possible after one becomes physically fit. For them, maintenance is considered only after many years of training.

● Specificity

Ample evidence exists to support the contention that the body adapts according to the specific type of stress placed upon it. The muscles used in any given activity are the ones that adapt, and they do so in the specific way in which they are used. Jogging does not prepare one for swimming, and swimming does not prepare one for cycling. The legs are stressed in jogging in a manner unique to that activity. Those adaptations that occur from jogging provide very little carryover to the leg kick for swimming.

Triathalon training is a good example of the influence of specificity. To achieve their potential in this sport, competitors must train vigorously in all three events of the triathlon, because no combination of training for two of them will result in significant improvement in the third.

Specificity of training was demonstrated when two groups of subjects were tested maximally on a treadmill and then in the swimming pool.[18] One of the groups then received 12 weeks of swim training, while the other group was excluded from this activity. Both groups were retested at the end of the 12 weeks. The swim-trained group improved significantly in swimming capacity, as indicated by the difference between their pretest and posttest scores, and they were also significantly better than the nontrained group on the posttest. However, the swim-trained group did not improve on the treadmill test, indicating that specific adaptations were made to the swim-training program. Task-specific training involves repetitive overloading of the muscles that are to be used in the event in the way that they are to be used to enhance performance.

The application of specificity is extremely important for competitive athletes who are attempting to maximize the returns from their investment in training. Therefore, swimmers must train by swimming, distance runners must run, and cyclists must cycle to train the body in the specific manner in which it is to perform. Although this locks athletes into set training programs, people who exercise for health reasons are not under such constraints. They can vary the activities in their program, averting the boredom and tedium of doing the same thing week after week.

Varying and combining different activities in the fitness program is called **cross-training.** People who employ cross-training techniques may not become highly fit or skilled in any of the activities, but if that is not a major concern, this

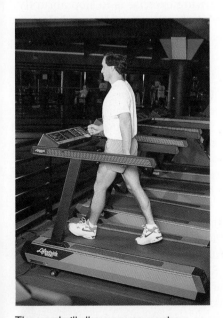

The treadmill allows one to set the speed and incline for a steady state workout.

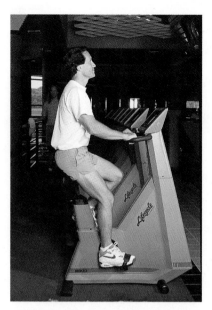

Stationary cycling is a safe way to exercise and requires minimal physical skill.

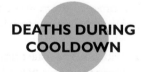

DEATHS DURING COOLDOWN

may be the training method of choice. Moderate elevation of the heart rate and a perceived exertion level of about 12 to 13 is sufficient to promote health and well-being. Cross-training allows for the inclusion of fun and diversity in the exercise program. You may employ cycling, jogging, swimming, racquetball, cross-country skiing, rope jumping, weight training, and so on, in the development of fitness and in any combination or order you may dictate. You may take into account weather conditions, availability of equipment and facilities, and what activity you feel like pursuing on any given day. You also might choose to combine two or more activities in the same exercise session.

Cross-training enables one to maintain a high volume of training with less likelihood of injury, staleness, and burnout. The different activities tend to spread the stress imposed by training to the different muscle groups, limiting the possibility of overworking any one group of muscles.

Many people enjoy more than one activity, while other people exclusively pursue one activity. Exercising for health does not preclude either approach for those who desire it. More options are available to people who exercise for health purposes than to competitive athletes. The important point is to select an activity or activities that give both pleasure and the desired training effect.

Cooling Down from Exercise

Cooling down from exercise is as important as warming up. Just as the body was allowed to speed up gradually, it must be allowed to slow down gradually. The body is not analogous to an auto engine that can be turned on and off with the turn of a key. Cooldown should last about 8 to 10 minutes.

The first phase of cooling down should consist of walking or some other light activity to prevent blood from pooling in the active muscles. Five minutes of continuous light activity causes rhythmical muscle contractions that prevent the pooling of blood and helps to move blood back to the heart for redistribution to the vital organs. This boost to circulation after exercise is an essential component of the cooldown period. Inactivity during this time forces the heart to compensate for the reduced volume of blood returning to it by maintaining a high pumping rate. The exerciser runs the risk of dizziness, fainting, and perhaps more serious consequences associated with diminished blood flow. Light activity also speeds up the removal of lactic acid that has accumulated in the muscles.

The worst possible cooldown procedure following exercise is to stop abruptly and sit or stand still. This will cause blood to pool in the muscles used during exercise that in turn will cause the blood pressure to drop and the heart rate to remain high.

Researchers have investigated several possibilities regarding the incidence of sudden death associated with vigorous physical activity. Sudden death of an exerciser is a rare event and one that tends to occur during the cool-down phase immediately after the workout. One of the viable theories as to why this occurs involves the relationship between blood pressure and epinephrine and norepinephrine. All three of these values increase as the intensity of exercise increases. Epinephrine and norepinephrine are hormones produced by the body that stimulate the heart to beat faster.

When exercise stops, blood pressure begins to drop but epinephrine and norepinephrine continue to rise for a few minutes. The marked increase in norepinephrine after exercise might be a reflex attempt to maintain the high blood pressure rate attained during peak exercise. Researchers have speculated that this may be the mechanism that triggers the potentially dangerous irregular heart beats after exercise that can lead to sudden death.

It takes a while for norepinephrine to return to normal levels after exercise. Circulation is out of balance during this time because the flow of blood slows

Continued

—Continued
faster than the beating heart, unless one follows proper cool-down procedures that promote circulation without blood pooling. The key is to keep moving—don't sit down and especially don't stand still.

K. H. Cooper, *Running Without Fear*, New York: M. Evans and Company, 1985.

The second phase of cooldown should focus on the same stretching exercises that were used during the warm-up period. You will probably note that stretching is tolerated more comfortably after exercise because of the increase in muscle temperature. Stretching at this time helps prevent muscle soreness.

Backward locomotion is a new technique employed by some exercisers to supplement their stretching program. Backward walking (retro walking) and backward jogging (retro running) reduce the range of motion at the hip joint and increase it at the knee joint.[19] In backward locomotion, the maximum knee extension occurs late in the support phase (when each leg in turn supports most of the body weight). At this point, there is substantial stretch of the hamstring muscle group (muscles located in the back of the thighs). The hamstrings tighten up when one walks, jogs, sits, and so on; therefore, it is important to engage in activities that keep them flexible.

Retro walking is currently being applied in the rehabilitation of hip and hamstring injuries and in postsurgical knee therapy.[20] If you choose to experiment with retro walking or running, follow these guidelines:

1. Choose a flat smooth surface such as that found on running tracks or, if available, a treadmill.

2. Begin slowly to avert muscle soreness, particularly of the calf muscle.

3. Walk or run backwards for brief periods—25 to 50 yards at a time—and increase the distance slowly.

4. When looking over your shoulder, alternate sides to prevent cramping of the neck.

5. Retro activity should be a supplement to your usual stretching exercise.

 OINTS TO PONDER

1. Trace the production of ATP both anaerobically and aerobically. Which results in the development of the most ATP?

2. Discuss active versus passive warm-up, general versus specific warm-up, and the effectiveness of warm-up in enhancing performance and decreasing the incidence of injury.

3. Discuss the ACSM guidelines for frequency, duration, and intensity of exercise.

4. What is a plausible explanation for the occurrence of sudden death during the cooldown after exercise?

5. Compute a training heart rate for a 28-year-old man with a resting heart rate of 76 beats per minute by the Karvonen formula. Use 65% as the intensity level. Then turn to Self-Assessment 3.1 in Appendix C and calculate your own training heart rate on the form provided.

EXERCISE DURING PREGNANCY

Considerable controversy exists regarding the benefits and possible harmful effects of exercise to expectant mothers and their fetuses. Experts are lined up on both sides of the issue, since no definitive study has occurred to provide substantive guidelines for maternal exercise during pregnancy. In lieu of such a study, the American College of Obstetricians and Gynecologists (ACOG) has developed

Facts, Fallacies, and Timely Tidbits

1. Lean, physically fit people do not die of heart disease.
This would be wonderful if it were true, but there is nothing known that is guaranteed to prevent heart disease. The good news is that those who are lean and physically fit have a lower probability of having a heart attack and a better chance of surviving should one occur.

2. It is a good idea to drink beer while recovering from exercise as many exercisers do.
Actually, this is a bad idea. Alcohol is a diuretic that stimulates the production of urine. The key to fluid replacement after exercise is to consume liquids that will migrate to the tissues rather than those that encourage removal by the kidneys.

3. Children don't need to make a conscious effort to exercise because they are naturally active and get all the exercise they need from these activities.
This was correct at one time but today there are so many competing activities of a nonphysical nature that many children are underexercised. Today's children are fatter and less fit than at any other time during this century. Video games, television, bussing, and reductions in

physical education programs in the public schools have all contributed to the decline in the fitness level of children. Children need at least an hour of vigorous physical activity every day.

4. Females should discontinue exercising while menstruating.
There is no evidence indicating that women should stop exercising during this time. However, since menstruation affects women in different ways, women should make their decision to exercise or not based on the degree of discomfort associated with physical exertion at this time. Many women find that exercise helps to reduce the pain, swelling, and discomfort during menstruation.

5. The solution to the problem of chafing during exercise from clothing rubbing the skin or skin rubbing against the skin is quite simple.
Apply a generous coat of petroleum jelly to the affected areas. If you have a history of skin irritation, for example, your thighs rub together as you walk or run, apply petroleum jelly to the area prior to the workout to prevent irritation from occurring.

Clinical experience and recent research challenge the current standards of exercise duration and intensity for pregnant women. By carefully assessing a patient's exercise history and teaching self-monitoring techniques, the physician can work with an active woman to create a safe exercise program during her pregnancy.
—J. White

guidelines for exercise during pregnancy (presented in Table 3.4). The ACOG guidelines have been criticized because they were written primarily by one physician, Raul Artal, based upon his own research, with little input from other experts. Since there was little available research at the time of their development, the ACOG guidelines represent the best guesses of Artal and a few others.

The concerns for women who exercise during pregnancy include reduction of blood flow to the uterus, overheating of the fetus, reduction in maternal and fetal blood sugar levels, and risk of musculoskeletal injury to the prospective mother. While reduced blood flow to the uterus, elevated temperature during exercise, and lowered blood sugar levels in mother and fetus are genuine concerns, no hard data exist indicating that they are harmful to the fetus or the mother.

An additional source of concern is associated with pregnant women engaging in exercise while lying on their backs. The ACOG guidelines recommend that women refrain from this practice because the weight of the fetus in this position squeezes the aorta and causes a reduction in blood supply and oxygen to the uterus. However, some gynecologists have noted that most pregnant women can tolerate lying on their backs unless they are at high risk for complications.

Another issue involves the effect of weight training for pregnant women. The same diversion of opinion exists.[21] Opponents state that the increased laxity (slackness) of ligaments and joints during pregnancy increases the probability of injury to these tissues. Weight training may be too stressful during this time, particularly for those who have not participated in it prior to pregnancy. Proponents of weight training point out that it strengthens muscles, tendons, and ligaments, thereby assisting pregnant women to more easily tolerate their altered center of gravity and increasing body weight. Low-back pain is rampant during pregnancy, and strengthening the back muscles produces less discomfort.

The type of weight training suggested for pregnant women consists of lifting light to moderate weights three days a week. Weight machines and free weights are acceptable. Proponents also suggest that women who have never trained with weights may begin during pregnancy provided they receive instruction from

TABLE 3.4	American College of Obstetricians and Gynecologists Guidelines for Exercise During Pregnancy and Postpartum

1. Regular exercise (at least three times per week) is preferable to intermittent activity. Competitive activities should be discouraged.
2. Vigorous exercise should not be performed in hot, humid weather or during a period of febrile illness.
3. Ballistic movements (jerky, bouncy motions) should be avoided. Exercise should be done on a wooden floor or a tightly carpeted surface to reduce shock and provide a sure footing.
4. Deep flexion or extension of joints should be avoided because of connective tissue laxity. Activities that require jumping, jarring motions or rapid changes in direction should be avoided because of joint instability.
5. Vigorous exercise should be preceded by a five-minute period of muscle warm-up. This can be accomplished by slow walking or stationary cycling with low resistance.
6. Vigorous exercise should be followed by a period of gradually declining activity that includes gentle stationary stretching. Because connective tissue laxity increases the risk of joint injury, stretches should not be taken to the point of maximum resistance.
7. Heart rate should be measured at times of peak activity. Target heart rates and limits established in consultation with the physician should not be exceeded.
8. Care should be taken to gradually rise from the floor to avoid orthostatic hypotension (a drop in blood pressure as one changes body position from lying down to standing up). Some form of activity involving the legs should be continued for a brief period.
9. Liquids should be taken liberally before and after exercise to prevent dehydration. If necessary, activity should be interrupted to replenish fluids.
10. Women who have led sedentary life-styles should begin with physical activity of very low intensity and advance activity levels very gradually.
11. Activity should be stopped and the physician consulted if any unusual symptoms appear.

Pregnancy only

1. Maternal heart rate should not exceed 140 beats per minute.
2. Strenuous activities should not exceed 15 minutes in duration.
3. No exercise should be performed in the supine position after the fourth month of gestation is completed.
4. Exercises that employ the Valsalva maneuver should be avoided.
5. Calorie intake should be adequate to meet not only the extra energy needs of pregnancy, but also of the exercise performed.
6. Maternal core temperature should not exceed 38 degrees C.

Source: Reprinted with permission from the American College of Obstetricians and Gynecologists: Exercise During Pregnancy and the Postnatal Period (ACOG Home Exercise Programs), Washington, D.C.: ACOG, 1985.

someone who is qualified, such as an exercise specialist certified by the American College of Sports Medicine.[22]

The debate regarding exercise for pregnant women centers around the identification of a safety zone for physical exertion that all pregnant women should observe. The problem is that pregnant women all have different needs for and attitudes about exercise and cannot be pigeon-holed by a set of generic guidelines. For instance, a competitive runner who trains by running 40 to 60 miles a week does not want to be told to reduce her exercise level to 20 minutes a day because she has become pregnant. By the same token, a sedentary woman may not want to begin exercising after she becomes pregnant.

Research indicates that active women may continue to train during pregnancy. They should use the ACSM guidelines; that is, they should exercise 20 to 60 minutes, three to five days a week at 60 percent to 90 percent of their maximum heart rate.[23] Pregnant exercisers should taper down as the time of birth nears.

Researchers have found that women who exercise during pregnancy have similar birth experiences as nonexercisers with regard to type of delivery, gestational age at delivery, fetal birthweight, and Apgar scores (evaluation of a newborn infant's physical status based on heart rate, respiratory effort, muscle tone, response to stimulation, and skin color).

What about sedentary women starting to exercise after becoming pregnant? The current view, although not supported by everyone, indicates that pregnancy is a good time to establish healthy lifestyle changes that include exercise and better nutrition.[24] Caution is warranted for these novice exercisers, and the conservative guidelines developed by the ACOG are appropriate for them.

Most physical fitness activities are acceptable during the early months of pregnancy. Contact sports are not recommended. In the later months, non-weightbearing activities such as swimming, water aerobics, and stationary cycling might be preferable. The following advantages are associated with maternal exercises:

1. Development and maintenance of physical fitness.
2. Avoidance of excess weight gain.
3. Reduction in the usual symptoms of pregnancy.
4. Less likelihood of complications during labor and delivery.
5. Faster recovery after giving birth.

M. Shangold has developed her own guidelines for exercise during pregnancy, some of which are at odds with the ACOG guidelines.[25] They include the following:

1. Continue the same sport or activity at the same level of perceived exertion. Since exercise becomes more difficult as pregnancy progresses, the required level of perceived exertion will occur sooner at a lower level of intensity.
2. Body temperature should not exceed 101 degrees.
3. Maximal heart rate should be between 140 and 160 beats/minute but should not exceed 160 beats/minute.
4. Total weight gain should be 20 to 30 pounds.
5. Consume an adequate amount of calories, vitamins, iron, and calcium.
6. Drink plenty of fluids.
7. Do not exercise at high altitude or in high temperatures.
8. Consult a physician immediately if pain, bleeding, rupture of the membranes, or lack of fetal movement occurs.

This author suggests that exercise during pregnancy be prescribed on an individual basis. The benefits of sensible exercise based upon individual needs are worth the effort. The evidence does not support the notion that exercise is harmful to the fetus and prospective mother. For those who are ultraconservative, walking is still an excellent exercise for pregnant women.

THE EFFECTS OF CLIMATE

Human beings are compelled to function in a variety of environments. People live and work in frigid, temperate, and tropical zones, at sea level, and at high altitudes and have adapted to and learned to tolerate extremes in temperature. In cold weather, body temperature can be maintained by putting on more clothes or by increasing the body's production of heat through physical movement or shivering. In hot environments, heat can be lost through sweating—increasing the blood flow to the skin—and by wearing as little clothing as the law and culture will allow.

Humans are homeotherms (meaning "same heat") capable of maintaining the constant internal temperature necessary for the support of such life-sustaining processes as cellular metabolism, oxygen transport, and muscular contraction. They exist within a relatively narrow band of internal temperatures, ranging from 97 to 99 degrees, but a human's temperature may and often does rise to 104 degrees during exercise. Temperatures that rise above 106 degrees, if not rapidly reduced, often result in cellular deterioration, permanent brain damage, and death, while temperatures below 93 degrees slow metabolism to the extent that unconsciousness and cardiac arrhythmias (disturbances of normal heart rhythm that can be fatal) are likely to occur.

Since many activities occur in the outdoors, participants are confronted with varying weather conditions. People's safety and comfort depend upon their knowledge of how the body reacts to vigorous exercise in different climate conditions.

 ## MECHANISMS OF HEAT TRANSFER

Heat is generated in the body—at rest and during exercise—as a by-product of all of the body's biochemical reactions. Metabolism is the collective sum of these reactions. The heat produced from exercise must be removed before it accumulates beyond tolerable levels. The body's adaptive mechanisms, centered upon shunting blood to the skin, are mobilized for this purpose. The processes of heat removal involve conduction, radiation, convection, and evaporation (see Figure 3.7). It is worth noting that the first three of these mechanisms can increase the heat load in the body if the conditions are right. Also, these mechanisms do not work in isolation. In most cases, more than one of the these processes work together to rid the body of its heat load.

Conduction

Conduction is the transference of heat from one object to another by physical contact. Conductive heat exchange takes place when a warmer body comes into contact with a cooler body or object. This process contributes little to heat loss during most types of physical activity, swimming and other water sports being the exceptions.

Radiation

Radiation is the transference of heat from the body to the atmosphere by electromagnetic waves, provided the environmental temperature is below a skin temperature of 92 to 93 degrees. Since heat travels on a temperature gradient from a warmer to a cooler object, the greater the difference between skin and environmental temperatures, the greater the heat loss through radiation. Radiation occurs in the reverse direction when the environmental temperature is above skin temperature and the participant absorbs heat from the environment. Outdoor exercise in high temperatures in direct sunlight increases the absorption of environmental heat.

Convection

Convection is the transfer of heat from the body to a moving gas or liquid. Convective heat gain occurs when the gas or liquid is warmer than the body. A cool breeze will cool the body by removing heat from the body's surface; a hot breeze will do the opposite. Convective heat loss also occurs in the swimming pool accompanied by conductive heat loss, provided the water is cooler than body temperature.

Evaporation

Evaporative heat loss is the major means of ridding the body of the heat generated by exercise. **Evaporation** occurs when the liquid in sweat is converted to a gas at the skin level. This process removes large quantities of heat from the dilated blood vessels below the surface of the skin. This mechanism is effective even in high temperatures, provided the relative humidity is low. The evaporative process is impaired when the humidity reaches 65 percent, regardless of the temperature, and it is virtually nonoperational when the humidity reaches 75 percent. At this point, the environmental air is so saturated that it can no longer absorb moisture.

Each liter of sweat that evaporates at the skin level removes 580 Kcals of energy in the form of heat from your skin.

—B. Stanford

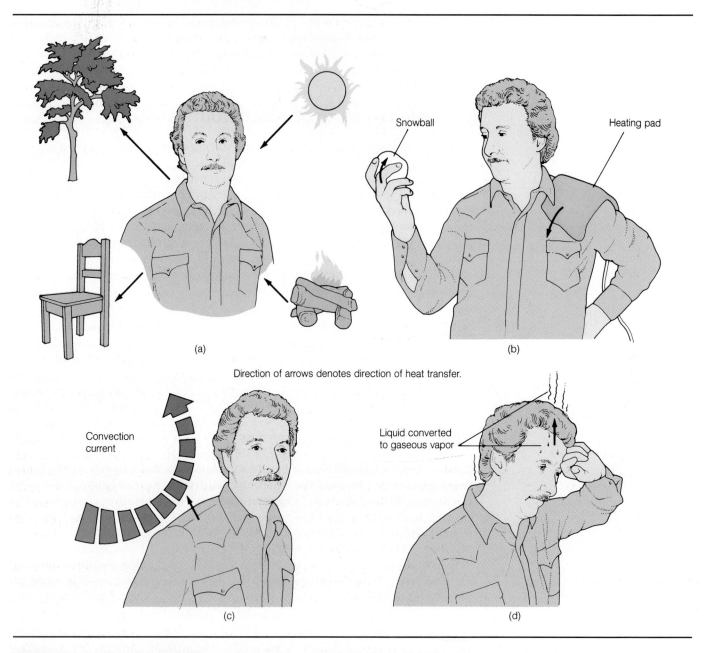

(a)

Snowball

Heating pad

(b)

Direction of arrows denotes direction of heat transfer.

Convection
current

Liquid converted
to gaseous vapor

(c)

(d)

FIGURE 3.7

Mechanisms of Heat Transfer (a) Radiation: heat is transferred by electromagnetic waves (heat waves) from warmer objects to cooler objects. (b) Conduction: heat is transferred from warmer objects to cooler ones by direct contact between the two. (c) Convection: the transfer of heat from objects to a circulating gas or liquid. (d) Evaporation: occurs where a liquid—such as sweat—is converted to a gaseous vapor.

Reprinted by permission. L. Sherwood, *Human Physiology*, St. Paul: West, 1993. Art rendered by Cyndie Wooley.

● Exercise in Hot Weather

Hazards Associated with Hot-Weather Exercise Hot, humid days present by far the greatest climatic challenge to the enthusiast who exercises outdoors. Since humid air, which is already saturated with moisture, cannot absorb much more moisture, sweat produced during exercise beads up and rolls off the body, providing minimal cooling effect. More blood than usual is diverted from the muscles to the skin in an effort to carry the heat accumulating in the deeper recesses of the body to its outer surface. The net result is that the exercising muscles are deprived of a full complement of blood and cannot work as long or as hard at a given task.

A loss of 1% of the body's water stores will increase rectal temperature; a 4 to 5% loss will impair physical work capacity.

—W. D. McArdle, F. I. Katch, V. L. Katch

Maximal aerobic power can be increased with training. However the degree of trainability in prepubescents seems somewhat lower than that of more mature age groups.

—O. Bar-Or

The high sweat rates that accompany vigorous exercise during hot and humid conditions promote the loss of a sizable quantity of the body's fluid, resulting in **dehydration** (excessive loss of body fluids). The most serious consequence of dehydration is the decrease in plasma volume (the liquid portion of the blood). The blood becomes more viscous (thick and sticky), lessening its ability to deliver oxygen to the active muscles. If the participant continues to exercise strenuously, body temperature will rise and may exceed the capacity of the temperature regulating mechanisms to remove heat.

Heat exhaustion or **heat stroke** occurs with the breakdown of the body's temperature-regulating mechanisms. Both conditions require immediate first aid, but heat stroke is a medical emergency that poses an imminent threat to life. It is the most severe of the heat-induced illnesses. Its symptoms include a high temperature (106° F or higher), generally the absence of sweating, and dry skin. Delirium, convulsions, and loss of consciousness often occur. The early warning signs include chills, nausea, headache, general weakness, and dry skin. The victim should be rushed to the nearest hospital immediately because death will probably occur without appropriate early treatment. Heat exhaustion, a serious condition but not an imminent threat to life, is characterized by dizziness, fainting, rapid pulse, and cool skin. The victim should be moved to a shady area or indoors, placed in a reclining position, and given cool fluids to drink.

Prepubescent children are more susceptible than adults to heat stress. Children who exercise continuously for 30 to 40 minutes become hyperthermic (overheated) much faster than adults exercising at the same rate in the same environmental conditions.[26] This is of interest because prepubescent children are participating in road races and triathlons, where they are exposed to the possibility of **hyperthermia** (abnormally high body temperature). Children are at risk for a number of reasons. First, their sweat glands produce only 40 percent as much sweat as adult sweat glands. The evaporation of sweat is the primary mechanism for cooling the body during exercise. The low sweat production of prepubescent children renders them more vulnerable to heat stress. Second, children absorb heat from the environment faster than adults through the mechanisms of convection, radiation, and conduction. Third, children produce more metabolic heat during exercise, probably because their movements are not as refined or efficient as those of adults. Fourth, children acclimate more slowly than adults to hot weather.

Successful performance in a hot environment is dependent upon the temperature, humidity, air movement, intensity and duration of exercise, the individual's level of fitness and previous exposure to heat (acclimatization), and whether the workout occurs in direct sunlight. Sharkey has developed a heat stress index for exercise based on temperature and humidity. Figure 3.8 indicates that heat stress can occur when the temperature is mild but the humidity is high. Since weather conditions such as these are deceptive, the danger in such a situation must be recognized.

Preventing Heat-Stress Illnesses   Heat-stress illness can be prevented by adhering to a few simple principles. Drink 12 to 20 ounces of a fluid that contains some salt 15 to 30 minutes before the workout.[27] Salt encourages the body to retain fluid so that more will be available for sweat production. Drinking plain water before the workout may stimulate urine production, thus defeating the attempt to conserve water and avoid dehydration.

The length of the workout will dictate the type of fluid needed during exercise to replace fluid lost through sweat. Plain water is the drink of choice when the workout lasts less than two hours. If the workout is longer than two hours, a beverage containing sugar and **electrolytes** (sodium chloride and potassium) is recommended. Such beverages are available in commercial sports drinks such as Gatorade, Exceed Fluid Replacement, and Energy Drink. They help to replace liquid as well as the body's carbohydrate stores. During exercise, you should drink 6 to 8 ounces of the appropriate beverage every 15 to 20 minutes.

FIGURE 3.8

Guidelines for Exercise in Heat and Humidity

Adapted from B. J. Sharkey, *Physiology of Fitness*, Champaign, Ill.: Human Kinetics, 1990.

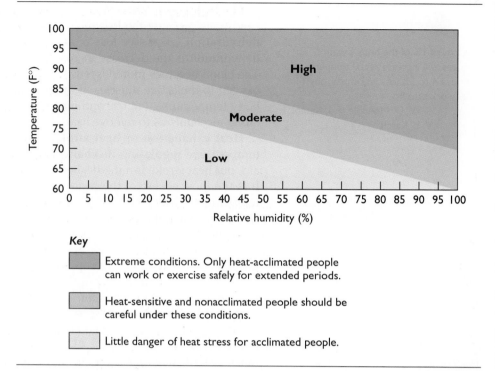

Key

Extreme conditions. Only heat-acclimated people can work or exercise safely for extended periods.

Heat-sensitive and nonacclimated people should be careful under these conditions.

Little danger of heat stress for acclimated people.

The fluids consumed during the period after exercise should contain salt and sugar in a continued effort to replace lost body fluids and to delay urine production. Commercial drinks fit the bill very nicely because they taste good and will probably entice the exerciser to drink more than if plain water were to be ingested.[28] This is important because our thirst mechanism is not a good barometer of our tissues' need for fluid. Plain water is not the drink of choice following exercise, because it extinguishes the thirst drive before the exerciser rehydrates. The thirst drive is maintained when salt is added to the drink.

Drinks that contain caffeine or alcohol should be avoided after exercise because they are diuretics (stimulate the production of urine). Carbonated beverages, such as soft drinks, are unacceptable because they produce a feeling of fullness before rehydration is complete.

The fluids ingested during and after exercise should be refrigerated because they will absorb some of the body's heat as they are warmed to body temperature. There is no physiological data contradicting the consumption of cold beverages for the dual purpose of replacing fluid and aiding in temperature control. Another benefit of using refrigerated fluids is that they tend to leave the stomach more rapidly, thereby meeting the tissues' needs sooner than unrefrigerated liquids.

Sweat is a filtrate of plasma, and it is hypotonic, which simply means that it is a diluted liquid containing little salt. Therefore, salt loss in sweat during exercise is very small unless exercise is prolonged for several hours. The average person who exercises 30 to 60 minutes, even in hot weather, should not be concerned with making a deliberate effort to replace the salt lost during exercise. The first postexercise meal will take care of salt replacement. Salt tablets are unacceptable as a method of salt replacement for the following reasons: they are stomach irritants that can produce nausea and vomiting, they can perforate the stomach lining, they sometimes pass through the body undissolved, and they attract fluid to the gut from other tissues where it is needed and thereby enhance dehydration.

Potassium is also lost in small quantities in sweat, but it is doubtful that supplements are necessary, even under extreme exercise conditions. Potassium is easily replaced by consuming citrus fruits or juices, bananas, potatoes, dates, nuts, and meats.

Modifications in the exercise program should be considered during hot weather. Participants should schedule their workout during the cooler times of the day. Shady locations where water can be obtained should be used. Clothing should be light, loose, and porous to facilitate the evaporation of sweat. It is wise to slow the pace and/or shorten the distance on particularly oppressive days. Be particularly alert for rapid weight loss because it may indicate an excessive loss of fluid.

Do not wear rubberized or plastic clothing while exercising because these garments promote sweating but retard its evaporation and seriously impede the cooling process. A supersaturated microenvironment is created between the skin and these garments that can lead very quickly to dehydration and heat illness.

Develop the habit of weighing yourself (dry nude weight) before and after exercise to assess water loss through sweating. The loss of each pound of body weight means the loss of one pint of fluid. After exercise, be sure to towel sweat off before weighing. If you do not enjoy exercising in hot weather and cannot make suggested schedule adjustments, try to move the program indoors into air-conditioned comfort. The health benefits of exercise can be achieved there just as well. The important point is to continue to exercise to maintain the gains you have made.

● Exercise in Cold Weather

Problems related to exercise in cold weather include frostbite, **hypothermia** (abnormally low body temperature), and occasionally hyperthermia (previously discussed). The most frequently occurring cold-weather injury to young healthy adults is frostbite, which can lead to permanent circulatory damage and the possible loss of the frostbitten part because of gangrene. Frostbite can be prevented by adequately protecting susceptible areas such as fingers, toes, nose, ears, and facial skin. Gloves, or preferably mittens, should be worn to protect the hands and fingers. A stocking or toboggan type of hat should be worn because it can be pulled down to protect the ears and to prevent significant heat loss through the bare head by radiation due to the poor vasoconstriction responses (clamping down of blood vessels) in the scalp. In very cold environments, participants may use surgical masks, ski masks, and scarves to keep facial skin warm and to moisten and warm inhaled air. All exposed flesh is vulnerable to frostbite when the temperature is very low and the wind chill factor is high (see Table 3.5).

Hypothermia occurs when body heat is lost faster than it can be produced. Exposure to cold temperatures, pain, and wind chill combine with fatigue to rob the body of heat. The body reacts with vasoconstriction of peripheral blood vessels as it attempts to conserve heat for the vital internal organs. Shivering, an involuntary contraction of the muscles, increases body heat. Since the shivering muscles produce no work, most of the expended energy appears as heat.

Hyperthermia is also possible during exercise in cold weather. It can occur when too much heavy clothing is worn and too few fluids are ingested. The problem can be avoided by following the guidelines for fluid replacement during hot weather and by wearing several layers of light clothing that will trap warm insulating air between the layers. Dressing in this manner allows the participant to peel off a layer or two as the metabolic heat produced by exercise increases. The amount and type of clothing worn should allow for the evaporation of sweat and help achieve a balance between the amount of heat produced and the amount of heat lost. Clothing that becomes saturated with sweat is rapidly cooled and can quickly chill a participant who is working or exercising in cold weather.

Very often, people may experience a hacking cough for a minute or two following exercise in cold weather. This is a normal response and should not cause alarm. Since very cold, dry air cannot be fully moistened when it is inhaled rapidly and in large volumes during exercise, the lining of the throat dries out. When exercise is discontinued, the respiratory rate slows and the volume of incoming air decreases, allowing the body to fully moisturize it. The lining is remoistened and coughing stops.

TABLE 3.5 Wind Chill Index

	Actual Thermometer Reading (0 F)											
	50	40	30	20	10	0	–10	–20	–30	–40	–50	–60
WIND SPEED	EQUIVALENT TEMPERATURE (0 F)											
Calm	50	40	30	20	10	0	–10	–20	–30	–40	–50	–60
5	48	37	27	16	6	–5	–15	–26	–36	–47	–57	–68
10	40	28	16	4	–9	–21	–33	–46	–58	–70	–83	–95
15	36	22	9	–5	–18	–36	–45	–58	–72	–85	–99	–112
20	32	18	4	–10	–25	–39	–53	–67	–82	–96	–110	–124
25	30	16	0	–15	–29	–44	–59	–74	–88	–104	–118	–133
30	28	13	–2	–18	–33	–48	–63	–79	–94	–109	–125	–140
35	27	11	–4	–20	–35	–49	–67	–82	–98	–113	–129	–145
40*	26	10	–6	–21	–37	–53	–69	–85	–100	–116	–132	–148

LITTLE DANGER	INCREASING DANGER	GREAT DANGER
For properly clothed person	Cover up fully (hands, ears, face, head, etc.)	Exercise Indoors

*Wind speeds greater than 40 mph have little additional effect.

Adapted from B. J. Sharkey, *Physiology of Fitness,* Champaign, Ill.: Human Kinetics, 1990, p. 236.

Some people develop chest pain while exercising in cold weather and fear that the blood vessels in the chest are being constricted or that the lungs are becoming frostbitten. But inhaled air is adequately warmed before it reaches the lungs. Even in very cold temperatures, the incoming air is warmed to at least 68 degrees F by the time it reaches the bronchi (large air passages that transport air to and from the lungs).[29]

Anyone who experiences chest pain upon exertion in the cold should consult a physician to determine whether an organic or physiological problem exists. If a medical problem is identified, the physician's recommendations regarding exercise should be followed. If a problem is not identified but chest pain in cold weather persists, the workout should be moved indoors. This simple act may be all that is necessary to continue the program during the winter months.

● Exercise at High Altitudes

The major problem associated with the performance of physical activities at high altitude is the reduced availability of oxygen at the cellular level. The percentage of oxygen at altitude is the same as it is at sea level (20.93). The total pressure of atmospheric air reduces as altitude increases, as does the pressure of oxygen (commonly referred to as the partial pressure of oxygen). Atmospheric pressure at sea level is 760 millimeters of mercury (mmHg), and the partial pressure of oxygen is 159 mmHg (760 mmHg × .2093 = 159 mmHg). At 8,200 feet of elevation, the atmospheric pressure drops to 560 mmHg, and the partial pressure of oxygen drops to 117 mmHg (560 mmHg × .2093 = 117 mmHg). Table 3.6 shows the effect of increasing altitude on the barometric pressure of the atmosphere and the corresponding partial pressure of oxygen.

High altitude produces physiological responses that reduce physical work capacity. For example, **hemoglobin** is 97 percent saturated with oxygen at sea level, but this value drops to 92 percent at 8,000 feet. This change is responsible for some of the decline in work capacity at high altitudes. The primary mechanism that seems to be responsible for the decline in performance relates to the decrease in the partial pressure of oxygen in arterial blood. At sea level, the arterial partial pressure of oxygen is 94 mmHg, but this drops to 60 mmHg at 8,000 feet. The par-

The symptoms of mountain sickness appear at 5,000 feet or above and include headache, shortness of breath, rapid heartbeat, and loss of appetite.

—B. J. Sharkey

TABLE 3.6 Barometric Pressure of the Atmosphere and Partial Pressure of Oxygen at Various Altitudes

ALTITUDE		ATMOSPHERIC PRESSURE (mmHg)	PARTIAL PRESSURE (O_2) (mmHg)
Meters	Feet		
0	0	760	159
500	1,640	716	150
1,000	3,280	674	141
1,500	4,920	634	133
2,000	6,560	596	125
2,500	8,200	560	117
3,000	9,840	526	110
4,000	13,120	462	97
5,000	16,400	405	85
6,000	19,690	354	74
7,000	22,970	308	64
8,000	26,250	267	56
9,000	29,530	230	48
10,000	32,800	198	41
19,215	63,000	47	10

tial pressure of oxygen in the tissues is approximately 20 mmHg. The difference between the oxygen pressure in arterial blood and the oxygen pressure in the tissues is the pressure gradient, which produces the force that drives oxygen from the bloodstream to the tissues. The higher the gradient, the more powerful the drive. At sea level, the pressure gradient is 74 mmHg (94 mmHg – 20 mmHg = 74 mmHg), but at 8,000 feet, the gradient drops to 40 mmHg (60 mmHg – 20 mmHg = 40 mmHg). This represents a 46 percent reduction in the driving force needed to deliver oxygen to the tissues, resulting in a decrement in aerobic performance.

Acclimation to high altitude begins within the first few days of exposure, but it takes approximately three weeks to make a good adjustment.[30] Full acclimation may take several months. The process of acclimation involves (1) an increase in the number of red blood cells and an increase in hemoglobin, which binds oxygen for transport in the circulatory system, (2) an increase in the number of capillaries in the lungs and skeletal muscles, and (3) increases in tissue myoglobin (the oxygen-transporting protein of muscle). All of these changes enhance oxygen intake and carrying capacity so that the transport systems may facilitate the supply of oxygen to the muscles. While these adjustments lessen the effects of high altitude, they never fully compensate for it. Endurance performance at high altitude is never as good as that at sea level, regardless of the degree of acclimation that has been attained. The adjustments to high altitude reverse completely when one returns to sea level for a couple of weeks.

Practical implications are associated with the effects of high altitude upon the human body. People with cardiovascular and/or respiratory disease who live at sea level need to understand the impact of higher altitudes upon these conditions. People suffering from these conditions should seek medical advice before going to that mountain retreat or on a skiing weekend. Even healthy young people need to reduce the intensity of exercise at high altitudes. Vacationers who go to the mountains need to realize that they will be unable to perform as they did at sea level. Those whose cardiovascular and respiratory systems are compromised at sea level must be especially careful at higher altitudes.

Prolonged exposure to extremely high altitudes (19,685 ft) leads to progressive deterioration that can eventually cause death unless the person is moved to a lower altitude.

—G. Brooks

Exercise in Polluted Air

Are residents of large cities—New York City, Chicago, Detroit, Los Angeles, etc.—at increased risk from industrial and traffic pollutants when they exercise outdoors? The answer is an unqualified yes. Carbon monoxide and ozone pose the

EXERCISE

1. Start slowly if you are sedentary. Be patient; fitness is not attained in two weeks.
2. Warm up before exercise to slowly raise heart rate and circulation. If done properly, you will avoid oxygen deprivation of the myocardium (heart muscle).
3. Follow the ACSM recommendations for exercise:
   a. Intensity
      - aerobic exercise—60 percent to 90% of maximum heart rate
      - weight training—8 to 12 repetitions to near maximum fatigue
      - perceived exertion of 12 to 13 (approximately 60% of the maximum heart rate) to 16 (approximately 85% of the maximum heart rate)
   b. Duration—20 to 60 minutes per workout. More than 60 minutes increases the chance of injury.
   c. Frequency—3 to 5 days per week. More than 5 days a week produces diminishing returns and increases the likelihood of injury.
4. Do not overload the cardiorespiratory and musculoskeletal systems too rapidly, because this also increases the likelihood of injury.
5. Cross-training is excellent for those whose major exercise objective is health enhancement. Cross-training enables one to maintain a high volume of training with less chance of injury, staleness, and burnout.
6. Cooling down after exercise is important to (1) prevent blood from pooling in the muscles that have been working, (2) speed up recovery from exercise, (3) remove the lactic acid that has accumulated in the exercising muscles, and (4) provide a good opportunity to stretch warm muscles.
7. Dress for the weather and be sure to consume liquids before, during, and after exercise.

greatest threat to outdoor exercisers, but hydrocarbons, industrial wastes, and particulate matter also contribute to the risk.

Hemoglobin has a much greater affinity for carbon monoxide than for oxygen. As a result, molecules of carbon monoxide competing with molecules of oxygen for hemoglobin attachment sites win hands down. Consequently, less oxygen is transported per unit volume of blood. The heart must work harder to deliver blood to the cells to compensate for the lower blood concentration of oxygen. Work output and aerobic capacity decrease because of reductions in maximum cardiac output and arterial venous oxygen difference.

A study completed in New York City examined the effect of air pollutants on runners versus nonrunners. The runners jogged a designated course for 30 minutes, while the nonrunners were stationed at various points along the course.[31] Thirty minutes of exposure by each group increased carbon monoxide levels five times above normal for the nonrunners, while the values increased ten times among the runners. This was the equivalent to smoking half a pack of cigarettes for the runners. Another problem related to carbon monoxide inhalation is that it does not easily disassociate from hemoglobin. In fact, it takes about five hours to remove half of the carbon monoxide in the blood.

Ozone, a primary component of smog, occurs from the action of the sun on nitrogen dioxide and hydrocarbons. The major effect of ozone exposure is that it increases the energy cost of breathing by increasing airway resistance. Bright, sunny days produce high doses of radiant heat, which increases the ozone level of the atmosphere and raises the difficulty of outdoor exercise. Aerobic capacity may decline as much as 10 percent when exercise occurs during peak levels of ozone in smog-prone cities.

Those who exercise outdoors should follow the following guidelines to minimize the risks associated with air pollution:[32]

1. Do not exercise during peak traffic hours.
2. Do not exercise when the sun is at its brightest.

3. Be aware of air pollution alerts and proceed cautiously with exercise.

4. Choose open areas for exercise so that wind currents may disperse pollutants.

5. When pollution is high, do not rest or run in the shade of trees, since trees, although they do provide shade, also trap pollutants.

6. Avoid as much as possible sidestream smoke emanating from cigarette, pipe, and cigar smoke.

POINTS TO PONDER

1. Why are prepubescent children at greater risk than adults when exercising in hot weather?
2. What are the potential harmful effects of exercise to pregnant women and their fetuses?
3. What are the benefits of exercise to pregnant women?
4. Define each of the mechanisms of heat loss.
5. What is the major mechanism through which we lose heat generated during exercise?
6. What is a heat stroke, and what are its symptoms? How should it be treated?
7. Should the fluid that exercisers drink during hot weather contain salt? Would you recommend salt tablets? Why or why not?
8. How should one dress for cold-weather exercise?
9. Why does aerobic performance suffer at higher altitudes?
10. What is the partial pressure of oxygen at a barometric pressure of 450 mmHg?
11. Identify the major air pollutants and describe their effect on people who are exposed to them during exercise.

CHAPTER HIGHLIGHTS

- The splitting of ATP into ADP & P provides the energy for muscular contraction.
- The anaerobic energy production pathway produces minimum ATP from glycogen without oxygen; the aerobic energy production pathway produces significant amounts of ATP from glycogen with oxygen.
- Carbohydrate is the preferred source of fuel during high-intensity exercise.
- The primary reason to warm up before exercising is to increase heart rate and circulation gradually so as to minimize oxygen deprivation to the heart muscle and other active tissues.
- The appropriate intensity for aerobic exercise is 60% to 90% of the maximum heart rate.
- The intensity of exercise can be monitored with the training heart rate or perceived exertion.
- To develop physical fitness, one must exercise at least three days a week. For most people, it is not necessary to exercise more than five days a week.
- Each bout of aerobic exercise should last 20 to 60 minutes.
- Overload involves a gradual increase in the exercise workload so as to improve the fitness level.
- Progression is the schedule of the application of overload.
- Task-specific training involves repetitive overloading of the muscles to be used in the activity.
- Proper cooldown after exercise is important for the safety of the exerciser.
- Exercise is beneficial for pregnant women and thus far has not shown to be harmful to their fetuses.
- Heat developed in the body during exercise must be removed. The mechanisms involved are conduction, radiation, convection, and evaporation of sweat.

- For exercise in hot weather, you should (1) drink 12 to 20 ounces of fluid that contains some salt 15 to 30 minutes before exercise, (2) drink plain water if exercising less than 2 hours and a beverage containing some sugar and salt if exercise will last longer than 2 hours, (3) drink 6 to 8 ounces every 15 to 20 minutes during exercise, (4) drink a beverage that contains sugar and salt after exercise.
- The dangers of exercise in cold weather can be minimized by taking several precautions—cover exposed skin, wear a hat, wear several layers of clothing, and drink fluids.
- Higher altitudes significantly impair physical exertion until one becomes acclimatized.
- The reduced partial pressure of oxygen is responsible for the performance decrement for aerobic activities at higher altitudes.
- Exercising and working outdoors in polluted environments may increase the risk of illness for some people.

● REFERENCES

1. B. J. Sharkey, *Physiology of Fitness,* Champaign, Ill.: Human Kinetics, 1990.
2. American College of Sports Medicine, *Guidelines for Exercise Testing and Prescription,* Philadelphia: Lea and Febinger, 1991.
3. R. J. Barnard, et al., "Cardiovascular Responses to Sudden Strenuous Exercise-Heart Rate, Blood Pressure, and ECG," *Journal of Applied Physiology* 34 (1973): 833.
4. American College of Sports Medicine, "The Recommended Quantity and Quality Exercise for Developing and Maintaining Cardiorespiratory and Muscular Fitness in Healthy Adults," *Medicine in Science and Sport* 22, no. 2 (April 1990): 265.
5. S. J. Fleck and W. J. Kraemer, "Resistance Training: Basic Principles (Part 1 of 4)," *The Physician and Sportsmedicine* 16, no. 3 (March 1988): 160.
6. American College of Sports Medicine, "The Recommended Quantity," April 1990, p. 265.
7. J. A. Davis, et al., "A Comparison of Heart Rate Methods for Predicting Endurance Training Intensity," *Medicine in Science and Sports* 7 (1975): 295.
8. M. L. Pollock et al., *Exercise in Health and Disease,* Philadelphia: W. B. Saunders, 1984.
9. G. A. V. Borg, "Perceived Exertion: A Note on History and Methods," *Medicine and Science in Sports* 5 (1973): 90.
10. W. P. Morgan and G. A. V. Borg, "Perception of Effort and the Prescription of Physical Activity," In T. Craig (Ed.), *Mental Health and Emotional Aspects of Sport,* Chicago: American Medical Association, 1976.
11. American College of Sports Medicine, *Guidelines,* 1991.
12. American College of Sports Medicine, "The Recommended Quantity," April 1990, p. 265.
13. S. J. Jacobs and B. L. Bernson, "Injuries to Runners: A Study of Entrants to a 10,000 Meter Race," *American Journal of Sports Medicine* 14 (1986): 151; Y. Mutoh et al., "Aerobic Dance Injuries Among Instructors and Students," *The Physician and Sportsmedicine* 16 (1988): 80.
14. "The 10-Minute Shape-Up," *The Walking Magazine* 6, no. 2 (March/April 1991): 14.
15. S. Levin, "Overtraining Causes Olympic-Sized Problems," *The Physician and Sportsmedicine* 19, no. 5 (May 1991): 112.
16. American College of Sports Medicine, "The Recommended Quantity," April 1990, p. 265.
17. R. S. Paffenbarger et al. "Physical Activity, All Cause Mortality and Longevity of College Alumni," *New England Journal of Medicine* 314 (1986): 605; S. N. Blair et al, "Physical Fitness and All-Cause Mortality—A Perspective Study of Healthy Men and Women," *Journal of the American Medical Association,* November 3, 1989, p. 2395.
18. J. R. Magalel et al., "Specificity of Swim-Training On Maximum Oxygen Uptake," *Journal of Applied Physiology* 38 (1975): 151.
19. "Put Your Best Foot Backward," *The Walking Magazine* 6, no. 3 (May/June 1991): 10.
20. C. Morton, "Running Backward May Help Athletes Move Forward," *The Physician and Sportsmedicine* 14 (1986): 149.
21. J. A. Work, "Is Weight Training Safe During Pregnancy?" *The Physician and Sportsmedicine* 17 (1989): 256.
22. Ibid.
23. P. J. Kulpa et al., "Aerobic Exercise in Pregnancy," *American Journal of Obstetrics and Gynecology* 156 (1987): 1395; D. C. Hall and D. A. Kaufmann, "Effects of Aerobic and Strength Conditioning on Pregnancy Outcomes," *American Journal of Obstetrics and Gynecology* 157 (1987): 1199.
24. J. White, "Exercising For Two," *The Physician and Sportsmedicine* 20, no. 5 (May 1992): 179.
25. M. Shangold and G. Mirkin, *The Complete Sports Medicine Book for Women,* New York: Simon & Schuster, 1985.
26. O. Bar-Or, "Climate and the Exercising Child—A Review," *International Journal of Sports Medicine* 1 (1980): 53.
27. B. Stamford, "How to Avoid Dehydration," *The Physician and Sportsmedicine* 18, no. 7 (July 1990): 135.
28. "Are Sports Drinks Better Than Water?" *The Physician and Sportsmedicine* 20, no. 2 (February 1992): 33.
29. W. D. McArdle, F. I. Katch, and V. L. Katch, *Exercise Physiology,* Philadelphia: Lea and Febiger, 1991.
30. B. J. Sharkey, *Physiology of Fitness,* Champaign, Ill.: Human Kinetics, 1990.
31. J. B. Nicholson and D. B. Case, "Carboxyhemoglobin Levels in New York City Runners," *The Physician and Sportsmedicine* 11, no. 3 (March 1983): 135.
32. "Exercising in Bad Air," *University of California at Berkeley Wellness Letter* 8, no. 11 (August 1992): 7.

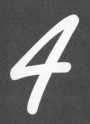

CHAPTER

4

Flexibility

CHAPTER OUTLINE

INTRODUCTION
Miniglossary
FLEXIBILITY AND WELLNESS
DEVELOPING THE FLEXIBILITY COMPONENT
Facts, Fallacies, and Timely Tidbits
TECHNIQUES FOR IMPROVING FLEXIBILITY
Ballistic (Dynamic) Versus Static Stretching
Proprioceptive Neuromuscular Facilitation (PNF)

EXERCISES TO ENHANCE FLEXIBILITY
Safety Tips: Developing Flexibility
ASSESSING FLEXIBILITY
FIELD TESTS
Points to Ponder
CHAPTER HIGHLIGHTS
REFERENCES

INTRODUCTION

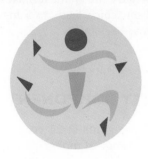

Flexibility is defined as "the range of possible movement in a joint (as in the hip joint) or series of joints (as when the spinal column is involved)."[1] Flexibility is not a general component; that is, the flexibility of one joint cannot be predicted accurately from a measurement made at another joint. This implies that the capacity for movement may differ from joint to joint. Flexibility, then, is specific to each individual joint.

Motion is limited at a given joint by its bony structure, accompanying muscle size, and soft connective tissues—the tendons, ligaments, and joint capsules.[2] Additionally, the skin may be involved to some degree in the resistance to movement. The skeletal structure of joints constitutes one of the unalterable limitations to movement. It is not amenable to change. Therefore, improvement in flexibility is accomplished by increasing the elastic properties of the soft tissues—the muscles and their facial sheaths, tendons, ligaments, and connective tissue.

Three Self-Assessment activities appear in Appendix C that apply directly to the contents of this chapter:

4.1 Sit-and-Reach

4.2 Back Extension

4.3 Shoulder Flexion

Females of all ages were more flexible than males, but males outperformed females on strength tests.
—The Canadian Fitness Study

FLEXIBILITY AND WELLNESS

Flexibility is recognized as one of the important health-related components of physical fitness. Its major contribution to health is related to the prevention of low back pain and injury. A healthy low back is dependent upon abdominal strength,

Miniglossary

Ballistic Stretching Also known as dynamic stretching, ballistic stretching employs repetitive contractions of agonist muscles to produce rapid stretches of antagonist muscles.

Flexibility The range of motion (ROM) around a joint or series of joints.

Flexometer An instrument for measuring static flexibility.

Golgi Tendon Organ A specialized receptor located in the muscles that responds to changes in muscle length and tension.

Goniometer A protractorlike device used to measure the flexibility of various joints.

Myotatic Reflex Stretch reflex.

Muscle Spindle A specialized receptor located in the muscles that is sensitive to changes in muscle length.

Proprioceptive Neuromuscular Facilitation (PNF) Several stretching techniques that involve some combination of contraction and static stretching of agonist and antagonist muscle groups.

Static Stretching Passive stretching of antagonist muscles by slowly stretching and holding terminal positions for 15 to 30 seconds.

Stretch Reflex Reflexive contraction of a muscle that is being stretched.

Prevention of back disorders should be the goal of all exercisers. Flexibility and muscle strengthening must be integral parts of the training program.
—Carl L. Stanitshi, M.D.

good posture, and flexibility of the hamstrings and back extensors.[3] The vertical and transverse layers of the abdominal muscles brace and provide stability for the trunk. The transverse layers are contiguous with lumbar connective tissue, resulting in a "bracing and corseting effect analogous to a Chinese finger trap."[4] If the strength of the abdominals is not maintained, posture will be negatively affected and low back pain may be the result.

Flexibility wanes with age and inactivity. Active individuals tend to be more flexible than sedentary individuals.[5] Although range of motion diminishes with passing years, there appears to be no evidence that the biological processes associated with aging are responsible.[6] Inactivity rather than aging seems to be implicated in the loss of flexibility, since muscles and other soft tissues lose their elasticity when they are not used. For example, a sedentary life characterized by sitting maintains the hamstrings in a shortened position which leads to a loss in their range of motion and increases susceptibility to low-back injury.

DEVELOPING THE FLEXIBILITY COMPONENT

Flexibility appears to reach a peak in most of the joints at 24 years of age for males[7] and 25 to 29 years of age for females.[8] The range of motion for most movements begins to decline in the mid-twenties for males and about 30 years of age for females. As the range of motion declines, so too does the ability to perform in an unrestricted way some essential movements, such as bending, stooping, and climbing stairs as well as some occupational and recreational movements.

Flexibility can be improved through exercises that promote the elasticity of the soft tissues of the joints. Chapman showed that 20 young men (ages 15 to 19) and 20 older men (ages 63 to 88) responded similarly to an exercise program designed to enhance finger-joint flexibility.[9] The older subjects exhibited greater joint stiffness at the inception of the program, but the amount of their improvement equaled that of the younger subjects. Several researchers investigated the effects of dance exercise on flexibility.[10] Subjects who participated in the exercise program significantly improved their flexibility compared to control groups who did not exercise. Research data regarding the effectiveness of physical activity in improving and maintaining flexibility are limited, but the few studies that have been attempted have found a positive relationship between the two.

 Facts, Fallacies, and Timely Tidbits

1. Lack of flexibility can lead to poor posture and increase the likelihood of certain types of injuries. But is it possible to be too flexible? There is some evidence that supports this phenomenon. Extreme flexibility is referred to in the vernacular as "loose jointed," which may increase vulnerability to injury, particularly from impact. Participation in a sound program of resistance training would be very helpful for those who are "loose jointed."

2. Should stretching exercises be performed every day? The ideal approach to the development and maintenance of flexibility is that stretching exercises should be performed

every day. Flexibility is lost very quickly when the stretching exercise program is discontinued. The maintenance of flexibility is dependent upon consistent effort. Ten minutes a day is about all that is required to keep from losing this important fitness component.

3. Factors that limit flexibility:
   - skeletal structure of the joints
   - skin
   - connective tissue (ligaments and tendons)
   - muscles
   - fat

Three popular methods are used for improving flexibility: ballistic or dynamic stretching, static stretching, and proprioceptive neuromuscular facilitation (PNF). When performed regularly, each of the three methods is effective in improving flexibility, but ballistic techniques are no longer recommended. An understanding of the neurophysiological bases of stretching is important for one to appreciate the differences and similarities among the methods.

Most of the joints of the body are capable of more than one movement. For example, the elbow joint is capable of flexion and extension. Complete flexion occurs in the elbow joint when the elbow bends, bringing the hand toward the shoulder. This movement represents a full range of motion (ROM). Complete extension occurs when the elbow straightens out, producing a 180-degree angle at the elbow. The elbow is capable of this type of motion because two sets of muscle groups, the biceps (flexors) and the triceps (extensors) work together to create movement. When one set contracts, the other relaxes and allows movement to occur. For example, reaching up to place an item on an overhead shelf requires contraction of the triceps muscle and relaxation of the biceps at the same time. Muscles that work together in this way are synergistic. If the biceps did not relax in the preceding example, no movement could occur.

The muscle that contracts and produces movement is the prime mover, or the agonist. Its opposite muscle, which relaxes, allowing the movement to occur, is the antagonist. A muscle can be an agonist for one type of movement and an antagonist for another. The triceps is the agonist and the biceps the antagonist for movements that extend the elbow joint; the biceps is the agonist and the triceps the antagonist for movements that flex or bend the elbow joint.

Muscles contain specialized receptors that are sensitive to change in their length and tension. These receptors—the muscle spindle and the Golgi tendon organ—inform the central nervous system regarding the stimulus that is applied to the muscles in which they are located. The **muscle spindle** responds to stretching of the muscle, while the **Golgi tendon organ** responds to both stretch and tension. Now you are ready to tackle the three types of stretching procedures previously mentioned.

> When a muscle is stretched, the muscle spindles (part of the stretch reflex) are also stretched, sending a volley of sensory impulses to the spinal cord that inform the central nervous system that the muscle is being stretched. Impulses return to the muscle from the spinal cord, which causes it to contract reflexively, thus resisting the stretch.
>
> —William E. Prentise

Ballistic (Dynamic) Versus Static Stretching

In the past, ballistic or dynamic stretching was used as a loosening up procedure before physical activity. Today, however, ballistic stretching is recognized as being counterproductive and may actually be harmful. **Ballistic stretching** employs bouncing and bobbing movements, such as when individuals try to touch their toes by bending from the waist with a series of bobbing movements, each of which takes the fingertips closer to the toes. Most people have stretched in this manner, and some continue to do so. It is counterproductive because ballistic movements stimulate the stretch reflex (the **myotatic reflex** originating in the muscle spindle), which responds by sending signals for the muscle to contract rather than stretch. Each bob or bounce stimulates the stretch reflex which, in turn, signals the muscle to contract with a force that is proportional to the force generated by bobbing and bouncing.[11] If you have dozed off while sitting upright in a chair, you have experienced the results of the stretch reflex doing its work. Your head drops forward as you nod off, causing the neck muscles to stretch rapidly and dynamically. This sudden and unexpected stretch stimulates the **stretch reflex,** which signals the central nervous system to order those muscles to contract, thereby snapping the head back to the upright position. Soreness may occur because the muscle is forced to pull against itself. Each bounce ends suddenly and forcefully, thereby applying substantial stress to muscle tissue. This technique can lead to injury because it is possible to exceed the elastic limits of the muscles. Such an occurrence is even more likely if cold muscles are stretched in this manner.

There is a theory that developing strength in the antagonist muscles of the tight muscle or muscle group has the potential for increasing flexibility.[12] If the hamstrings are tight, their antagonists, the quadriceps muscles, are strengthened to provide for greater range of motion. Although research evidence in support of this approach to the enhancement of flexibility is lacking at this time, greater elasticity is one of the properties of stronger muscles. This approach will probably improve range of motion in the target muscle.

Static stretching is preferred to dynamic forms of stretching. **Static stretching** features slow, controlled movements for 15 to 30 seconds that lead to the end point in the joint's range of motion. The final position should produce a feeling of discomfort but not pain. When the position of mild discomfort is reached, it is held for 15 to 30 seconds and then slowly released. This technique does not stimulate the stretch reflex, allowing the muscles to stretch essentially free of opposition. Each exercise may be repeated several times. Unlike ballistic stretching, static stretching is less likely to cause injuries, produces no muscle soreness (and is, in fact, advocated as an antidote to soreness), and consumes less energy. One must perform stretching exercises on a regular basis to receive optimal benefits.

The bouncing and bobbing movements employed in ballistic stretching send conflicting signals that cause the muscle to pull against itself. But if the stretch is continuous—that is, it is held for a minimum of six seconds—the Golgi tendon organ has time to respond to the change in muscle length and tension. It sends a volley of signals to the spinal cord that result in reflexive relaxation of the antagonist muscles. This is a protective mechanism that allows the muscle to stretch farther before reaching its limits of extensibility.

Static stretching gives the Golgi tendon organ time to react to the increase in muscle tension. Its signals override those of the muscle spindle, thus allowing the muscle to relax and lengthen. Holding a stretch for at least six seconds is not likely to result in injury to muscle tissue. However, rapid, repetitive movements keep the muscle spindle activated so that it resists stretch.

Proprioceptive Neuromuscular Facilitation (PNF)

A third form of stretching, **proprioceptive neuromuscular facilitation (PNF),** has been slowly infiltrating the fitness movement as a technique for increasing flexibility. Physical therapists have for many years been employing PNF stretching techniques for patients with neuromuscular disorders. Several studies have shown that PNF stretching techniques are usually more effective in improving flexibility than the other two methods.[13]

PNF stretching uses three common techniques: (1) hold-relax, (2) contract-relax, and (3) slow-reversal-hold-relax. All three methods require the assistance of a partner and employ some combination of contraction and static stretching of agonist and antagonist muscle groups.

PNF techniques are a bit more complex than conventional stretching procedures. The three PNF techniques are illustrated in Figures 4.1, 4.2, and 4.3. For

FIGURE 4.1

The Hold-Relax Technique

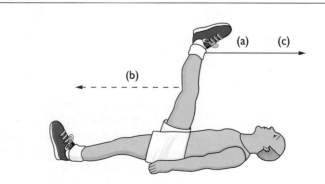

FIGURE 4.2

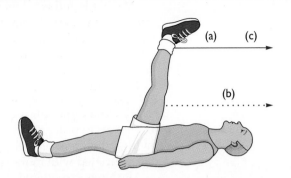

comparison purposes, all three figures illustrate how the hamstring muscles are stretched with each of the three PNF techniques. For this exercise, the hamstring muscle group (located in the back of the thighs) is the antagonist, while the quadricep muscle group (located in the front of the thighs) is the agonist. All of the contractions and stretches are held for a minimum of six seconds (the minimum time required by the Golgi tendon organ to produce its relaxation effect). A 10- to 15-second hold in each phase produces better results. The contraction and stretching phases of each of these techniques should be repeated at least three times.

The hold-relax technique (Figure 4.1) is performed in the following way:

1. A partner pushes the subject's outstretched leg in the direction of arrow (a). This is a passive prestretch of the antagonist (hamstrings).

2. This is followed by a voluntary contraction by the subject of the hamstrings, arrow (b). This phase is resisted by the partner.

3. This is followed by another partner push in the direction of arrow (c) which once again stretches the hamstrings.

The contract-relax method (Figure 4.2) is performed in the following way:

1. Same as no. 1 in the hold-relax method.

2. This is followed by a voluntary contraction of the agonist (quadriceps) in the direction of arrow (b).

3. This is followed by another partner push in the direction of arrow (c) which once again stretches the hamstrings.

The slow-reversal-hold-relax technique is performed in the following way:

1. Same as no. 1 in the previous two descriptions.

2. This is followed by a voluntary contraction of the antagonist (hamstrings) in the direction of arrow (b). This is resisted by the partner.

FIGURE 4.3

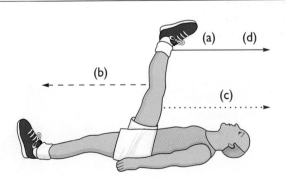

3. This is followed by a voluntary contraction of the agonist (quadriceps) which is gently assisted by the partner in the direction of arrow (c).

4. This is followed by another partner push in the direction of arrow (d) which stretches the hamstrings.

Although PNF stretching techniques appear to be the most effective for the purpose of improving flexibility, they are not without limitations. First, all three techniques require the assistance of a partner who needs to be competent in these techniques in order to perform the stretches correctly and reduce the likelihood of injuring the exerciser. Second, it takes more time to stretch in this manner. Third, it is associated with more pain and muscle stiffness.[14]

All things considered, I would recommend static stretching as the method of choice for practicality (it requires no assistance), ease of performance, safety, and effectiveness.

The stretching component of the physical fitness program may be incorporated as a segment of the warmup and cooldown phases of aerobic exercise. For the stretching exercises to be most effective, they should follow exercises in the warmup phase that stimulate circulation and heat up the muscles. Stretching during cooldown should follow a few minutes of walking. Flexibility exercises performed at this time afford the best opportunity to stretch those muscles that have been contracting vigorously during the workout. Stretching after the workout is very important because it helps prevent the muscle shortening associated with loss of flexibility and it prevents or decreases muscle soreness.

EXERCISES TO ENHANCE FLEXIBILITY

The exercises presented in this section are a sample of the many exercises that have been devised to enhance flexibility. Figures 4.4 through 4.27 are samples of stretching exercises for major joints and soft tissues of the body. Choose one exercise from each group of exercises.

There are many exercises that stretch the major muscle groups of the body. Some of these are inherently dangerous, while others are dangerous because they often are performed incorrectly. Movements that are potentially hazardous involve poor body alignment or ballistic movements during performance. Figure 4.28 presents some high-risk flexibility exercises that have the potential to be harmful to some people. Alternative exercises are presented that work the same muscles and joints but are considered to be safe. Before engaging in any of the stretching exercises, read the box entitled Safety Tips for Developing Flexibility.

FIGURE 4.4

Stretching the Neck Rotate your head downward and to the extreme left. Hold this position for 5 seconds and then rotate your head upward and to the extreme right. Hold for 5 seconds and then look downward. Hold for 5 seconds and rotate your head upward and to the extreme left and hold for 5 seconds. Repeat the sequence in reverse order.

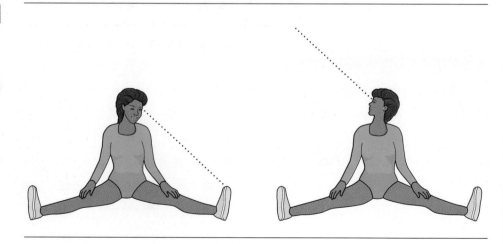

Safety Tips ✓

DEVELOPING FLEXIBILITY

What to do:

1. Warm up before stretching. Exercise to the point that you start sweating before stretching. Stretching is safer and more effective when the muscles are warm.
2. Static stretching is preferable.
3. Stretch to the point of discomfort but not pain. Pain is a sign that you are dangerously close to exceeding the muscle's elastic capacity.
4. Hold each stretch for 15 to 30 seconds. Move slowly and control movement from one position to the next.
5. Do two to three sets of each stretch.
6. Static stretches may be performed daily.

What not to do:

1. Do not overflex a joint.
2. Do not excessively arch the back or neck.
3. Do not stretch the neck by swinging the head in a circle. The neck is not a ball and socket joint and is not constructed for rotational movements.
4. Do not twist or flex suddenly.
5. Do not employ bouncing or bobbing movements.
6. Do not swing the arms or legs rapidly.
7. Do not attempt to stretch the hamstring muscles by placing the foot of the outstretched leg higher than the hips because this puts pressure on the sciatic nerve.

FIGURE 4.5

Stretching the Neck   Gently pull your head forward until a stretch is felt in the back of the neck and hold for 15 to 30 seconds.

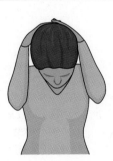

FIGURE 4.6

Stretching the Neck   Bend your neck from side to side and then from front to back. Do not roll your head in a circle.

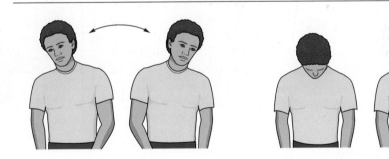

FIGURE 4.7

Stretching the Shoulders and Arms   With the left elbow up and the right elbow down, try to clasp your hands behind your back. If you cannot clasp them, reach as far as possible and hold for 15 seconds and then reverse arms.

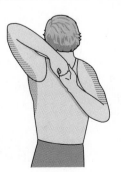

FIGURE 4.8

Stretching the Shoulders and Arms Gently pull your right arm behind your head and hold for 15 seconds. Then pull the left arm in the same manner.

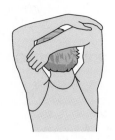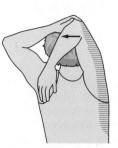

FIGURE 4.9

Stretching the Shoulders and Arms Stretch your arms forward to full extension with both palms on the floor and press down with your chest. Hold 15 to 30 seconds.

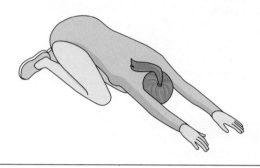

FIGURE 4.10

Stretching the Shoulders and Arms Place your hands on opposite sides of a doorjam and lean forward and straighten your arms. Hold 15 to 30 seconds.

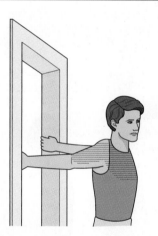

FIGURE 4.11

Stretching the Upper Back Sit in a chair with feet separated greater than shoulder width. Place your arms to the inside of the thighs and bring your chest down toward the floor. At the same time, attempt to reach back as far as you can with your arms.

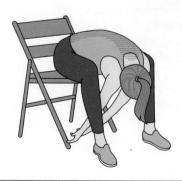

FIGURE 4.12

Stretching the Upper Back
Interlace your fingers behind your head and gently pull forward until you feel a comfortable stretch. Hold 15 to 30 seconds.

FIGURE 4.13

Stretching the Lower Back
Cross your legs and lean forward extending your arms to the front. Hold 15 to 30 seconds.

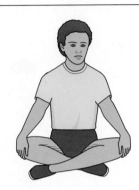

FIGURE 4.14

Stretching the Lower Back
Pull your left knee to your chest while simultaneously raising your head. Hold 15 to 30 seconds and repeat with the other leg.

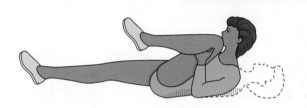

FIGURE 4.15

Stretching the Lower Back
Pull both knees to the chest while simultaneously raising your head. Hold 15 to 30 seconds.

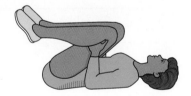
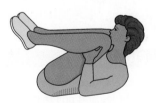

FIGURE 4.16

Stretching the Chest   Clasp your hands behind your back, straighten your arms, and lift them in the direction of the arrow.

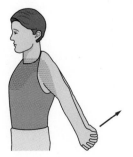

FIGURE 4.17

Stretching the Chest Stretch your arms forward to full extension with both palms on the floor and press down with your chest. Hold 15 to 30 seconds.

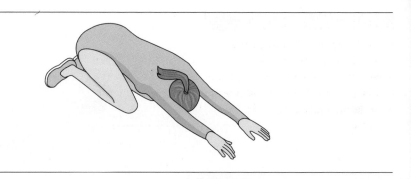

FIGURE 4.18

Stretching the Groin Place the soles of your feet together and lean forward. Hold for 30 seconds. A variation of this exercise is to push down gently on both knees until a stretch is felt and hold 15 to 30 seconds.

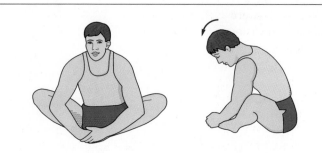

FIGURE 4.19

Stretching the Groin Keep your legs straight, rest your heels against a wall, and slowly let your feet slide downward so that your legs spread apart. Stop when you feel a good stretch and hold for 15 to 30 seconds.

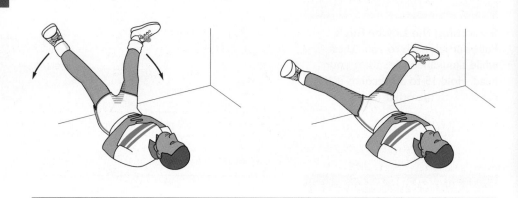

FIGURE 4.20

Stretching the Quadriceps Bend your right leg and pull that foot upward toward the buttocks with the opposite hand until a stretch is felt in the front of the thigh. Hold for 15 to 30 seconds and repeat with the other leg.

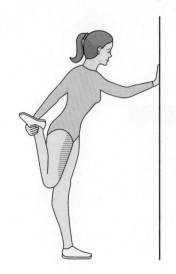

FIGURE 4.21

Stretching the Quadriceps
Assume the above position and lower your hips to create a stretch in the front of the thigh and hold 15 to 30 seconds. Repeat with the other leg.

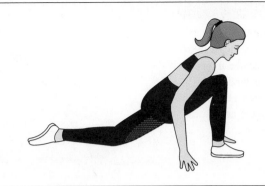

FIGURE 4.22

Stretching the Quadriceps
Extend your left leg to the rear and place your foot on a chair or other object at a comfortable height. Press down until a stretch is felt. Hold 15 to 30 seconds and repeat with the other leg.

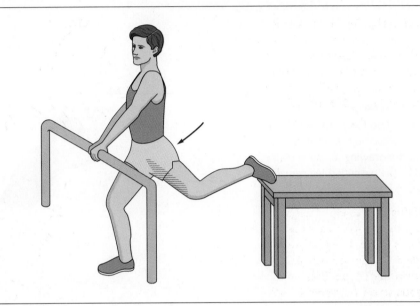

FIGURE 4.23

Stretching the Hamstrings
Extend one leg and place the sole of the opposite foot against the thigh of the extended leg. Lean forward and pull the toes back to exert a stretch in the calf and hamstrings. Hold 15 to 30 seconds and repeat with the other leg.

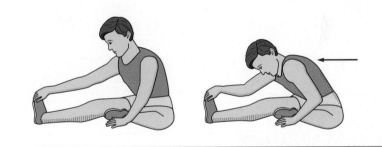

FIGURE 4.24

Stretching the Hamstrings
Bend your knees slightly and slowly lean forward from the waist until a stretch is felt in the hamstrings. Hold 15 to 30 seconds.

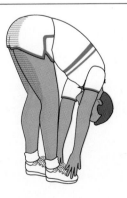

FIGURE 4.25

Stretching the Hamstrings
Extend both legs and lean forward.
Pull back on the toes (b) to exert a
stretch in the calves as well as the
hamstrings. If you cannot reach your
toes reach as far forward as you can
(a). Hold for 15 to 30 seconds.

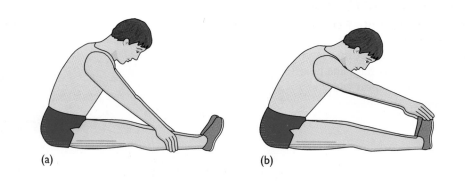

(a)　　　　　　(b)

FIGURE 4.26

**Stretching the Calf and Achilles
Tendon**　Assume the position
shown in the drawing. Be sure that
the heel of the extended leg remains
in contact with the floor and that
both feet are pointed straight ahead.
Slowly move your hips forward until
you feel a stretch in the calf of the
extended leg. Hold 15 to 30 seconds
and repeat with the other leg.

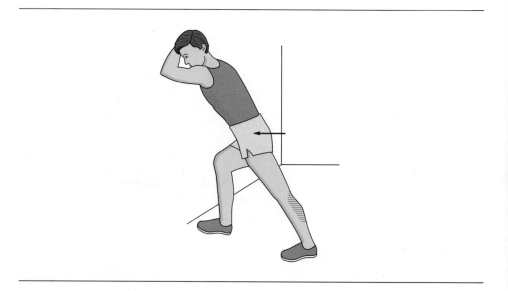

FIGURE 4.27

**Stretching the Calf and Achilles
Tendon**　Bend the knee of the
extended leg in this variation of
Figure 4.26. This places the stretch
upon the Achilles tendon. Hold 15
to 30 seconds and repeat with the
other leg.

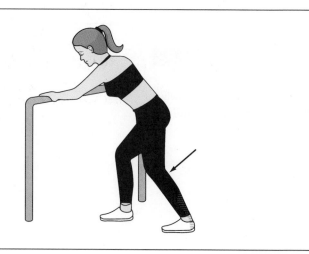

FIGURE 4.28

**High-Risk Flexibility Exercises:
Dont's and Do's**

Don't

Do

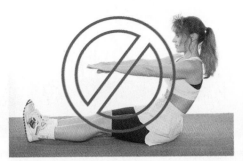

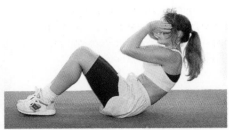

Straight-leg sit-up Sit-ups done in this manner stress the low back by forcing it to arch. Muscles other than the abdominals do a significant amount of the work.

Bent-leg sit-ups Keep your knees bent and your feet flat on the floor. Sit up 30 to 45 degrees and keep your low back pressed to the floor.

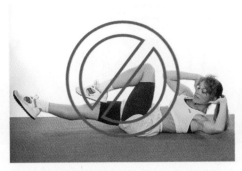

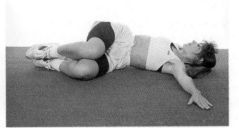

Alternating bent-leg sit-ups Asymmetric pull on the pelvis occurs when you hold one leg straight out and touch the elbow opposite to the bent knee. This puts a strain on the low back.

Knee rolls This exercise strengthens the oblique abdominal muscles more safely. Lie on your back with knees tightly tucked, arms out flat at shoulder level. Slowly roll to the right, hold for 2–3 seconds, return to the starting position, and then roll to the left and hold. All movements are to be done slowly and under control.

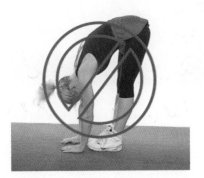

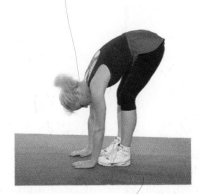

Toe touches Toe touches with locked knees may overstress the back, hamstring muscles, and knees.

Bent-knee hang downs Bend your knees slightly and slowly roll forward until stretch is felt in the hamstrings. Hold for 10–15 seconds. Do not bounce or try to touch the floor.

Continued

Flexibility   **85**

FIGURE 4.28

**High-Risk Flexibility Exercises:
Dont's and Do's—Continued**

Don't

Do

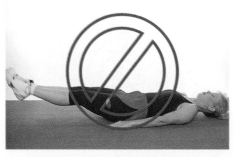

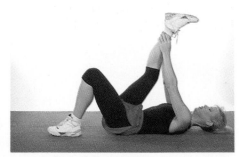

Double-leg lifts   This exercise forces the back to arch and increases the risk of injury.

Raised-leg crunches   One leg is bent with the foot flat on the floor; the other leg is straight up. Raise your shoulders and upper back and reach toward the upraised ankle.

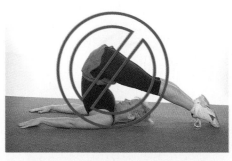

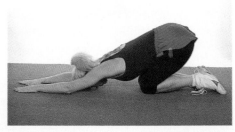

Yoga plow   Places considerable stress on the neck and its underlying structures. Any exercise that assumes this position is potentially hazardous.

Fold-up stretch   Sit back on your heels, press your chest to the thighs, and reach forward with both hands. This is a safer way to stretch the upper and lower back.

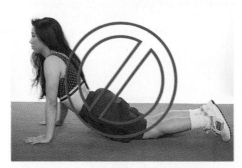

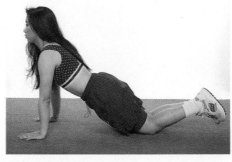

Arched-back push-ups   This incorrect method of doing push-ups will strain and possibly injure the low back.

Straight-back push-ups   Hold your body in a straight line and slowly lower your chest to the floor by bending your arms and elbows. Provides greater workout for the arms, shoulders, and chest.

Continued

FIGURE 4.28

High-Risk Flexibility Exercises: Dont's and Do's—Continued

Don't

Do

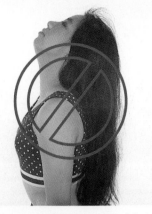

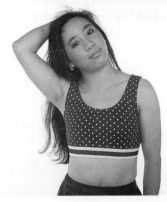

360° head rolls Rolling the head in a full circle may injure the spinal disks in the neck.

Side neck stretches Pull your head gently to one side, forward, to the other side, and back. You may also pull diagonally.

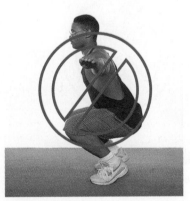

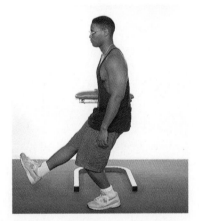

Full squats Stretches ligaments in the knees and may result in injury.

Partial squats Use the back of a chair or other object for balance and squat one-quarter on one leg while the other leg is extended forward.

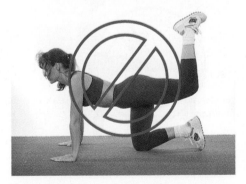

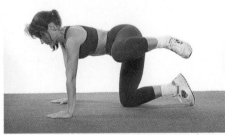

Donkey kicks These force the back to arch and place the shoulders and neck in a contorted position.

Rear thigh lifts Keep your back straight and slowly raise your leg straight up until the thigh is parallel to the torso.

Continued

Flexibility   **87**

FIGURE 4.28

**High-Risk Flexibility Exercises:
Dont's and Do's—Continued**

Don't

Do

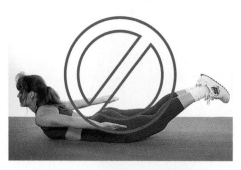

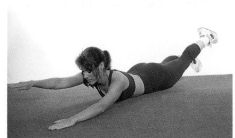

Swan stretch Lifting your chest and legs simultaneously may put excessive stress on the low back.

Prone arm/leg raise Place one or two pillows under your stomach and raise the right arm and left leg 4–6 inches and hold for 5 seconds. Repeat with left arm and right leg.

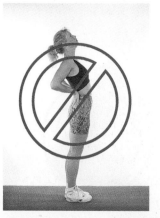

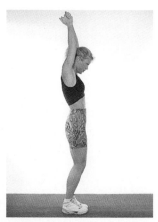

Trunk rolls Puts pressure on the low back and sciatic nerve when knees are straight.

Bent knee trunk rolls Bend your knees, pull in your stomach, and draw the pelvis forward. Slowly lean to the left, forward, and right.

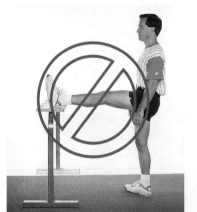

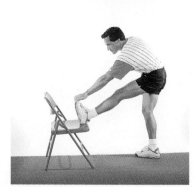

Hamstring stretch When the foot is higher than the hips it excessively stretches the sciatic nerve, lower back, and muscles in the back of the leg.

Hamstring stretch Lead leg is slightly bent at the knee, and the foot is well below the height of the hips. Bend forward slowly until stretch is felt in the hamstrings. Hold 15–20 seconds. Repeat with other leg.

Continued

FIGURE 4.28

**High-Risk Flexibility Exercises:
Dont's and Do's—Continued**

Don't

Do

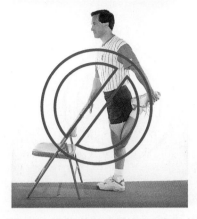

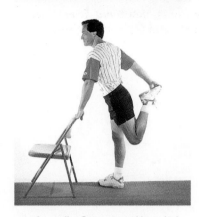

Quadriceps stretch If the ankle is pulled too hard, there may be excessive pressure applied to the knee, possibly resulting in ligament or muscle damage.

Opposite leg pull Grasp one ankle with the opposite hand and attempt to straighten the leg.

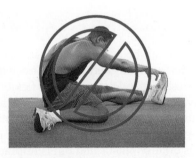

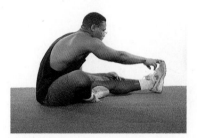

Hurdler's stretch This position puts great stress on the hip, knee, and ankle.

Modified hurdler's stretch Bend the right knee and place the right foot up against the left thigh. Lean forward until the stretch is felt in the left hamstring and hold for 15–20 seconds. Repeat with the other leg.

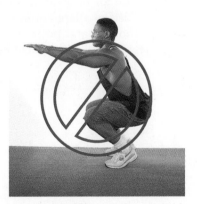

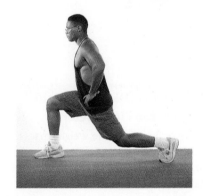

Deep knee bend Places excessive pressure on the ligaments of the knee.

Single knee lunge Place one leg in front and extend the other to the rear. Bend the lead leg 90° and hold for 5 seconds. Repeat with other leg.

Continued

FIGURE 4.28

High-Risk Flexibility Exercises: Dont's and Do's—Continued

Don't

Do

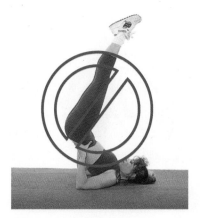

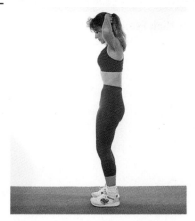

Shoulder stand Excessive pressure on neck may cause injury to muscles or disks.

Neck stretch Gently pull head forward and hold for 10 seconds.

 ASSESSING FLEXIBILITY

Flexibility can be assessed both statically and dynamically. Static measurements are easier to obtain and require less expertise but are less realistic than dynamic measures. Dynamic measures of flexibility are made while subjects are involved in physical activity. A device known as an electrogoniometer is fastened to the joint to be measured. It provides a continuous stream of electrical signals regarding the movement of that joint during physical activity.[15] This measuring instrument is quite sophisticated but is impractical for use with groups of people.

Static measurements are more practical although less functional. The most effective, versatile, and objective device for measuring static flexibility is the Leighton Flexometer[16] (see Figure 4.29). The **flexometer** is attached to the joint to be measured and records the joint's range of motion from full flexion to full extension. Thirty joint movements can be reliably measured with this device.

A second device for measuring static flexibility is the **goniometer** (see Figure 4.30), which consists of a large protractor and two 15-inch straight edges. One of the edges is stationary and positioned at the zero line, while the other rotates through 180 degrees. This instrument not only is inexpensive but also can be con-

FIGURE 4.29

The Leighton Flexometer

(a) The pointer, (b) The weight that keeps the pointer in a vertical position, and (c) The housing that rotates as the body part moves.

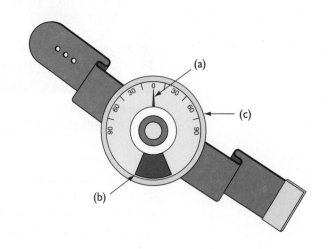

FIGURE 4.30

Large Goniometer

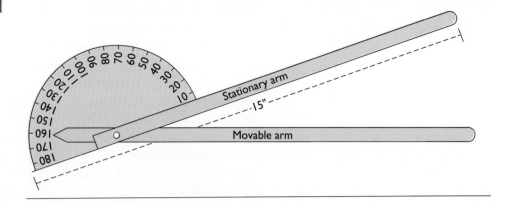

structed with simple materials and a few tools. The major disadvantage of the goniometer is the subjective process of determining the long axes of the bones that comprise the joints, but the device is inexpensive, and measurements using it can be rapidly made.

FIELD TESTS

Field tests to measure flexibility can be employed in the absence of more sophisticated devices. Three commonly used field tests are the sit-and-reach, back extension, and shoulder flexion. Self-Assessments 4.1, 4.2, and 4.3 in Appendix C describe these tests. The tables in the Self-Assessments will help you interpret your performance on the tests.

POINTS TO PONDER

1. Describe the relationship between flexibility and wellness.
2. Identify the techniques for improving flexibility.
3. What are the advantages and disadvantages of ballistic stretching, static stretching, and PNF stretching?
4. Which of the three techniques is the most effective?
5. Which of the techniques has the most potential for harm?
6. Describe the roles of the muscle spindle and the Golgi tendon organ with regard to stretching the muscles and joints.
7. What is an agonist?
8. What is an antagonist?
9. Identify 10 exercises that may be harmful to perform.
10. What does the sit-and-reach test measure?

CHAPTER HIGHLIGHTS

- Flexibility refers to the range of motion about a joint or series of joints.
- Flexibility is improved by increasing the elastic properties of muscles, tendons, ligaments, and connective tissue.
- Inactivity tends to diminish flexibility.
- A muscle that contracts and produces movement is an agonist.
- A muscle that relaxes and allows movement to occur is an antagonist.

- The muscle spindle is responsive to muscle stretch, the Golgi tendon organ is responsive to stretch and tension.
- Ballistic stretching employs repetitive contractions of agonist muscles to produce rapid stretches of antagonist muscles.
- Static stretching features passive stretching of antagonist muscles by slowly stretching and holding terminal positions for 15 to 30 seconds.
- PNF stretching consists of several techniques that involve some combination of contraction and static stretching of agonist and antagonist muscle groups.
- Flexometers and goniometers are instruments used for measuring the flexibility of a variety of joints.
- Field tests for measuring flexibility include sit-and-reach, back-extension, and shoulder flexion.

● REFERENCES

1. H. A. deVries, *Physiology of Exercise,* Dubuque, Iowa: Wm. C. Brown, 1986.
2. B. Stamford, "Flexibility and Stretching," *The Physician and Sportsmedicine* 12 (1984): 171.
3. C. L. Stanitski, "Low Back Pain in Young Athletes," *The Physician and Sportsmedicine* 10 (1982): 77.
4. W. Liemohn and G. Sharpe, "Muscular Strength and Endurance, Flexibility, and Low Back Function" in E. T. Howley and B. D. Frank, *Health/Fitness Instructor's Handbook,* Champaign, Ill: Human Kinetics, 1992.
5. W. E. Prentice and C. A. Bucher, *Fitness for College and Life,* St. Louis: Times Mirror/Mosby, 1988.
6. M. J. Adrian, "Flexibility in the Aging Adult," in E. L. Smith and R. C. Serfass (Eds.), *Exercise and Aging,* Hillside, N.J.: Enslow, 1981.
7. G. W. Grey, "A Study of Flexibility in Selected Joints of Adult Males Ages 18–72," (University of Michigan: Doctoral Dissertation, 1955).
8. A. Jervey, "A Study of Flexibility of Selected Joints in Specified Groups of Adult Females" (University of Michigan: Doctoral Dissertation, 1961).
9. E. A. Chapman et al., "Joint Stiffness: Effects of Exercise on Young and Old Men," *Journal of Gerontology* 27 (1972): 218.
10. K. Munns, "Effects of Exercise on the Range of Joint Motion in Elderly Subjects," in E. L. Smith and R. C. Serfass (Eds.),

Exercise and Aging, Hillside, N.J.: Enslow, 1981; M. Lesser, "The Effects of Rhythmic Exercise on the Range of Motion in Older Adults," *American Corrective Therapy Journal* 32 (1978): 4.
11. E. T. Howley and B. D. Franks, *Health/Fitness Instructor's Handbook,* Champaign, Ill.: Human Kinetics, 1992.
12. S. J. Hartley-O'Brien, "Six Mobilization Exercises for Active Range of Hip Flexion," *Research Quarterly for Exercise and Sport* 51 (1980): 625.
13. B. R. Entyre and E. J. Lee, "Comments on Proprioceptive Neuromuscular Facilitation Stretching Techniques," *Research Quarterly for Exercise and Sport* 58 (1987): 184; B. R. Entyre and L. D. Abraham, "Antagonist Muscle Activity During Stretching: A Paradox Re-Assessed," *Medicine and Science in Sports and Exercise* 20 (1988) 285.
14. D. C. Nieman, *Fitness and Sports Medicine, An Introduction,* Palo Alto, Calif.: Bull, 1990.
15. P. V. Karpovich and W. E Sinning, *Physiology of Muscular Activity,* Philadelphia: W. B. Saunders, 1971.
16. J. R. Leighton, "An Instrument and Technic for the Measurement of Range of Joint Motion," *Archives of Physical and Medical Rehabilitation* 36 (1955): 571.

CHAPTER 5

Developing the Muscular Component

CHAPTER OUTLINE

INTRODUCTION

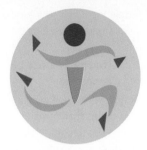

Few fitness authorities would disagree with the idea that aerobic exercises—those that increase the fitness of the heart and lungs—should be the centerpiece of an exercise program for the purposes of health enhancement and physical fitness. Nor would few authorities disagree with the inclusion of exercises for muscular development as an adjunct to the aerobics program. The growing support for muscle-building exercise is reflected in the newest guidelines for exercise developed by the American College of Sports Medicine. For the first time, this organization is recommending a well-rounded exercise program that includes strength training along with aerobic training.[1]

The body contains more than 600 muscles, each of which is imprinted with a physiologic decree: use it or lose it. Most Americans lose it as they leave an active youth and progress to a less active middle age and finally to a sedentary old age. The muscles shrink in size and strength as they receive progressively less stimulation. This change is not the result of age; it is the result of the physical inactivity that accompanies aging.

Approximately 65 percent of the body's muscles are located above the waist. The majority of this muscle mass is virtually unstressed by most aerobic exercises and thoroughly neglected by sedentary living. The result is a predictable loss of muscle mass and strength with the passing years. Surveys have shown that after the age of 74, 28 percent of the men and 65 percent of the women of this nation do not have enough strength to lift objects that weigh more than ten pounds.[2] As a result, the simplest everyday chores—carrying groceries, opening bottles and jars,

Miniglossary

Agonist The muscle that contracts to produce a specific movement; the prime mover.

Anabolic Steroid A drug with tissue-building or growth-stimulating properties.

Androgen Male sex hormone produced in the testes and, to a limited extent, from the adrenal cortex.

Antagonist The muscle that stretches in response to the contraction of the agonist muscle.

Cardiac Muscle Specialized muscle tissue found only in the heart.

Circuit Training A series of six to ten exercises performed in sequence and as rapidly as one's fitness level allows.

Concentric Muscular Contraction That phase of muscular contraction in which the muscle shortens.

Eccentric Muscular Contraction That phase of a muscular contraction in which the muscle lengthens.

Fast-Twitch Muscle Fiber A type of muscle fiber that contracts rapidly but fatigues rapidly. Also referred to as white muscle fibers.

Hyperplasia An increase in size caused by an increase in the number of cells.

Hypertrophy An increase in size caused by an increase in the thickness of fibers.

Isokinetic Muscular Contraction A dynamic contraction in which the muscles generate force against a variable resistance that moves at a constant rate of speed.

Isometric Muscular Contraction A static contraction in which the muscles generate force against an immovable object with no observable shortening.

Isotonic Muscular Contraction A dynamic contraction in which the muscles generate force against a

Continued

—Continued

constant resistance. Movement occurs as the muscles shorten and lengthen with each repetition.

Locomotor Movement Movements that bring about a change in location, including walking, jogging, climbing, cycling, and swimming, to name but a few.

Lordosis Swayback; abnormal curvature of the low back.

Motor Unit A motor nerve and all of the muscle fibers that it innervates.

Muscular Endurance The ability of a muscle to sustain repeated contractions or to apply a constant force for a period of time.

Nonlocomotor Movement Movements that take place around the axis of the body. The subject remains in one place, creating dynamic movement by means of stretching, bending, stooping, pushing, pulling, and twisting, among numerous other motions.

Overload Periodically stressing the body with greater loads than those usually experienced.

Periodization A way to provide variety in training. The training period is divided into different cycles in which the volume is periodically reduced and the intensity is concomitantly increased.

Skeletal Muscle Voluntary muscles whose attachments to the bones of the skeletal system provide the basis for human movement.

Slow-Twitch Muscle Fiber A type of muscle fiber that contracts slowly but is difficult to fatigue. Also referred to as red muscle fibers.

Smooth Muscle Muscle located in the blood vessels and digestive system; not under conscious or voluntary control.

Strength The force exerted by a muscle or muscle group in a single maximal contraction.

Testosterone A sex hormone appearing in much higher concentrations in males than females.

Valsalva Maneuver Occurs when individuals lift heavy weights and hold their breath. The glottis closes and intrathoracic pressure increases, hindering the flow of blood to the heart.

and carrying out the trash—become challenges that may exceed the capabilities of older people. Eventually, muscle weakness can progress to the point that even walking without assistance becomes very difficult, if not impossible.

POLE WALKING—WORKING THE UPPER BODY

Walking is great exercise for the legs, cardiorespiratory and muscle endurance, and weight loss. What is great about walking is that it is easy to do, requires very little motor skill, and can be done anywhere. But like most aerobic activities, it fails to significantly activate upper-body musculature. Pole walking is an effort to stimulate the upper-body muscles.

Specially designed shock-absorbing poles have been developed that enable walkers to achieve the same muscle-toning benefits as cross-country skiing. Each time you press down on the poles and push off during each stride, you contract abdominal, triceps, back, shoulder, and chest muscles. This provides about 2,000 contractions of these muscles per mile walked.

Pole walking increases calorie expenditure per mile by approximately 36% as a result of the use of extensive body musculature. Pole walking also reduces the stress on ankles, knees, hips, and lower back because the upper body is also working to support the body weight.

Source: R. Sweetgall, "How to Design the Perfect Personal Walking Program," *Walking* 8, no. 2 (April 1993): 37.

This chapter explains how you can delay or avoid these consequences. Including progressive resistance exercises two to three times a week will profoundly prolong your ability to manage musculoskeletal challenges throughout your lifetime. The chapter also covers how you can develop muscular strength and endurance and discusses the health implications of muscle training, the strength differences between the sexes, and the principles associated with progressive resistance exercise. Exercises for developing the major muscle groups of the body are illustrated.

Three Self-Assessment activities appear in Appendix C that apply directly to the contents of this chapter:

HUMAN LOCOMOTION

All human movement is dependent on appropriate muscular contractions and relaxations. **Locomotor movements** are those that bring about a change in location, including walking, jogging, climbing, cycling, and swimming, to name but a few. **Nonlocomotor movements** are those that take place around the axis of the body. The subject remains in one place, creating dynamic movement by means of stretching, bending, stooping, pushing, pulling, and twisting, among numerous other motions. Movement can be categorized as fine or precision-oriented, such as typing or playing the piano, or gross (involving contractions of large muscles), such as punting a football or hitting a baseball. Movements can be job related, recreational, rhythmical, athletic, or associated with daily living, but they all require the contraction and relaxation of appropriate muscles.

The muscular system consists of three types of muscle: smooth, cardiac, and skeletal. **Smooth muscles,** such as those located in the digestive system and blood vessels, are not under conscious control. They are involuntary muscles that are under autonomic (nonvoluntary) neural control. **Cardiac muscle,** which appears in the heart only, is also under nonvoluntary control. Some practitioners of yoga—the ancient philosophy of India that emphasizes mental attitude, diet, and posture—as well as others who are trained in biofeedback are able to influence their heart rate through meditation and will power, but by and large, cardiac muscle responds to automatic control processes. The **skeletal muscles,** on the other hand, are voluntary muscles whose attachments to the bones of the skeletal system provide the basis for human movements. Their origins and insertions on the bones provide a lever system in which small contractions of the muscles produce large movements of the extremities.

> The human body has over 600 muscles containing more than 6 billion microscopic muscle fibers. Each fiber is so strong that it can support more than 1000 times its own weight.
>
> —C. Moore

FIGURE 5.1

Isometric Contraction   Force is exerted against both sides of an immovable door jam.

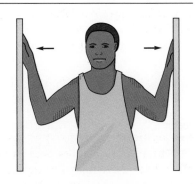

MUSCULAR STRENGTH AND MUSCULAR ENDURANCE

Muscular **strength** can be defined as the force exerted by a muscle or muscle group in a single maximal isotonic, isometric, or isokinetic contraction. Isometric strength is developed through muscular contractions against an immovable object (see Figure 5.1). The muscles contract statically for 6 to 10 seconds without shortening. Isometric strength is measured with dynamometers and cable tensiometers.

Isotonic muscular contractions consist of dynamic movement as a result of muscle shortening. Isotonic movements involve **concentric** and **eccentric muscular contractions.** The dumbbell curl in Figure 5.2 exemplifies both types of isotonic contractions. The concentric phase of this exercise occurs when the flexor muscles of the arm contract and lift the weight to the chest. The eccentric phase occurs as the weight is *slowly* lowered to the starting position against the force of gravity. Lowering the weight rapidly will limit the potential for strength development in the eccentric phase of exercise.

FIGURE 5.2

Isotonic Dumbbell Curl
Concentric phase—the weight is lifted toward the shoulder; eccentric phase—the weight is returned to the starting position.

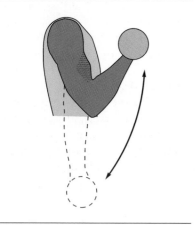

Most dynamic exercises consist of both types of contractions. **Strength** may be developed by either type of dynamic muscular contraction, but little is known about the effects of exercise programs that feature eccentric movements exclusively. Since systems of isotonic exercises (and most exercise equipment) as well as movements made in daily life involve both types of contraction, for practical reasons, the two types of contractions will not be treated separately. It should be noted that of the two types of contraction, eccentric contractions generate the greater amount of muscular force. For the optimal development of isotonic strength, however, the muscles must be exercised and fatigued both concentrically and eccentrically.

Isokinetic muscular contractions are dynamic movements requiring specialized equipment, such as the Cybex or Minigym, that adjusts the resistance so that it will be maximum throughout the full range of motion (see Figure 5.3). Regardless of the amount of force applied, these devices allow movement to occur at a constant rate of speed.

Muscles that are activated or in the process of contracting produce tension and may or may not react by changing their length. Contraction may produce a shortening of the muscle fibers (concentric movement) or a lengthening of the fibers (eccentric action) or no change in the length of the fibers **(isometric muscular contraction)**. Muscles that contract dynamically change their length because they are able to overcome a resistance. A muscle or group of muscles at a joint that produce concentric movement are the prime movers of the joint. For example, the prime mover, or **agonist,** in Figure 5.2 is the biceps muscle. Its contraction produces muscle shortening, thereby moving the weight from thigh to shoulder. For this movement to occur efficiently, the triceps muscle must relax and lengthen. In this exercise, the triceps is the **antagonist** of the biceps. The biceps and the triceps function synergistically so that as one muscle—the biceps—contracts and does the work, the other muscle—the triceps—relaxes and permits the work to occur. In Figure 5.3, the roles of these two muscles are reversed as the triceps becomes the prime mover, or agonist, and the biceps becomes the antagonist.

Muscular endurance is the ability of a muscle or muscle group to sustain repeated contractions (isotonic) or the ability to apply a constant force for a period of time (isometric). Muscular endurance is developed through exercise programs that emphasize many repetitions with relatively light weights. Muscular strength

FIGURE 5.3

Isokinetic Training and Testing Device

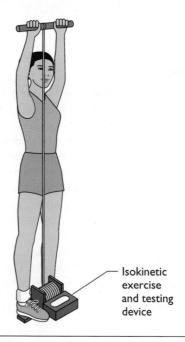

Isokinetic exercise and testing device

is highly correlated with absolute muscular endurance, which involves lifting a specified amount of weight a maximum number of times. This is dependent upon the maximum contractile force of the muscles involved. For example, two people of unequal strength attempt to lift 100 pounds as many times as possible. One is capable of a maximum lift of 200 pounds, while the other can lift only 150 pounds. One hundred pounds represents one half of the capacity of the first person but two thirds of the capacity for the second person. Two thirds of the weaker person's total strength must be used on every lift, while only one half of the stronger person's total strength is used. Each lift is more difficult for the weaker person. Because a greater percentage of the weaker person's total number of motor units per lift must be used, the weaker person will fatigue more rapidly than the stronger person. (A **motor unit** is a nerve and all of the muscle fibers that it stimulates.) To increase absolute endurance, one must increase strength.

Muscular endurance can also be measured on a relative basis by testing people at a given percentage of their maximal strength for selected lifts. Returning to the two weightlifters, if they were each to be tested at 50 percent of their capacity, the stronger one would lift 100 pounds, while the weaker one would lift 75 pounds. Under this protocol, it is conceivable that the weaker person could outperform the stronger one in muscular endurance.

THE MUSCULAR COMPONENT AND THE WELLNESS CONNECTION

● The Effect of Muscle Training on Body Composition

Training with moderate weights increases muscle tissue while decreasing the amount of stored body fat, as documented by several short-term studies. The largest increase in lean body mass was seven pounds, and the largest decrease in the amount of fat was 9.4 percent.[3] This favorable change in body composition leads to an increase in the resting metabolic rate (referring to the amount of energy used by the body during the resting state). The addition of muscle tissue increases the body's energy requirements because muscle uses more calories than fat tissue, both during rest and during physical activity. Jogging burns more calories during the workout than weight training. The effect of jogging is cumulative; that is, x number of calories are burned during every workout. On the other hand, weight training increases muscle mass, while jogging increases muscle mass little, if at all. An increase of three to four pounds of muscle tissue with a year of weight training will increase energy expenditure by 120 to 200 calories every 24 hours, because a pound of muscle burns 40 to 50 more calories a day than fat. One may conclude that aerobic exercise combined with weight training is an excellent and effective approach to losing excess body fat and keeping it off.

Since we spend more time resting than in activity, the increase in muscle tissue becomes an aid in the effort to control body weight. The change in body composition results in a restructuring of body contour as males and females acquire more muscle tissue, lose some fat, and develop more fit and trim silhouettes. This change in body composition occurs because muscle is denser than fat: one pound of muscle takes up less room in the body than one pound of fat. These changes in the body contribute to better mental health through the enhancement of a positive self-concept.

FAT MEASURES: A POUND OF LEAN—18% SMALLER

> When you start to slide out of shape, you get to look really out of shape before your friends or your bathroom scales give you clear warning. That's because each pound of fat you put on bulges out 18% bigger than a pound of lean (1.1 liters compared with 0.9).
>
> *American Health*, September/October 1982, p. 17.

The Effect of Muscle Training on Posture and Injury Prevention

Appropriate resistance exercises develop the antigravity muscles of the abdomen and lower back, thereby decreasing the likelihood of back pain and injury. The development of these muscle groups provides the support needed by the spinal column to hold up the torso and to maintain good posture. Strengthening other antigravity muscles (those of the hips, front and back of the thighs, and both calves) also helps maintain good posture. Proper posture reduces stress upon the spinal column and the low back. **Lordosis** (swayback) is an exaggerated curve of the lower back related to weak abdominals, poor posture, tight hamstrings, and excess weight—all of which lead to back pain and injury and all of which are beneficially affected by exercise.

Resistance training strengthens the ligaments, which attach one bone to another, and the tendons, which attach muscle to bone. Cartilage and connective tissue become thicker and stronger. The joints are better protected from injury and much more stable when their muscles and surrounding structures are well developed and strong.

The Effect of Muscle Training on the Skeletal System

The bones, as living organs, also respond to resistance training in healthful ways according to the specific demands placed upon them. A study of 3,000 adult laborers and sports participants showed that the characteristic shapes and structures of bones were significantly influenced by the stress placed upon them.[4] Changes in bone sizes and shapes were noted on shifts in occupation and sports participation. A classic example of the adaptation of bone to stress was reported by J.A. Ross.[5] A subject who had lost all but the little finger of his right hand showed remarkable **hypertrophy** (an increase in size caused by in increase in the thickness of fibers) of that digit. In the 32 years since the amputation, his little finger had grown in size to that of the middle finger of his left hand. This was measured and confirmed by x-ray examination of both hands. In another study, nationally ranked athletes were compared with nonathlete controls for bone mineral content.[6] The athletes had significantly more bone mineral content, and they demonstrated bone hypertrophy consistent with the demands of their specific sport. The greatest amount of hypertrophy among the athletes was achieved by the weightlifters. The implications of studies such as these are that resistance as well as aerobic exercises strengthen and maintain the integrity of bony tissue.

Osteoporosis, a disease characterized by bone demineralization, may be prevented, delayed, or alleviated by long-term adherence to resistance exercises coupled with some form of aerobic training, proper nutrition, and hormonal supplementation for postmenopausal women. "Regular exercise is essential. Bones that are not used are automatically thinned out by the remodeling process."[7]

Twenty-five million Americans have osteoporosis and 80 percent of them are elderly women.[8] While there is no cure for osteoporosis, most authorities are convinced that it can be prevented provided that preventive efforts begin in adolescence. It is during this period of life that the body stores the calcium reserves that will be drawn upon during later life. If the body is inadequately nourished during the adolescent years, particularly with regard to calcium intake, osteoporosis is more likely to occur later on.

Bone is living tissue that responds to exercise. Two categories of exercise are particularly beneficial: (1) weight-bearing aerobic exercises, such as walking and jogging, because supporting and moving one's body mass against the force of gravity stresses the muscles and strengthens the bones to some extent and (2) progressive resistance exercises, such as weight training, because the best way to strengthen a bone is to sufficiently stimulate the muscle that pulls on it. Both categories of exercise cause the bone to maintain and even increase its calcium density. Exercises that are combined with calcium and/or hormonal therapy for postmenopausal women can slow or prevent bone loss.[9]

The Effect of Muscle Training on Older Adults

Reporting on the effects of exercise for older people, the *Harvard Medical School Health Letter* indicated that approached with caution, weight training can protect bone and soft tissue from injury.[10] Several recent studies have indicated that the elderly are more responsive to resistance exercises than was previously thought. In one study, 12 men aged 60–72 participated in 12 weeks of strength conditioning of the quadricep and hamstring muscle groups.[11] The strength and size of these muscle groups increased significantly during the training period. The ability of the muscles to perform aerobically to utilize oxygen also increased as a result of increased muscle size and strength.

Subjects in another study consisted of 10 frail men and women whose average age was 90.[12] They participated in eight weeks of resistance training designed to increase the strength of the quadriceps muscle group. By the end of the study, strength gains averaged 174 percent, while midthigh muscle area increased an average of 9 percent. Compared to pretraining values, the subjects were able to walk a specified distance 48 percent faster, two subjects were able to discard their walking canes, and one of the three subjects who could not rise from a chair without an assist from the arms was able to do so.

Both of these studies show that muscle hypertrophy (enlargement) can occur in older subjects and accounts for at least some of the strength gains achieved. Think of the implications this has for living and moving independently in old age. Increased muscle mass that improves strength and aerobic efficiency has a significant impact on the quality of life during the later years. Muscle development should definitely be an integral part of one's fitness program.

The Effect of Muscle Training on Blood Pressure and Serum Cholesterol

Several researchers have investigated the effect of weight training on resting blood pressure. High blood pressure (hypertension) is a primary risk factor for heart attacks and strokes. One study found no change in blood pressure,[13] two studies found significant decreases in systolic pressure,[14] and another found a significant decrease in both systolic and diastolic pressures.[15] Weight training lowered resting blood pressure in the majority of the studies and did not negatively impact it in any of the studies.

Weight training also seems to have a beneficial effect on serum cholesterol. A high circulating level of cholesterol in the blood is a primary risk factor for heart attack and stroke. This topic is covered in some detail in a later chapter, but for the purposes of this chapter, you should know that cholesterol can be both good and bad. Cholesterol is bad if the total blood level is too high and one of its subfractions—high-density lipoprotein (HDL)—is too low. A certain amount of cholesterol is necessary for several important body functions, such as the construction of cell membranes, synthesis of vitamin D, development of male and female sex hormones, and the formulation of bile for the emulsification of fat (a process by which fat globules break down to smaller droplets).

Cholesterol in the blood in levels below the average risk is good and is needed. It is also good if its HDL component represents a significant portion of its total as indicated by a ratio of total cholesterol to HDL of less than 3.4. Several studies have indicated that weight training with moderate resistance tends to increase the HDL fraction.[16] In general, the higher the HDL, the better.

Power lifters—those who lift extremely heavy weight competitively—seem to have lower HDL levels than normal.[17] This suggests that the amount of resistance and the number of repetitions may affect the cholesterol profile. Although further investigation is needed, the available data indicate that cholesterol is favorably affected by weight-training programs featuring *moderate* resistance and 10 to 12 repetitions.

From a health and aesthetic perspective, it seems prudent to include resistance exercises in the fitness program because they increase strength, favorably change

1. **If I exercise my stomach muscles, my waist will get smaller.**

   Spot reduction is an idea that persists in spite of evidence to the contrary. Many people do abdominal exercises to lose fat from the abdominal area. The effectiveness of such a practice has been examined. In one study, subjects participated in 27 days of intense sit-up training. Biopsies performed on levels of abdominal fat before and after training showed no difference between the two measurements. The current theory of fat usage is that it is mobilized either from areas of greatest concentration or it is removed equally from all storage areas. In either case, the body is incapable of specifically targeting fat only from those areas that are being exercised.

2. **If I stop exercising, my muscles will turn to fat.**

   What actually happens if you stop exercising is that the muscles will atrophy because they are no longer receiving the amount of stimulation required to maintain their size and strength. If at the same time the appetite remains at or near exercise levels, you will gain weight in the form of fat. The muscles are shrinking in size while fat is accumulating. This gives the appearance that the muscles are turning to fat, but this does not occur—muscle tissue and fat tissue are not interchangeable.

3. **Exercising with weights makes females look masculine.**

   Actually, weight training properly performed has the potential to produce females that look more female with well-toned, firm bodies. It takes the male hormone testosterone to develop large muscles. Women produce testosterone naturally but in quantities too small to result in significant muscle enlargement.

4. **If I exercise with weights, I will become musclebound.**

   Muscle-boundness implies some restriction of movement due to enlarged tight muscles. Some range of motion may be lost for those who become super muscular because excessively large muscles get in the way of each other during movement. But for the majority of weight trainers, range of motion will more likely increase because greater elasticity is one of the characteristics of stronger muscles. However, when performing resistance exercises, it is important to execute the movements throughout the full range of motion. This stimulates muscle elasticity and helps to maintain or develop suppleness.

body composition, increase resting metabolism through the addition of muscle, contribute to the enhancement of self-concept, help prevent low-back and joint injury, strengthen and thicken the bones (which may delay or prevent osteoporosis), have the potential for favorably changing blood lipid and lipoprotein levels in ways consistent with lowering the risk for coronary artery disease, and have produced beneficial changes in systolic and diastolic blood pressures.

GENETIC AND GENDER CONSIDERATIONS

Gender Differences

Several factors contribute to the differences in strength between males and females. Prior to puberty, the differences between the sexes are small, but they become substantially greater after puberty. The average male can generate 30 percent to 40 percent more force than the average female. The disparity is great when the sexes are compared for arm and upper-body strength but much less when leg strength is compared.

One factor responsible for the sex difference in strength is the male sex hormone **testosterone.** This substance stimulates the protein-synthesizing mechanisms and is responsible for the muscle **hypertrophy** seen in males. Females also produce testosterone, but at a rate of one-twentieth to one-thirtieth that of males, accounting for their lessened ability to gain substantial muscle size.[18] Research has shown that females can make significant gains in strength without developing large muscles. The masculinizing effect of weight training is a myth that has persisted despite substantial evidence to the contrary. It is a fact that women do develop muscle tissue with resistance exercises, but muscular development in women is limited by insufficient quantities of testosterone. J. H. Wilmore's study indicated quite nicely that college women could gain significant amounts of strength with ten weeks of weight training without significant increases in muscle size.[19] Male subjects in the same study improved significantly in both strength and muscle size.

K. J. Cureton agrees that women's muscles don't grow as large as those of males, but for a different reason.[20] He hypothesized that the "absolute changes in muscle hypertrophy following weight training do tend to be larger in men than in women, probably because the initial size of muscle fibers is larger and the number of fibers undergoing hypertrophy in some muscles is greater." He further indicated that women can and do get stronger, and on a percentage basis, they can achieve the same muscle hypertrophy as men without looking like men.

Sex differences in muscle size are readily discernible by observing contestants in mixed pairs body-building contests. Despite similar training philosophies and procedures, males develop extraordinary muscularity, while females develop well-defined but significantly less muscularity. The differences between the sexes is considerable, but when compared to the average woman, female body builders have more muscle tissue, much more muscle definition, and considerably less body fat.

Strength differences between the sexes essentially disappear when strength is measured by cross-sectional area of muscle tissue. Human skeletal muscle is capable of generating 3 to 8 kilograms of force per centimeter squared ($3–8 \, kg/cm^2$) of muscle cross-section regardless of gender. Since the quality of muscle between males and females appears to be similar, the differences in strength seem to be due to the total muscle mass of males. Males may have as much as 50 percent more muscle tissue than females.

Hypertrophy of muscle fibers, total amount of muscle mass, and recruitment of motor units are associated with strength gains. Under ordinary circumstances, we are unable to mobilize all of the motor units in a given muscle. Training and emotionally charged situations increase our ability to recruit more motor units, thereby producing a more forceful muscular contraction.

Neural Factors

Neural and cultural factors are also involved in the development of strength. The evidence of the neural influence comes from cases of superhuman feats of strength that have been observed and documented from time to time. Workers trapped under heavy steel girders as a result of construction cave-ins or children trapped beneath automobiles have provided some of the settings in which phenomenal feats of strength have occurred in both sexes. As a result of these extreme emotional conditions, rescuers have ignored body signals regarding their own safety and have been capable of expressions of strength that substantially exceed the ordinary. The victims of these unfortunate accidents are often spared by the heroic efforts of their rescuers. These efforts often result in muscle and skeletal damage because the average human is not trained or equipped to handle such heavy loads. People generally learn their strength limits through experience with heavy objects. But the urgency of a rescue situation is characterized by a surge in the flow of adrenaline accompanied by suppression of the inhibitory neural impulses that formulate our safety system. A combination of both neural and chemical input produces superhuman strength for the brief interval needed for an extraordinary performance.

Neural factors are responsible for the rapid gains in strength achieved during the first two to six weeks of resistance training. These increases occur without muscle growth in fiber size or cross-sectional area and provide additional evidence supporting the neural influence associated with expressions of strength. Some of the neural mechanisms include (1) recruitment of motor units, (2) increased motor neuron excitability, (3) effective inhibition of antagonists, and

(4) inhibition of neural protective mechanisms. The mechanisms designed to protect us from injury may be suppressed to some extent in highly emotionally charged situations. Weight training is another vehicle through which the body is trained to inhibit the safety system. For example, untrained subjects were able to generate 17 percent more force in the muscles responsible for elbow flexion under hypnosis, while trained subjects experienced no improvement. The trained group was unable to improve because their weight-training programs had already taught their bodies to repress the safety systems and hypnosis was unable to add to the effects achieved by training.

Sex role expectations and cultural dictates have discouraged women from participating in strength development programs. However, many of today's females, and indeed many female watchers, consider attractiveness to be synonymous with a firm, healthy-looking, fit body. It is indeed encouraging to find women, both young and old, who devote a portion of their fitness time to weight training because they have come to understand its contribution to physical appearance and health. Unfortunately, the myth that women will build masculine-looking bulging muscles with resistance exercise persists in spite of evidence to the contrary. Proponents of this myth cite examples of female athletes who are muscularly well-developed as proof of the effect of training. In reality, these athletes are successful performers because they have the genetic endowment to capitalize on training—they had a head start.

All women—indeed, all people—respond to training, but in differing degrees. Well-muscled female athletes might be producing above-average levels of testosterone, which would account for their adaptation to training. Others might combine training with the ingestion of **anabolic steroids**—drugs that have similar muscle-building qualities as testosterone. The term *anabolic* implies that these substances promote the development of tissue, particularly muscle tissue. Because these drugs are considered to be harmful, the dosage that can be safely studied in laboratory experiments with humans is only a fraction of the dosage taken by competitive athletes. The laboratory experiments have not confirmed the alleged acceleration of muscle tissue growth with steroids, but many athletes attribute their muscle growth and strength increases directly to steroid use.

Anabolic Steroids

Steroids are a health hazard and illegal when used for the purposes of athletic enhancement. The medical risks associated with long-term usage include potential cancer, damage to the liver and kidneys, and sterility, to name a few. After studying the worldwide literature on this subject, the American College of Sports Medicine produced a position paper on the use and abuse of steroids.[21] The effect of steroid usage in men "often, but not always reduces the output of testosterone and gonadotropins and reduces spermatogenesis." The effects of steroids on females, particularly prepubertal adolescents or those who have not completed full growth, is especially hazardous. Steroid use disrupts the normal pattern of growth, promotes the development of acne, and produces such masculinizing effects as a deepening of the voice and growth of facial and body hair. Steroid use significantly increases aggressive behavior. Users refer to this as "roid rage." Steroids have been implicated in at least one psychotic episode that ended in homicide,[22] and it has been linked to at least one case of suicide.[23] While cause and effect is difficult to establish between steroid use and this type of violent and self-destructive behavior, the circumstantial and anecdotal evidence continues to accumulate, thus giving credence to the possibility.

The long-term risks of steroid use far outweigh the short-term benefits that might be achieved. The purpose of this text is to present the necessity of exercise and physical fitness as an integral part of a wellness lifestyle. The use of steroids is to be deplored for competitors and noncompetitors alike because it is the antithesis of wellness.

Muscle Fiber Types

In humans, it appears that the total number of muscle fibers and the fiber type are set genetically and that both are fully established at birth. Current research indicates that the number of muscle fibers probably cannot be increased, nor can fiber type be changed. If this precept is accurate, the increases in muscle size resulting from training must be caused by hypertrophy of the existing fibers. Muscle **hyperplasia** (an increase in the number of muscle fibers) has been shown to occur in several species of animals with heavy resistance exercise. Muscle hyperplasia has not been verified in humans, but at this time, the possibility cannot be ruled out.

Two types of muscle fibers have been identified—slow-twitch and fast-twitch. **Slow-twitch muscle fibers** function aerobically and are richly supplied with blood, slow to fatigue, and relatively slow in contractile speed. **Fast-twitch muscle fibers** function anaerobically and are poorly supplied with blood, rapid to fatigue, and fast in contractile speed. Fast-twitch fibers are larger, contract with more force, and are well equipped for short-duration, high-intensity work. On the other hand, slow-twitch fibers, with their abundant blood supply, are well-adapted for endurance work.

Muscle fibers do not cross over: slow-twitch fibers remain slow-twitch and fast-twitch fibers remain fast-twitch regardless of the type of training to which they are exposed.[24] To produce a change in muscle fiber type would require a structural change in the motor nerve that supplies it with electrical impulses. A motor nerve stimulates either all slow-twitch or all fast-twitch fibers, and when the electrical impulse is delivered, all fibers in the motor unit contract.

The ratio between the fiber types appears to be set genetically. Changing one fiber type to another under normal conditions is probably impossible because the motor nerve that innervates the muscle determines its function.

The ratio of slow-twitch to fast-twitch muscle fibers can be determined by examining muscle biopsies from selected sites The muscle composition of world-class aerobic athletes (distance runners, cyclists, cross-country skiiers) is predominantly slow-twitch, while the muscle compositions of the world-class power or anaerobic-event athletes (shot-putters, sprinters, power and Olympic weightlifters) is primarily fast-twitch. Knowing the ratio of fiber type could be important for these competitors, but it is relatively unimportant when one exercises for health reasons. Health enthusiasts can participate in a variety of activities with some degree of success and satisfaction regardless of fiber type.

> Variety and innovation are important in training programs. Prepubescent children are immature psychologically and physiologically and need the elements of fun and play.
>
> —L. Totten

WEIGHT TRAINING FOR CHILDREN AND ADOLESCENTS

What about the effectiveness of resistance training for young children? Can they benefit from such training, or are they exposing their immature musculoskeletal systems to possible harm? The American Academy of Pediatrics (AAP) developed a position paper on weight training and weightlifting for youngsters in 1983. It essentially endorsed weight training for sports performance for adolescents but stated that prepubescent children would receive minimum benefits. This was based on the premise that circulating **androgens** in prepubescent children are not sufficiently high to stimulate muscle growth. A number of independent investigations since the publication of the AAP position have refuted the basic premise that prepubescent children cannot attain strength with weight training. These studies were well conceived; control groups were used to account for the natural effects of growth; and weight-training regimens similar in intensity, frequency, duration, and training techniques to those prescribed for adults were used.

Each of the studies demonstrated significant strength gains for the exercised groups compared to nonexercising controls. The gains were even more remarkable considering the short length of training time in three of the four studies (5 to 9 weeks). These data, which are in conflict with the AAP position, prompted the National Strength and Conditioning Association (NSCA) to formulate a position endorsing weight training for prepubescent youngsters. The group also

Continued

—Continued

addressed the need for precautions in developing and implementing weight-training programs for this age group. Both organizations discourage weightlifting (a sport in which contestants lift maximal weights) until the age of 16 or 17, at which time the skeletal system is mature enough to withstand such loads. On the other hand, weight training is an activity in which light to moderate weights are used to exercise the major muscle groups of the body.

Nationwide samples of children typically show that they are poorly fit and particularly weak in upper-body strength. This is often accompanied by excessive fat or poor body composition. Weight-training programs guided by well-qualified instructors would help rectify this situation.

TRAINING CONSIDERATIONS

Achieving optimum results safely with progressive resistance exercises requires some knowledge. You should know the following:

1. How often to work out.
2. The length of each workout.
3. Proper lifting and spotting techniques
4. The amount of weight with which to begin each lift.
5. The number of times (repetitions) that the weight should be lifted.
6. The number of times an exercise should be repeated (sets).
7. Proper warmup and cooldown procedures.
8. The order of the exercises.
9. The length of the rest periods between repetitions and sets.

The next step is to select the mode of training that best suits your needs. You may select from isometric, isotonic, or isokinetic training systems or combine them. The selection should be based upon your objectives, the availability of equipment and space, and the amount of time you wish to invest.

Isometric Training

Isometric exercises train the muscular system by a series of static contractions where no change in muscle length occurs. Force is applied against an unyielding object so that the affected muscles contract in a fixed position. The term *isometric* literally means equal tension.

Figure 5.4 illustrates an isometric contraction. In this illustration, the top of the doorjam is the unyielding object. By repeating this exercise regularly, the affected muscles will gain in strength at the angle in which the joint is stressed. The development of strength through isometrics is joint angle specific; that is, maximal strength occurs at the angle of contraction. There is a training carryover of approximately 20 degrees from that angle. Isometric contraction at four different angles throughout the range of motion of elbow flexion increases strength at each angle and significantly increases the dynamic power of the elbow flexors (see Figure 5.5).

To optimize the results from isometric training, one should adhere to the following guidelines:

1. The total contraction time should be greater than 30 seconds. This can be accomplished by a few contractions of long duration or many contractions of short duration.
2. Maximal contractions are superior to submaximal contractions.
3. Daily isometric training produces greater results than the usual 3 to 4 times per week.

FIGURE 5.4

Isometric Contraction

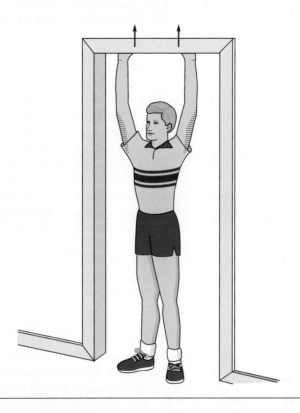

FIGURE 5.5

Isometric Curl Performed at Different Joint Angles Each dot represents a joint angle where an isometric contraction should occur to work the bicep muscle through a full range of motion.

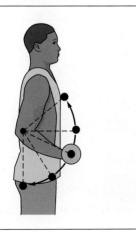

Isometrics can be performed quickly with little or no equipment and in very little space, but they tend to raise blood pressure because the statically contracting muscles squeeze the blood vessels. This increases the resistance to blood flow, forcing the heart to pump with greater force. These exercises are particularly unsuitable for older people, hypertensives, and people with heart disease, atherosclerosis, or any form of compromised circulation. Since most Americans above age 35 have some degree of atherosclerosis, it would be wise to choose another means of developing the muscular system.

Improvement in strength is difficult to assess isometrically because the resistance does not change throughout the program. Knowledge of results remains a mystery unless you have access to equipment that records the amount of force exerted. Motivation is difficult to sustain in the absence of feedback.

The time savings associated with isometrics compared to other forms of resistance training diminishes when you attempt, and correctly so, to develop strength throughout the full range of movement for each exercise. This requires 5 to 10 sets of each exercise. The nature of isometric exercises is such that it stimulates the development of strength but does not develop muscular endurance.

No measurable work is accomplished through isometric training. According to a principle in physics, work is defined as force multiplied by distance (Work = Force × Distance). In an isometric contraction, the distance that the resistance moves is equal to zero. In this equation, zero distance multiplied by any amount of force still equals zero amount of work performed.

The disadvantages of isometrics tend to outweigh the advantages. Minimal health benefits seem to be associated with this type of exercise. However, this is the only type of exercise that can be performed to limit the muscular atrophy that occurs when a limb is immobilized. With the approval of the physician, the muscles of a leg placed in a cast because of a bone break can be exercised isometrically to reduce atrophy.

In terms of practicality, there is some transferability from isometric training to ordinary daily chores. Carrying the groceries, a small child, or any object in a fixed position requires isometric strength. Pushing, pulling, or lifting objects that require the muscles to contract statically also requires isometric strength.

Isotonic Training

Isotonic exercises feature dynamic muscle movement against a constant resistance. When executed correctly, the affected muscles shorten and move the resistance through a full range of motion around a joint. An isotonic muscular contraction is one in which the muscle exerts a constant force throughout the entire movement.[25] The term *isotonic,* which literally means equal tension, may soon be replaced by the term *dynamic constant external resistance,* since lifting a specific weight through a range of motion is not truly isotonic.[26] The actual force exerted by the muscle is not constant. At some point in the movement, the position of the joint will produce a mechanical advantage, resulting in less force needed to overcome the resistance. For example, the two-arm biceps curl begins with a barbell held at arm's length resting on the thighs (Figure 5.6). The object is to lift the weight in a semicircular motion to the chest by contracting the biceps muscles. This constitutes the concentric phase of the two-arm curl. Slowly lowering the weight to the starting position represents the eccentric phase of the lift. The amount of force required to complete this lift is greatest at approximately 90 degrees and less at other joint angles in the movement. The application of force in isotonic exercise is constantly changing throughout the range of motion, and the muscle is stressed unequally. If a maximum lift is attempted in the biceps curl, the amount of weight successfully accomplished would be limited by the weakest point (approximately 90 degrees) in the range of motion.

Both concentric and eccentric movements develop strength in the affected muscles. Researchers have investigated the effectiveness of both movements in developing strength and have found that neither is superior to the other.[27] Most dynamic exercises require both concentric and eccentric contractions, and most training equipment incorporates both types of movement so that participants receive the benefits of both.

One negative feature is associated with the eccentric phase of exercise: muscle soreness that occurs following a workout. Therefore, isotonic training sessions should be held every other day to allow for muscle recovery between sessions. Three to four workouts per week are sufficient for developing strength in the novice lifter. Frequency may be increased as one becomes trained and can tolerate the increased stresses.

Weight training is more effective than calisthenics for developing strength because the resistance can be adjusted as strength increases. Body weight is the resistance in calisthenic exercises. It can be increased by strapping on weight or by

FIGURE 5.6

Isotonic Barbell Curl

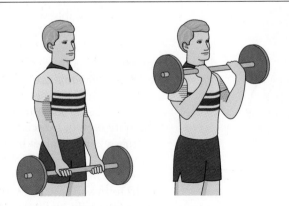

having a partner apply resistance, and it can be reduced by modifying some of the exercises. These techniques tend to be too inconvenient for the average participant.

The starting weight in weight training is determined by trial and error. Find a weight that you can lift no more than 10 to 12 times (repetitions) and then perform three sets of each exercise. Add weight when you are able to execute 15 to 16 repetitions for three sets. At this point, add enough weight to bring you back to 10 repetitions and continue with that weight until you can perform 15 to 16 repetitions and repeat the cycle by adding weight once again.

Each repetition should be executed slowly, rhythmically, and in strict form. You should not throw the weight during the concentric phase or drop it rapidly during the eccentric phase. Move slowly enough (approximately 2 to 3 seconds for each phase) so as to maintain control of the weight and be sure to fully contract and extend the muscles during each repetition. Generally, the heaviest weight that can be lifted for 10 to 12 repetitions represents approximately 75 percent of one repetition maximum (1 RM). This represents a sufficient stimulus for developing muscles and improving strength.

Bear in mind that the weight-training program suggested here is a supplement to the aerobic program and is not intended to produce a champion weightlifter or a Mr. or Miss Universe. It is intended to develop some strength and to increase muscle tissue. Understand, too, the optimum number of sets, repetitions, and amount of weight to be lifted are not fully known for meeting various objectives. The program suggested in this text is only one of many that have produced results.

The American College of Sports Medicine has develop minimum guidelines for weight training. This organization suggests that participants select 8 to 10 exercises that collectively stress the major muscle groups of the body, perform 8 to 12 repetitions of each exercise to near maximum fatigue, and perform this routine two times a week.[28]

For those who prefer to leave the health benefits to the aerobic portion of their training in order to concentrate on the strength development properties of weight training, the optimum routine is to lift heavy weights for four to six repetitions maximum, do more sets, and take ample rest time (two to three minutes) between sets.[29] It is a generally accepted principle that strength is best developed by utilizing heavy resistance which will, in turn, limit the number of repetitions performed. Heavy resistance programs do not contribute to health in the same way as resistance programs of a moderate nature that work many muscle groups. If the resistance program is a weightlifting program designed to develop strength primarily, an aerobics program is where the health benefits will be obtained.

Students interested in more information regarding strength development may read the following:

- M. H. Stone and H. O'Bryant, *Weight Training: A Scientific Approach*, Minneapolis: Burgess, 1986.
- T. R. Baechle and B. R. Groves, *Weight Training—Steps To Success*, Champaign, Ill: Human Kinetics, 1992.

Always warm up prior to weight training or any other resistance exercises and cool down after the workout. The warmup should consist of stretching exercises and some activities that elevate the heart rate, such as jogging in place, rope skipping, or jumping jacks. According to W. L. Westcott, programs that utilize sets of 10 to 12 repetitions do not require warmup sets with lighter weights.[30] That is, it is not necessary to perform a set with a weight lighter than the weight that will ultimately be used for each exercise. Westcott states that "under normal circumstances, a weightload that can be lifted ten times should not cause injury or require special preparation."[31]

The cooldown procedure is important because what occurs during this time will affect recovery from the workout. Lactic acid produced during the workout seems to be most effectively removed from the muscles by 15 minutes of moderate aerobic activity. Rhythmic and continuous activities that stimulate circulation seem to accelerate the removal of lactic acid from the muscles. Quick removal allows the rebuilding process to occur and readies the individual for the next workout. The length of each workout will depend on program objectives, number of exercises, number of repetitions and sets performed, and the amount of rest taken between exercises. Beginners can benefit from one to two sets of each exercise.[32] The number of sets can increase to as many as five as fitness improves.

Rest periods less than one minute result in very high blood lactate levels and will impair one's ability to produce maximum force because the next exercise begins before recovery from the previous one is complete.[33]

Some evidence exists indicating that large-muscle exercises should precede exercises affecting the smaller muscle groups. Work the muscles of the legs, chest, and back first because they require the lifting of heavier loads. If the smaller muscles are exercised first, such as those of the arms, they will fatigue, making exercises for the larger muscles that require arm movement (bench press) more difficult.

You may wish to alternate muscle groups with each exercise. The bench press would not be followed by the standing press, because both of these exercises work the extensor muscles of the arms as well as the deltoids of the shoulders. You will be fresher if you separate these two exercises with one or two others for different muscle groups.

Vary the program to maintain interest. You can change the order of the exercises for different days and change the days that you exercise from Monday, Wednesday, Friday, to Tuesday, Thursday, Saturday. You can change the workload as well. One of the latest techniques for including variety is **periodization,** a basic concept which involves starting with high volumes of exercise at low intensity. The training period is divided into different cycles in which the volume is periodically reduced and the intensity is concomitantly increased. This system has been effective in developing strength. It can be accomplished by alternating light, moderate, and heavy workout days during the week. Another option is to perform light sets of 12 to 15 RM for two or three weeks, moderate sets of 8 to 10 RM for the next two or three weeks, and heavy sets of 3 to 5 RM for the last two or three weeks of the period.

Unlike isometrics, isotonic exercises develop strength throughout the full range of muscular movement. Progress is easily and objectively measured because a known quantity of weight is added as strength increases. Motivation is more easily maintained when results are readily available. One further advantage of isotonic training systems is that they are adaptable to free weights or exercise machines.

One of the disadvantages of isotonic exercise is that is produces delayed muscle soreness as a result of the eccentric phase of the contraction. It takes the body approximately 4 to 6 weeks to adapt to weight-training exercises. At this point, delayed muscle soreness is minimized or no longer occurs unless the program is expanded by substantially increasing intensity, frequency, or duration. A second disadvantage of isotonic exercise systems is that the maximum amount of weight that can be lifted is dependent upon the weakest point of contraction during the range of motion. However, variable resistance equipment has been developed that minimizes this problem. The Universal Variable Resistance exercise machines increase resistance by shortening the lever arm at the point where the exerciser is at a mechanical lifting advantage. In effect, greater force is required to complete the lift because the resistance increases.

Isokinetic Training

Isokinetic (equal speed) training, which involves a unique system of dynamic exercises, was introduced in 1968 by James Perrine, a bioengineer who developed an exercise device that allowed for maximum resistance at a constant speed throughout the full range of movement. As a result, this revolutionary device theoretically improves upon traditional dynamic exercises where maximum resistance can be experienced only at the weakest point in the muscular contraction.

Isokinetic devices accommodate to the applied force by adjusting the resistance to equal the force. The greater the application of force by the participant, the greater the resistance by the device. Highly motivated participants who apply maximum force throughout the full range of motion will be met with maximum resistance throughout. Isokinetic exercise's potential for strength development has generated much interest from athletes and the general public. Research in the next few years should determine the effectiveness of isokinetic training.

The major advantage of isokinetic training is that the resistance is maximum throughout the range of motion. Theoretically then, maximal strength can be obtained throughout the range of motion. The newer isokinetic devices allow one to select the speed of exercise movement. This has important implications for those who wish to develop strength for transfer to a specific sport or physical activity, such as football or basketball.

The disadvantage of isokinetic training is that it requires specialized equipment designed to produce isokinetic loading, such as the Mini-Gym Corporation's Leaper and Charger. This equipment is very expensive and may be found in weight rooms in some colleges and universities, health clubs, and health spas.

In summary, all three exercise training systems—isometrics, isotonics, and isokinetics—are effective in building and maintaining strength. However, the static nature of isometric exercises limits their capacity to enhance muscular endurance. The three exercise systems are compared on ten factors in Table 5.1

CIRCUIT TRAINING

Circuit Training is a relatively new concept developed in England approximately 35 years ago. This versatile training method promotes the development of muscular strength and endurance as well as cardiorespiratory endurance. Training goals must be established to construct an appropriate circuit.

Typical circuits consists of a minimum of 6 to a maximum of 12 exercises. Each exercise represents a different station in the circuit. The object of this type of training is to complete each circuit rapidly. Each completion is followed by a short rest period of approximately two minutes. The entire workout includes three complete routes through the circuit.

Different components of fitness can be developed simultaneously with circuit training. The number of stations devoted to each component should be determined at the outset. The stations should be arranged so that the same muscle group is not exercised at two consecutive stations. When possible, exercises for each of the components of fitness should be alternated; that is, a cardiorespiratory exercise should

Eight to 12 weeks of circuit weight training increases VO$_2$ max 5 percent in men and 8 percent in women.
—L. R. Gettman

TABLE 5.1 **Summary of Isometric, Isotonic, and Isokinetic Training Methods***

FACTORS	ISOMETRIC	ISOTONIC	ISOKINETIC
1. Rate of strength gain	3	2	1
2. Strength gain throughout the range of motion	3	2	1
3. Time per training session	1	3	2
4. Expense	1	2	2–3
5. Ease of performance	1	3	2
6. Ease of progress assessment	3	1	3
7. Probability of soreness	Little	Great	Little
8. Probability of musculoskeletal injury	Slight	Moderate	Slight
9. Cardiac risk	Moderate	Slight	Some
10. Skill improvement	None	Slight	Some

*A rating of 1 is superior, 2 is intermediate, 3 is inferior.

Source: Adapted from D. R. Lamb, *Physiology of Exercise*, New York: Macmillan, 1978.

not be followed by another cardiorespiratory exercise. For group participation, each station should be numbered and labeled with a concise set of instructions. A sample circuit combining the development of strength, muscular endurance, and cardiorespiratory endurance is presented in Table 5.2. For the weightlifting exercises, each weight selected should be heavy enough so that no more than 12 repetitions can be completed. Improvement is reflected by the amount of time needed to complete each circuit or by the amount of work accomplished at each station or by both concurrently. Overload (discussed in the following section) is initiated only when appropriate.

Circuit training has several advantages over conventional training systems. First, it is not boring, because it incorporates a variety of activities. Second, different fitness components can be developed together. Third, circuits do not require large amounts of space, nor are they confined to the indoors. Fourth, this system can accommodate groups of people, since any station can be an entry point into the circuit. Fifth, the entire workout can be completed in less than 40 minutes.

Circuit training has few disadvantages for people whose major interest is the use of exercise for health enhancement. It can be employed as an adjunct to an aerobic program, or it can be the primary vehicle for developing aerobic fitness. This is easily accomplished by loading the circuit with aerobic activities.

As with all forms of exercise, beginners should approach circuit training cautiously and slowly. It is best to utilize the circuit system after a degree of physical fitness has been developed through less demanding training systems. Enter circuit training with the following guidelines: (1) take at least one minute of rest between stations, (2) select weights that allow you to perform the suggested number of repetitions without straining, and (3) do the aerobic exercises slowly or reduce the suggested time for performing each. Training will result in progress, and you will be able to reduce the rest period between stations to approximately 15 seconds, increase the weight and/or number of repetitions for each exercise, and increase the length and/or speed of the aerobic activities.

Another method for going through the circuit involves performing as many repetitions as you can for 15 seconds at each station until the circuit is complete. As you become trained, you can increase the time spent at each station to a maximum of 30 seconds. You can also decrease rest time between stations.

PRINCIPLES FOR TRAINING THE MUSCULAR SYSTEM

Overload, Progression, and Maintenance

Muscles grow in strength and size in response to the amount of overload placed upon them. **Overload** can be accomplished by increasing the resistance or by increasing the number of repetitions completed for each exercise. For strength development, maximum results are attained with few repetitions (4 to 6) and heavy weights. Muscular endurance occurs with 20 to 30 repetitions and light to

TABLE 5.2	Circuit Training		
STATION	EXERCISE	REPETITIONS OR TIME	FITNESS COMPONENT DEVELOPED
1	Bench press	12	Strength & endurance
2	Rope skipping	2 min	Cardiorespiratory endurance
3	Two-arm curl	12	Strength & endurance
4	Half-squat	15	Strength & endurance
5	Stationary bike	2 min	Cardiorespiratory endurance
6	Sit-ups	20	Strength & endurance
7	Standing press	12	Strength & endurance
8	Running in place	2 min	Cardiorespiratory endurance
9	Upright rowing	12	Strength & endurance
10	Toe raises	15	Strength & endurance

moderate weights. Programs that attempt to develop both strength and endurance represent a compromise between the two, with resistance selected to elicit 10 to 12 repetitions per exercise. The resistance is increased when the num-

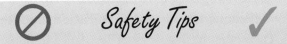

PERFORMING RESISTANCE EXERCISES

The risk of injury is increased when people progress from sedentary habits to vigorous physical activity. Karpovich studied the rate of injury associated with weight training and found it to be one of the safest forms of physical activity. This study was completed more than 30 years ago, but a European study in 1970 reaffirmed these results. Familiarization and practice of simple safety procedures will sharply minimize the incidence of injury. The following suggestions will help to decrease the risk associated with resistance training:

1. Warm up prior to working out. The warmup should include stretching and exercises of moderate intensity that cause sweating and an increase in muscle temperature (refer to Figures 4.4 to 4.27 in Chapter 4). The evidence regarding the effectiveness of warming up for improved performance and injury prevention is inconclusive, but it should also be emphasized that the evidence against it is not compelling.

2. Learn correct lifting techniques, especially if you use free weights. The movement of free weights is unrestricted; that is, the weights can be moved in any direction. As a result, their use requires greater control by the user, who must exert force not only from the primary muscles but also from supporting musculature in order to move the weights in the desired direction. Any deviation from the desired path reduces the amount of weight that can be lifted and increases the chance of injury. When using free weights, make sure that you

   • Keep the weight close to your body during the lift.

   • Lift all weights resting on the floor with your legs rather than with the lower back. This is accomplished by placing your feet close to the bar, bending your knees and lowering your hips into a half-squat position. Keep your back straight and your head up. (This technique applies to lifting a barbell, a child, a piece of furniture, or any other object.

   • Avoid excessive backward lean (hyperextension of the low back) when pressing a weight overhead.

3. Make sure that the collars securing the metal plates to dumbbells and barbells are tightly bound to the bar and that pins are fully inserted if you use weight machines.

4. Use rubber-soled shoes for secure footing.

5. Gloves are effective in protecting against blisters and calluses and decrease the likelihood of slippage from perspiration. Chalk dust can be used if you do not wish to wear gloves.

6. Work out with a partner for safety and mutual motivation. Partners are especially handy as spotters for such lifts as bench presses and half-squats.

Exercises performed on weight machines are generally safer than exercises using free weights. Weight machines are constructed so that a stack of plates is restricted to motion in one plane. Spotters or exercise partners are not necessary, because the plates are supported by the stack. Weight machines offer convenience because they eliminate the need to stack and unstack barbells and dumbbells for the different exercises. All that is required is the insertion of a pin to obtain the appropriate resistance. Weight machines are convenient, simple, and safe to use and require very little energy to set up for the next exercise.

Regardless of the exercise system or the equipment used, you should NEVER hold your breath while lifting a weight. Breath holding precipitates a potentially dangerous chain of physiological events. If an exerciser inhales deeply and then lifts a heavy weight without first releasing the inspired air, the glottis (a narrow opening between the vocal cords) closes, trapping the air in the chest cavity. The chest is fully expanded, which maximally activates the expiratory muscles, and the individual forcefully attempts to exhale against the closed glottis. The forceful expiration of air against the closed glottis is the **Valsalva maneuver,** which results in greatly increased pressure in both the chest and the abdominal cavities. The pressure in the chest is great enough to compress or collapse the large vein, bringing blood back to the heart. This significantly reduces blood flow to the heart, which in turn reduces the amount of blood that it ejects. Initially, an abrupt rise in blood pressure occurs, but if the exertion is sustained, blood pressure declines sharply. Diminished blood flow to all bodily tissues, including the brain, leads to dizziness and the phenomenon of "seeing spots before one's eyes."

The Valsalva maneuver usually accompanies a straining type of muscular exertion. When the exertion ends, normal cardiovascular dynamics are quickly restored. This maneuver is particularly dangerous for people with high blood pressure and for those with heart or blood vessel disease. Straining types of exercises that induce breath holding should be avoided. One way to inhibit the Valsalva maneuver is to exhale on the concentric phase of a contraction and inhale on the eccentric phase. Keep the weight moving and breathe rhythmically, never holding your breath.

ber of repetitions increases to 15 to 16. This represents a safe and effective means of applying overload according to a set schedule of progression. This schedule may be continued until you reach a level of muscular strength and endurance satisfactory for your needs. At this point, you merely exercise to preserve the gains that you have achieved. Two workouts per week are sufficient for maintenance.

● Frequency, Intensity, Duration, and Rest

The optimum frequency of resistance training depends on the system selected. Isometric exercises may be practiced daily because muscle soreness does not occur, but because of motivational concerns and the need for muscles to recover, it would be best to take one or two days off each week. Since dynamic systems of training

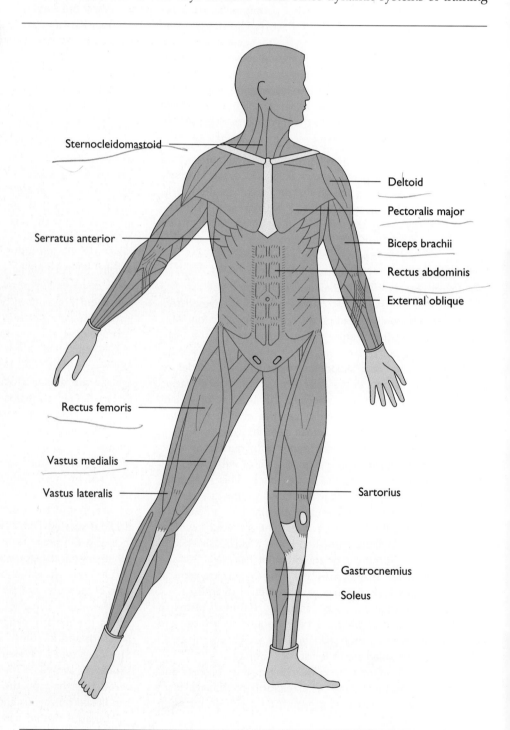

FIGURE 5.7

Selected Muscles of the Body—Front View (Shaded areas indicate bone.)

initially lead to considerable muscle soreness, at least one day of rest is needed between workouts. Adequate rest is as important as consistent exercise because muscles need time to recuperate to meet the challenge of the next workout.

Muscle soreness that persists into the next scheduled workout reflects inadequate rest or an intensity of exercise greater than can be tolerated at this point in the training program. The following provides more information on muscle soreness.

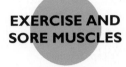

EXERCISE AND SORE MUSCLES

Muscles may become sore during exercise (acute soreness) or one to two days later (delayed soreness). Acute soreness is probably the result of reduced blood flow to exercising muscles. When muscles contract vigorously—as in weight training—blood vessels constrict, inhibiting the delivery of oxygen and nutrients as well as the removal of waste products.

Delayed muscle soreness occurs 24 to 48 hours after a workout. There are several possible explanations for this phenomenon. The most widely accepted is the tissue damage theory, proponents of which state that exercise damages muscle fibers and connective tissue, which in turn respond by swelling and impinging upon nerves, resulting in soreness.

Lactic acid accumulation in the muscles was thought to be involved in delayed soreness, but this is unlikely because lactic acid is removed from muscles long before soreness occurs. Secondly, activities that produce lactic acid do not necessarily result in muscle soreness, while other activities produce no lactic acid but result in considerable muscle soreness. Running on a level surface involves concentric contractions of the leg muscles, producing significant amounts of lactic acid but no delayed muscle soreness. On the other hand, running downhill—an activity consisting of eccentric contractions of the leg muscles—produces no lactic acid but considerable delayed muscle soreness.[34]

Delayed muscle soreness occurs to untrained beginners, but it also occurs to trained participants who overload excessively or who change from one activity to another. It can be prevented or minimized by exercising within your capacity and by overloading in small increments. People trained in one activity should approach new activities cautiously because their previous training may not carry over to the new activity.

The antidote to delayed muscle soreness involves stretching exercises, light workouts, or complete rest. The best treatment is prevention.

Optimal gains in strength occur with high-intensity training. This translates to near-maximum resistance for all exercises regardless of the training system. The duration of the workout will depend upon the program objectives, the number of exercises, and the training system. A well-conceived isometric or isokinetic program might take 30 to 45 minutes, compared to an hour for isotonic programs. If maximal strength development is the goal, the workout may take two hours or longer.

EXERCISES FOR DEVELOPING STRENGTH AND ENDURANCE

Programs for developing muscular strength and endurance for health purposes differ significantly from those utilized by athletes preparing for competition. Athletes attempt to develop strength and endurance in a manner specific to the sport in which they participate. They train their muscles to apply force in a manner similar to the demands of their sport. These programs are highly structured and leave little room for variety and fun. Those who engage in resistance exercises for the health benefits have a wide variety of exercises and several systems from which to choose. Isotonic and isokinetic exercises using free weights or weight machines are recommended. The major muscle groups of the body should be exercised in each session. Figures 5.7 and 5.8 show some of the major muscles of the body.

FIGURE 5.8

Selected Muscles of the Body— Back View (Shaded areas indicate bone.)

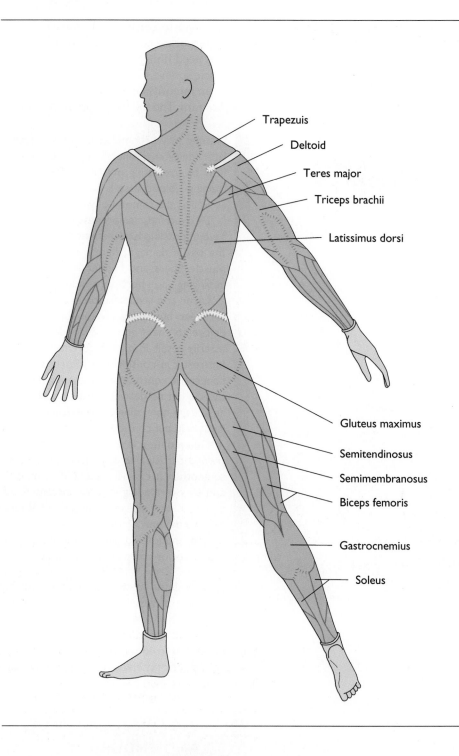

Trapezuis

Deltoid

Teres major

Triceps brachii

Latissimus dorsi

Gluteus maximus

Semitendinosus

Semimembranosus

Biceps femoris

Gastrocnemius

Soleus

Selected exercises for the major muscle groups are presented in Figures 5.9 to 5.18, illustrated with both free weights and machine weights. The muscles developed by each exercise are highlighted in the free-weight figures through the use of shading. (Refer to Figures 5.7 and 5.8 for the name and location of the muscles affected by each exercise.) The exercises in Figures 5.9 to 5.18 make up a good basic program for developing strength and endurance. Three sets can be completed in 30 to 45 minutes and would be an excellent supplement to your aerobic program. Either the free-weight or machine-weight method will develop the muscular system, and both methods have advantages and disadvantages.

FIGURE 5.9

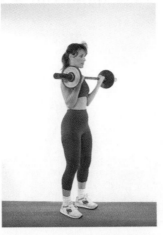

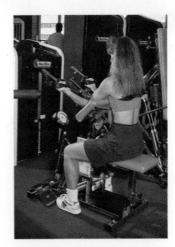

Two-Arm Curl—Free Weights

Starting position: the bar is resting against the thighs with the palms facing out. Curl the weight slowly to the shoulders and lower it slowly to the starting position. Do not lean back from the waist, do not swing the bar, and extend your arms fully each time the weight is lowered. Develops the biceps muscles.

Two-Arm Curl Performed on Nautilus Equipment

FIGURE 5.10

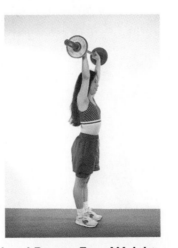

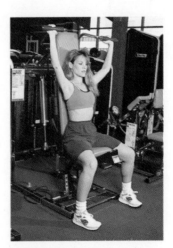

Overhead Press—Free Weights

The weight is pushed upward from the shoulders until the arms are fully extended overhead. Then it is lowered back to the starting position. Move the weight slowly and rhythmically. Avoid excessive backward lean and do not jerk the weight by bending and extending the knees. Develops the triceps, deltoids, and trapezius.

Overhead Press Performed on Nautilus Equipment

FIGURE 5.11

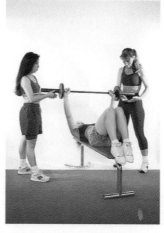

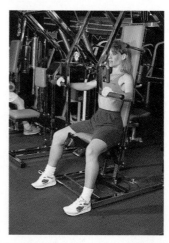

Bench Press—Free Weights

Lie on your back, knees bent, feet on the bench to prevent arching of the low back. Start with the weight on your chest, slowly push it to arm's length, and slowly lower to the starting position. There should be two spotters who can remove the weight at the completion of the exercise. Develops the pectoralis majors, deltoids, and triceps.

Bench Press Performed on Nautilus Equipment

FIGURE 5.12

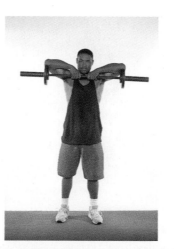

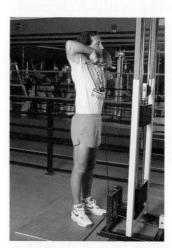

Two-Arm High Pulls—Free Weights

Starting position: the bar is held against the thighs, arms extended, palms facing inward, hands close together. Slowly pull the weight to the chin, ending with elbows high, and slowly lower to the starting position. Develops the trapezius, deltoids, and biceps.

Two-Arm High Pulls on Universal Equipment

FIGURE 5.13

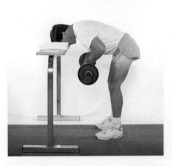

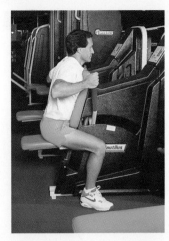

Bent-Over Rowing—Free Weights

Bend from the waist and rest your forehead on a table. This position minimizes the likelihood of back injury. Start with the weight held at arm's length, bend your knees slightly, slowly pull the weight to your chest, and lower it to the starting position. Develops the latissimus dorsi, deltoids, and biceps.

Seated Row Performed on Nautilus Equipment

FIGURE 5.14

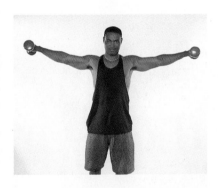

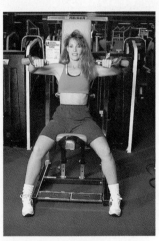

Lateral Raises—Free Weights

Start with the weights held at your sides, lift them laterally with straight arms to shoulder height, and lower them to the starting position. Both movements should be executed slowly. Develops the deltoids and triceps.

Lateral Raises Performed on Nautilus Equipment

FIGURE 5.15

Sit-ups and Crunches

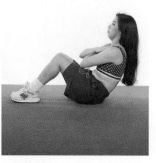

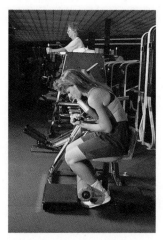

Bent-leg Sit-ups

Lie on the floor with your knees bent as shown. Fold your arms across your chest and sit up until your elbows touch your thighs and return to the starting position. Develops the abdominals.

Abdominal Crunches Performed on Nautilus Equipment

FIGURE 5.16

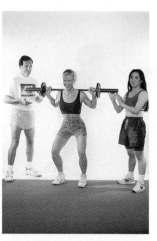

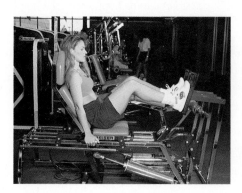

Half-Squat—Free Weights

Start in the standing position with the weight held across your shoulders behind the neck. Keeping your back straight and your head up, slowly bend your knees until you reach a half-squat position, and return to the starting position. Do not allow your hips to get lower than your knees. Be sure to have 2 spotters for assistance. Develops the quadriceps.

Leg Press Performed on Nautilus Equipment

FIGURE 5.17

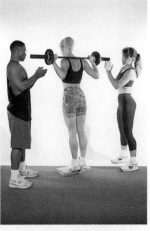

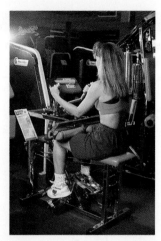

Heel Raises—Free Weights

With the weight across your shoulders, slowly raise and lower your heels. Be sure to have 2 spotters for assistance. Develops gastrocnemius.

Calf Press Performed on Nautilus Equipment

FIGURE 5.18

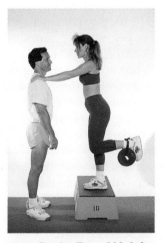

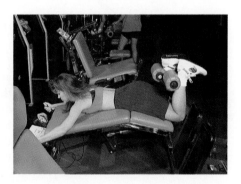

Hamstring Curl—Free Weights

Start with your exercise leg extended with a weight strapped to your ankle. Slowly bend your knee until your lower leg forms a 90 degree angle to your thigh and return to the starting position. Put your hands on a wall or on another person's shoulders for balance. Develops the hamstring group.

Hamstring Curl Performed on Nautilus Equipment

▶ ASSESSING MUSCULAR STRENGTH AND ENDURANCE

Muscular strength is measured by the amount of force a given muscle or muscle group is capable of exerting in a single maximum contraction. A number of tests measuring the strength of different muscle groups must be administered if one wishes to estimate total body strength. Several tests are needed because strength is not a general component. If it were, total strength could be accurately predicted by measuring any one muscle group, but in reality, the strength of different muscle groups is often disproportionate. This can be the result of body build or the physical demands of a person's occupation, or it might be due to fitness training that concentrates on particular parts of the body.

A good battery of strength tests should measure the strength of the arms, chest, shoulders, back, abdomen, and legs. These measurements can be made

FIGURE 5.19

Measurement of Back Strength with a Dynamometer

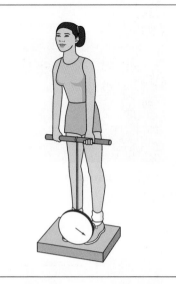

isometrically, isotonically, or isokinetically. But a word of warning: measuring the strength of novices is potentially hazardous because novices are not physically prepared to exert maximum force. The measurement of back strength is particularly perilous because of the body positions that must be assumed during these measurements. To help ensure safety, strength measurement should not occur until participants have been actively involved in resistance training for several months. For those interested in the health-related benefits of resistance training, the measurement of strength is unnecessary. Those who train isotonically and isokinetically will see the improvement that occurs with time and effort. To them, the measurement of strength might be viewed as an unnecessary hazard.

Muscular endurance involves repeated contractions or positions held for a certain length of time. It is a function of how long or how many times a muscle can contract. Once again, several tests must be administered to determine the endurance of various muscle groups.

● Isometric Assessment

The measurement of isometric strength requires devices that assess the tension exerted by different muscle groups in static positions. Back and leg dynamometers (Figures 5.19 and 5.20) measure leg and back strength. Cable tensiometers (Figures 5.21), used in conjunction with a specially constructed table, can be used to measure many muscle groups.

Figures 5.22 through 5.24 illustrate the measurements of the hamstrings, biceps, and quadriceps at specified angles using the cable tensiometer. The validity of these measurements is dependent upon the subject's ability to produce maximum exertions. All tests of strength, regardless of the method employed, should isolate the muscle or muscle group being tested. Precautions must be taken to minimize the possible assistance that might come from other muscle groups, since this would overestimate the strength of the test group.

Isometric muscular endurance can be evaluated with the same devices by measuring the amount of time that a contraction can be maintained at a specific percentage of maximum strength.

● Isotonic Assessment

Isotonic or dynamic strength can be assessed by measuring the maximum amount of weight (1 RM) that can be lifted by different muscle groups. These measurements can be made with free weights or weight machines. Figure 5.9 illustrates the biceps curl, which is a measurement of arm flexor strength; Figure 5.10 illustrates the standing press, which measures the strength of the extensors of the arms, deltoids, and trapezius; Figure 5.11 illustrates the bench press, which measures the strength of the pectorals, deltoids, and extensors of the arms; Figure 5.16 illustrates the half-squat, which measures the strength of the quadriceps and hip flexors; and Figure 5.18 illustrates the hamstring curl, which measures the strength of the hamstrings. The measurement of low-back strength is not included for reasons alluded to earlier in this chapter.

If you are interested in assessing your strength in these categories and comparing your performance to the values obtained from other college age students, see Self-Assessments 5.1 and 5.2 in Appendix C. A word of caution: Do not attempt to lift maximum amounts of weight until you have been in training for at least two months. It is not necessary to test yourself to achieve the health benefits of strength training.

The muscular endurance of these muscle groups is measured with the same exercises. The number of repetitions that can be performed at a selected percentage of 1 RM (70 percent is used in many cases) will provide this measurement.

Muscular endurance can also be measured with a variety of calisthenics. For males, the number of chin-ups (Figure 5.25), push-ups (Figure 5.26), parallel-bar

FIGURE 5.20

Measurement of Leg Strength with a Dynamometer

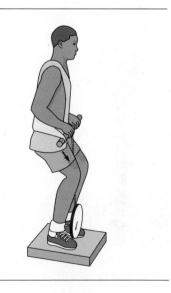

FIGURE 5.21

Cable Tensiometer

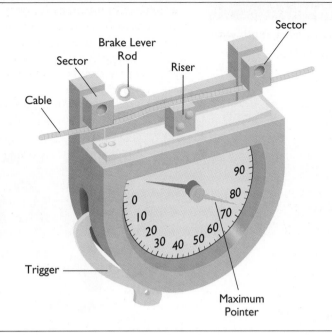

dips (Figure 5.27), and bent-leg sit-ups in 60 seconds (Figure 5.28) is commonly used to measure muscular endurance. For females, muscular endurance is usually measured by the number of modified push-ups (Figure 5.29), bent-leg sit-ups that can be done in 60 seconds (Figure 5.28), and the amount of time that the flexed-arm hang can be held (Figure 5.30).

Interested individuals can consult Table 5.3 in Appendix C for selected practical muscle endurance tests along with standards of performance for comparison.

Isokinetic Assessment

Isokinetic strength is assessed with accommodating resistance devices equipped with indicators that measure the amount of force being generated (Figure 5.3).

FIGURE 5.22

Measurement of Hamstring Strength with Cable Tensiometer

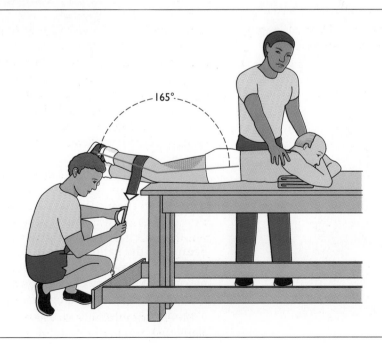

FIGURE 5.23

Measuring Biceps Strength with Cable Tensiometer

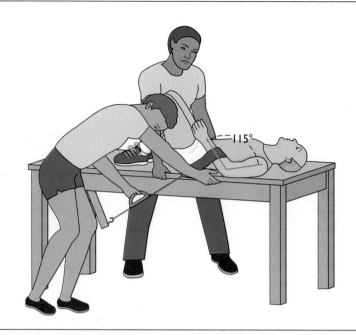

FIGURE 5.24

Measuring Quadriceps Strength with Cable Tensiometer

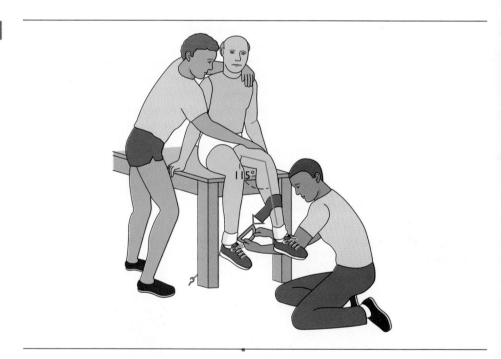

Because of the nature of these devices (they allow the contraction to be completed at any percent of maximum), several trials must be allowed to ensure that a maximum voluntary contraction has been attained. Once this has been achieved, muscular endurance can be measured by the number of repetitions performed at a specified percentage of maximum strength (70 percent of 1 RM is a common standard).

FIGURE 5.25

Chin-Ups Measures endurance of the arm flexors (primarily the biceps).

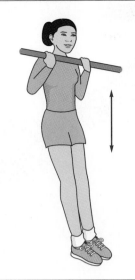

FIGURE 5.26

Push-Ups Measures endurance of the arm extensors (primarily the triceps).

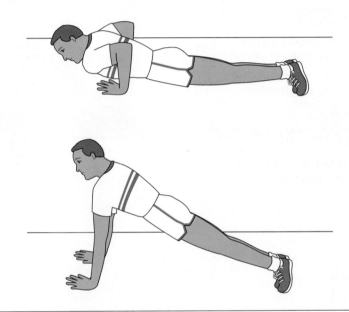

FIGURE 5.27

Parallel-Bar Dips An alternative way to measure endurance of the arm extensors.

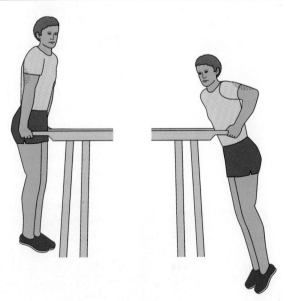

FIGURE 5.28

**Measurement of Abdominal
Endurance**

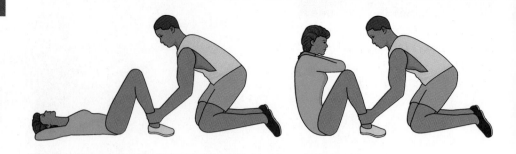

FIGURE 5.29

**Measuring Endurance of the
Arm Extensors**   This is one of
the modified versions of the push-
up, commonly used by females.

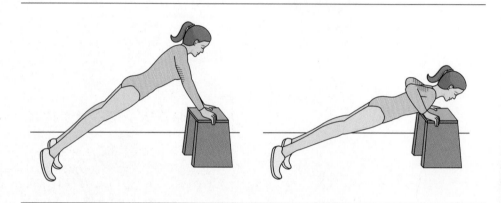

POINTS TO PONDER

1. Define isometric, isokinetic, and isotonic contraction.
2. Which of these is not dynamic and why?
3. What are concentric and eccentric contractions? Which of the two is involved in delayed muscle soreness?
4. Discuss fully the relationship between resistance training and health.
5. What is responsible for the difference in strength and muscle size between males and females?
6. Respond to this statement: Several years of heavy resistance exercise will convert slow-twitch muscle fibers to fast-twitch muscle fibers.
7. Weight training for prepubescent children is ineffective for the development of strength. Do you agree or disagree, and why?
8. Define hypertrophy and hyperplasia.
9. What seems to be most responsible for the delayed muscle soreness that accompanies resistance exercise?
10. What are the agonist and antagonist muscles for push-ups?

FIGURE 5.30

Flexed-Arm Hang Measures endurance of the arm flexors. This is a modified version of the chin-up, commonly used by females.

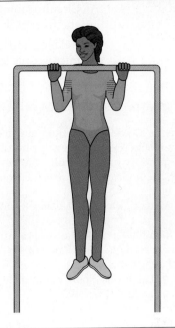

 CHAPTER HIGHLIGHTS

- Sixty-five percent of the body's muscles are located above the waist.
- In the United States, 28 percent of the men and 65 percent of the women over age 74 cannot lift objects that weigh more than ten pounds.
- The muscular system consists of three types of muscle: smooth, cardiac, and skeletal.
- Isotonic and isokinetic muscular contractions are dynamic; isometric muscle contractions are static.
- Dynamic movements feature concentric and eccentric muscle contractions.
- Progressive resistance exercise
    a. increases strength
    b. increases muscle mass
    c. increases metabolism
    d. enhances self-concept
    e. decreases the likelihood of low-back injury
    f. strengthens and thickens bones
    g. may increase HDL cholesterol
- The average male can generate 30% to 40% more force than the average female because men have about 40% more muscle mass than women.
- Women can gain substantial strength with weight training in the absence of a substantial gain in muscle tissue; men increase both.
- Consistent use of anabolic steroids produces aggressive, often psychotic behavior as well as other short and long-term risks to health and wellness.
- Slow-twitch muscle fibers are adapted for aerobic work, while fast-twitch muscle fibers are adapted for anaerobic work.
- Adolescents should not participate in weightlifting, but they can and should participate in weight training.

- Circuit training consists of a series of 6 to 12 exercises performed in sequence and as rapidly as one's fitness level allows.
- Delayed muscle soreness (24 to 48 hours after a workout) is probably due to microscopic tears in the muscles and connective tissue.

● REFERENCES

1. American College of Sports Medicine, "The Recommended Quantity and Quality of Exercise for Developing and Maintaining Cardiorespiratory and Muscular Fitness in Healthy Adults," *Medicine in Science and Sport* 22, no. 2 (April 1990): 265.

2. "Strength Training," *Mayo Clinic Health Letter* 8, no. 8 (August 1990): 2.

3. S. J. Fleck and W. J. Kraemer, "Resistance Training: Physiological Responses and Adaptations (Part 3 of 4)," *The Physician and Sportsmedicine* 16 (1988): 63.

4. M. Prives, "Influences of Labor and Sport upon Skeleton Structure in Man," *Anatomical Record* 136 (1960): 261.

5. J. A. Ross, "Hypertrophy of the Little Finger," *British Medical Journal* 2 (1950): 987.

6. B. Nilsson and N. Westline, "Bone Density in Athletes," *Clinical Orthopedics* 77 (1971): 179.

7. "Osteoporosis—A Silent Epidemic," *Harvard Medical School Health Letter* (November 1981): 4.

8. "Osteoporosis—The Silent Thief," *Worldview* 3, no. 2 (Summer 1991): 1.

9. R. L. Prince et al., "Prevention of Postmenopausal Osteoporosis—A Comparative Study of Exercise, Calcium Supplementation, and Hormone-Replacement Therapy," *New England Journal of Medicine,* October 24, 1991, p. 1189.

10. "Aging and Exercise," *Harvard Medical School Health Letter* (April 1983): 4.

11. W. R. Frontera et al., "Strength Training and Determinants of VO_2 Max in Older Men," *Journal of Applied Physiology* 68, no. 1 (1990): 329.

12. M. A. Fiatarone et al., "High Intensity Strength Training in Nonagenarians," *Journal of the American Medical Association,* June 13, 1990, p. 3029.

13. T. E. Allen et al., "Hemodynamic Consequences of Circuit Weight Training," *Research Quarterly AAHPER* 47 (1976): 299.

14. M. H. Stone et al., "Cardiovascular Responses to Short-Term Olympic Style Weight Training in Young Men," *Canadian Journal of Applied Sport Science* 8 (1983): 134; T. D. Fahey et al., "Body Composition and VO_2 Max of Exceptional Weight Trained Athletes," *Journal of Applied Physiology* 39 (1975): 559.

15. L. Goldberg et al., "Changes in Lipid and Lipoprotein Levels After Weight Training," *Journal of the American Medical Association* 252 (1984): 504.

16. L. Goldberg et al., "Changes in Lipid," 1984; M H. Stone and H. O'Bryant, *Weight Training: A Scientific Approach,* Minneapolis: Burgess, 1986; B. F. Hurley et al., "Resistive Training Can Reduce Coronary Risk Factors Without Altering VO_2 Max or Percent Body Fat," *Medicine and Science in Exercise and Sports* 20 (1988): 150.

17. B. F. Hurley et al., "High Density Lipoprotein Cholesterol in Body-builders Vs. Power Lifters, Negative Effects of Androgen Use," *Journal of the American Medical Association* 4 (1984): 507.

18. W. D. McArdle, F. I. Katch, and V. L. Katch, *Exercise Physiology, Energy, Nutrition, and Human Performance,* Philadelphia: Lea and Febiger, 1991.

19. J. H. Wilmore, "Alterations in Strength, Body Composition, and Anthropometric Measurements Consequent to a 10-Week Weight Training Program," *Medicine and Science in Sports and Exercise* 6 (1974): 33.

20. K. J. Cureton et al., "Muscle Hypertrophy in Men and Women," *Medicine and Science in Sports and Exercise* 20 (1988): 338.

21. American College of Sports Medicine, "Position Statement on the Use and Abuse of Anabolic-Androgenic Steroids in Sports," in R. H. Strauss (Ed), *Sports Medicine,* Philadelphia: W. B. Saunders, 1984.

22. A. Lubell, "Does Steroid Abuse—Cause—or Excuse—Violence?" *The Physician and Sportsmedicine* 17, no. 2 (February 1989): 176.

23. G. Elofson and S. Elofson, "Steroids Claimed Our Son's Life," *The Physician and Sportsmedicine* 18, no. 8 (August 1990): 15.

24. J. H. Wilmore and D. L. Costill, *Training for Sport and Activity,* Dubuque, Iowa: William C. Brown, 1988.

25. W. J. Kraemer et al., "A Review: Factors in Exercise Prescription of Resistance Training," *NSCA Journal* 10 (1988): 36.

26. H. G. Knuttgen and W. J. Kraemer, "Terminology and Measurement in Exercise Performance," *Journal of Applied Sport Science Research* 1 (1987): 1.

27. S. J. Fleck and R. C. Schutt, "Types of Strength Training," *Clinics in Sports Medicine* 4 (1985): 159.

28. American College of Sports Medicine, "The Recommended Quantity," April 1990.

29. S. J. Fleck and W. J. Kraemer, *Designing Resistance Training Programs,* Champaign, Ill.: Human Kinetics, 1987.

30. W. L. Westcott, *Strength Fitness—Physiological Principles and Training Techniques,* Boston: Allyn and Bacon, 1983, p. 49.

31. Ibid.

32. W. J. Kraemer, and S. J. Fleck, "Resistance Training: Exercise Prescription (Part 4 of 4)," *The Physician and Sportsmedicine* 16 (1988): 69.

33. W. J. Kraemer et al., "Physiologic Responses to Heavy-Resistance Exercise with Very Short Rest Periods," *International Journal of Sports Medicine* 8 (1987): 247.

34. J. A. Schwane et al., "Effects of Training on Delayed Muscle Soreness and Serum Creatine Kinase Activity After Running," *Medicine and Science in Sports and Exercise* 19 (1987): 584.

Developing the Cardiorespiratory Component

CHAPTER OUTLINE

INTRODUCTION

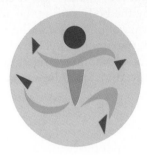

Exercise produces immediate but temporary physiological and metabolic changes. The acute effects of exercise are those that occur during and after every bout of exercise, regardless of whether or not the individual is trained. Physiology and metabolism return to normal when the bout of exercise is over. Recovery can take only a few minutes or as long as 24 hours, depending upon the length and intensity of the workout.

When exercise becomes a habit and is pursued for months or years, the physiological and metabolic changes that occur are longer lasting. These adaptations, which are the result of training, are the chronic effects of exercise. This chapter covers in an elementary way the basic changes the body makes as it adjusts to exercise. It is important to identify these changes and to understand how and why one's physical fitness improves with exercise.

Three Self-Assessment activities appear in Appendix C that apply directly to the contents of this chapter:

6.1 The Rockport Fitness Walking Test

6.2 Running Tests

6.3 Bench Step Test

Miniglossary

Aerobic Capacity The maximal ability to take in, deliver, and use oxygen; also referred to as cardiorespiratory endurance, or VO_2 max.

Alveoli Tiny air sacs in the lungs that are richly perfused with blood. Gaseous exchange between the lungs and blood occurs at these sites.

Anaerobic Threshold The point during exercise where blood lactate suddenly begins to increase.

Arterial-venous Oxygen Difference (a-vO_2 diff) The difference between the oxygen (O_2) content of arterial and mixed venous blood.

Body Composition The amount of lean versus fat tissue in the body.

Cardiac Output The amount of blood pumped by the heart in one minute.

Double Product or Rate Pressure Product (RPP) Heart rate multiplied by systolic blood pressure. It is an estimate of the oxygen required by the heart during aerobic exercise.

Metabolism The sum of the chemical reactions and processes that supply the energy used by the body.

Mitochondria Organelles within the cells that utilize oxygen to produce the ATP (refer to Chapter 3) needed by the muscles.

Oxygen Debt The amount of oxygen needed in recovery from exercise above that normally required during rest.

Oxygen Deficit The period of time when exercise begins during which the body does not supply all of the oxygen needed to support exercise.

Residual Volume The air remaining in the lungs following a maximum exhalation.

Stroke Volume The amount of blood pumped by the heart with each beat.

Tidal Volume The amount of air inhaled and exhaled with each breath.

Ventilation The amount of air inhaled and exhaled per minute.

Vital Capacity The amount of air that can be expired after a maximum inhalation.

The short-term effects of exercise—also referred to as the acute adaptations—involve those physiological changes that occur during a single bout of exercise. The adjustments to a single bout of exercise are temporary and include changes in heart rate, stroke volume, cardiac output, blood flow, blood pressure, blood volume, respiratory responses, and metabolic responses.

● Heart Rate

The heart's response to dynamic exercise is immediate. The rate of beating rises and continues to do so until a steady state is achieved. Steady state occurs when the oxygen demand of the activity can be met by the body during the activity. If the exercise intensity is such that a steady state cannot be achieved, the heart rate (HR) will continue to increase until it reaches its maximum level, at which point the effort can be sustained for only a few seconds. Elevating the heart rate represents the major vehicle for increasing blood flow, and therefore oxygen, to the muscles during moderate to intense exercise.

● Stroke Volume

Stroke Volume (SV) refers to the amount of blood that the heart can eject in one beat. The size of the stroke volume is dependent upon the amount of blood returning to the heart, the interior dimensions of the left ventricle, and the strength of ventricular contraction. Stroke volume rises with increases in workload up to 40 percent to 60 percent of capacity and then levels off.[1] From this point on, further increases in blood flow occur as the result of increases in heart rate (see Figure 6.1).

The higher stroke volumes of trained people represent one of the major differences between trained and untrained people and accounts for the ability of trained people to sustain endurance activities at a high level. Table 6.1 illustrates typical differences in the stroke volumes at rest and during maximum exertion of untrained, trained, and highly trained people. These differences are significant among the groups in their ability to supply blood and oxygen to the exercising muscles and associated organs.

● Cardiac Output

Cardiac Output (Q) represents the amount of blood pumped by the heart in one minute. It is the product of heart rate and stroke volume ($Q = HR \times SV$). The cardiac output increases as the intesity of exercise increases. Initially, it increases because both heart rate and stroke volume increase. Stroke volume levels off

---

FIGURE 6.1

Relationship Between Heart Rate and Stroke Volume During Maximum Exercise

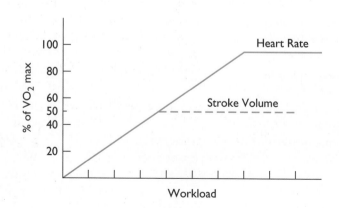

| TABLE 6.1 | Typical Stroke Volume Values for Untrained, Trained, and Highly Trained People |

Typical Stroke Volume Values for Untrained, Trained, and Highly Trained People

	UNTRAINED	TRAINED	HIGHLY TRAINED
At Rest	≤ 70 ml (2.4 oz)	≤ 90 ml (3 oz)	≥ 130 ml (4.4 oz)
During Maximum Exertion	≤ 125 ml	≤ 150 ml (5.1 oz)	≥ 220 ml (7.4 oz)

≤ equal to or less than
≥ equal to or greater than

when exercise reaches approximately 50 percent of capacity. Further increases in cardiac ouput are a result of elevations in heart rate (see Figure 6.1).

The average value for cardiac output at rest, regardless of one's physical fitness level, is 4 to 6 liters (L) of blood (approximately 4.2 to 6.3 quarts) pumped per minute. The differences in cardiac output between the trained and untrained appear during maximum exercise, as illustrated in Table 6.2.

Blood Flow

The body has the remarkable capacity to shunt blood to tissues that have the greatest need. For example, blood flow to the working muscles increases during physical activity. This is accomplished because blood flow to other tissues and organs such as the liver, kidneys, and digestive system is reduced. In the competition for available blood, the muscles take precedence during physical activity. Blood flow to the digestive system is increased after a meal because this represents the greatest area of need. However, if physical activity occurs immediately after eating, blood will be shunted away from the digestive system to the muscles. Digestion will slow down or stop depending upon the severity of the exercise. This is one of the major reasons why a workout should not begin until at least one hour after a meal.

More blood than usual is shunted to the skin during hot weather to help cool the body. The skin competes with the exercising muscles for the available blood, which results in the muscles' receiving slightly less than normal. Less blood means less oxygen and nutrients for exercise, and the workout becomes more difficult. This is why exercise in hot weather should be less vigorous and last for a shorter period of time.

Blood Pressure

Blood pressure is the force exerted by the heart as it pumps blood into the arteries. It is measured in millimeters of mercury (mmHg) with an instrument called a sphygmomanometer. Blood pressure is expressed in two values: systolic and diastolic. The systolic pressure is the pressure of the flow of blood when the heart beats. The diastolic pressure is between heart beats. A typical pressure for a young adult might by 120/70 (read as 120 over 70).

The systolic pressure rises during exercise—a normal and expected response that is due to an increase in cardiac output. Cardiac output increases to supply the blood and oxygen needed by the muscles and the organs (heart and lungs) that support

| TABLE 6.2 | Typical Cardiac Output Values for Untrained, Trained, and Highly Trained People |

Typical Cardiac Output Values for Untrained, Trained, and Highly Trained People

	UNTRAINED	TRAINED	HIGHLY TRAINED
At Rest	4 to 6 L	4 to 6 L	4 to 6 L
During Maximum Exercise	14 to 16 L	20 to 25 L	34 to 40 L

exercise. The blood vessels in these tissues dilate to accept the extra blood, but their ability to dilate is limited. Since the increase in cardiac output is greater than the stretching ability of the blood vessels, the systolic blood pressure rises. The increase in systolic blood pressure during exercise should not exceed 250 mmHg.[2] Such an increase is abnormal and symptomatic of a cardiovascular problem.

The diastolic blood pressure changes very little during dynamic or aerobic exercise. The change is usually less than 20 mmHg plus or minus. A rise in the diastolic blood pressure to 120 mmHg is excessive and considered an abnormal response to exercise.[3]

● Blood Volume

Fluid is removed from all areas of the body to produce the perspiration needed to cool the exerciser. Some of this fluid comes from the blood plasma, which reduces blood volume. As a result, the ratio of red blood cells to plasma volume increases. This increases the viscosity of the blood and inhibits the delivery of oxygen. Viscosity represents the thickness of the blood (more solids than liquid) which increases the blood's resistance to flow. The ratio of red blood cells to plasma volume returns to normal as fluids are consumed following the workout.

● Respiratory Responses

The average person breathes 12 to 16 times per minute at rest and 40 to 50 times per minute during maximum exertion. **Ventilation** (V)—the amount of air inhaled and exhaled per minute—is a product of the frequency of breathing (f) and the volume of air per breath, or **tidal volume** (TV). At rest, the lungs typically ventilate 5 to 6 liters of air each minute. For example, 14 breaths per minute at 0.4 liter per breath results in a ventilatory rate of 5.6 liters of air per minute.

$$V = f \times TV$$
$$= 14 \times 0.4 \text{ liter}$$
$$= 5.6 \text{ liters}$$

Ventilation can escalate to 100 liters or more during maximal exertion. Large, well-conditioned athletes can move as much as 200 liters per minute.

The movement of large volumes of air from the lungs during exercise places a burden upon the respiratory muscles. The energy cost of breathing during rest represents 2 percent of the total oxygen consumed, but during vigorous exercise the cost can rise to 10 percent.[4]

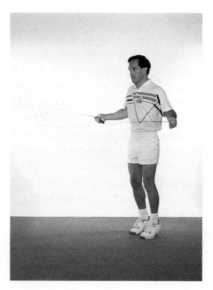

Rope Jumping

● Metabolic Responses

Aerobic Capacity Defined   Metabolism increases with the inception of exercise and continues to do so in direct proportion to increases in exercise intensity. **Metabolism**—the sum of the chemical reactions and processes that supply the energy used by the body—can be measured indirectly with appropriate equipment by the amount of oxygen consumed during exercise on such devices as a treadmill or a bicycle ergometer. When the intensity of exercise steadily increases, the individual's ability to supply the oxygen needed to keep pace will eventually plateau. This plateau represents the upper limit of endurance and is referred to as maximal oxygen consumption (VO_2 max). Also known as **aerobic capacity,** or circulorespiratory endurance, it defines a point at which further increases in exercise intensity do not elicit further increases in oxygen consumption (see Figure 6.2).

VO_2 max represents the body's peak ability to take in, devlier, and extract oxygen, and it is considered to be the best indicator of physical fitness. It is a well-defined exercise endpoint that can be measured and accurately reproduced in the laboratory. These procedures are not generally available to the public, but fortunately, field tests have been developed that correlate fairly well with the lab tests and may substitute for them (discussed later in this chapter).

FIGURE 6.2

Oxygen Uptake by Trained and Untrained People   This figure illustrates the difference in response to exercise between the trained and the untrained being exercised by a progressive treadmill protocol.

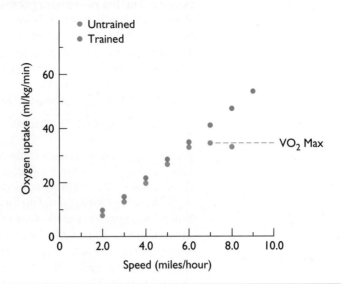

Body Mass and Oxygen Utilization

VO_2 max is measured in liters of oxygen utilized per minute—an absolute value influenced considerably by body size. Since oxygen is needed and used by all body tissues, larger people take in and use more oxygen both at rest and during exercise. Aerobic capacity, when expressed in liters of oxygen per minute, is not conducive to comparison, as it will yield false results. To eliminate the influence of size, aerobic capacity must be considered in terms of oxygen utilization per unit of body mass. This is accomplished by converting liters of oxygen to milliliters and then dividing by body weight in kilograms. For example, a 220-pound subject uses 4.5 liters of oxygen per minute during maximum exertion, while a 143-pound subject's capacity is 3.5 liters of oxygen per minute. From these data, it appears that the larger subject is more aerobically fit because of a greater capacity to use oxygen, but observe what occurs when these values are corrected for body size. Divide body weight in pounds by 2.205 to convert to kilograms:

Subject 1

$4.5 \text{ LO}_2/\text{min} = 4500 \text{ ml O}_2/\text{min}$
$4500 \text{ ml O}_2/\text{min} \div 100 \text{ kg} (220 \text{ lb.}) = 45 \text{ ml O}_2/\text{kg} \times \text{min}$

Subject 2

$3.5 \text{ LO}_2/\text{min} = 3500 \text{ ml O}_2)/\text{min}$
$3500 \text{ ml O}_2/\text{min} \div 65 \text{ kg}(143 \text{ lb.}) = 54 \text{ ml O}_2/\text{kg} \times \text{min}$

It's obvious from this example that the lighter subject can transport, extract, and use more oxygen per unit of body mass than the larger subject and is better equipped to perform endurance activities. VO_2 max values expressed in ml O_2/kg/min range from the mid-20s in sedentary older people to 94, the highest documented value recorded thus far. This enormous capacity belongs to an extremely well conditioned male cross-country skier. The highest value recorded for a female athlete, also by a cross-country skier is 74. College age males typically record values in the mid-40s, while college age females have values in the upper 30s to low 40s.

Gender Differences in Aerobic Capacity VO_2 max is affected by age, sex, body composition, heredity, and type of training. Sex differences in aerobic capacity become evident after puberty, with females exhibiting lower VO_2 max values. The difference is atributed to smaller heart size per unit of body weight, less oxygen-carrying capacity because of lower blood hemoglobin concentration, less muscle tissue, and more body fat. However, there is considerable overlap between the

sexes regarding aerobic capacity. World-class females competing in endurance events are aerobically superior to most males, although they have lower values than world-class male competitors. The differences between males and females are probably a combination of true physiological limitations and cultural restraints that have been placed upon females regarding endurance training and competition. The influence of culture and biology on female performance will become clearer during the next decade as more females train and compete.

Mechanisms of Aerobic Decline The decline in VO_2 max seems to parallel the functional losses as people age. Less than 50 percent of this loss is due to the aging process, with the remainder due to an inactive lifestyle. Maximum heart rate, cardiac output, and metabolism decrease during the adult years. **Body composition** changes as muscle tissue is lost, thus decreasing the body's energy-producing machinery. An increase in fat tissue is an impediment to physical performance. Breathing capacity decreases as the thoracic cage (chest) loses some of its elasticity caused by weakened intercostal muscles (muscles between the ribs), increased residual volume (air remaining in the lungs after expiration), and increased rigidity of lung structures. These changes can be significantly delayed by consistent participation in exercise and physical activity.[5]

Oxygen Deficit and Oxygen Debt When exercise begins, a short interval of time is needed for the body to adjust to the increased oxygen demand. This period when the oxygen demand of exercise exceeds the body's transport capability is referred to as the **oxygen deficit** (see Figure 6.3).

A second phenomenon—oxygen debt—occurs during both aerobic and anaerobic exercise (see Figure 6.3). **Oxygen debt** refers to the amount of oxygen consumed during the exercise recovery period above that normally consumed while at rest. It is measured at the end of exercise and includes the oxygen deficit. During anaerobic exercise, the body cannot supply all the oxygen needed, resulting in a deficiency between supply and demand that must be repaid at the end of exercise. A ten-second sprint or running up two or three flights of stairs elevates heart rate and ventilation. Both persist for a few moments following the activity before gradually returning to resting levels. The extra oxygen consumed during this interval represents the oxygen debt. Aerobic exercise also produces an oxygen debt that may be entirely due to the oxygen deficit, particularly in low-intensity exercise. Aerobic exercise in excess of 50 percent of the aerobic capacity will produce lactic acid and a further increase in oxygen debt.

FIGURE 6.3

Oxygen Deficit and Oxygen Debt (Energy Debt)

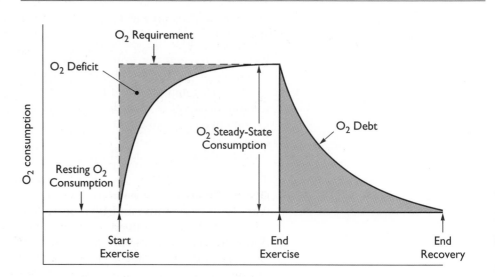

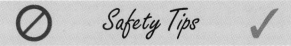
AEROBIC EXERCISE

1. The risk for serious medical complications during and after a bout of exercise is quite low, but it is higher than during sedentary activities. The risk is higher for the physically unfit than for the physcially fit.
2. Be aware of the symptoms during and after exercise that might indicate that heart disease is present. Two large studies of sudden deaths among marathon runners indicated that 81% had warning signals that they chose to ignore. Despite severe chest pain and shortness of breath, these people continued to train and race. Instead, they should have discontinued training and immediately sought medical evaluation. With proper and immediate medical intervention, many of these runners might be alive today.
3. People who experience any one of the following from the U.S. National Heart, Lung and Blood Institute should consult a physician before engaging in an exercise program:

- A family history of premature coronary heart disease (primary relatives under the age of 55).
- Frequent pains or pressure in the left or middle chest, left side of the neck, shoulder, or arm during or immediately after exercise.
- Fainting, spells of severe dizziness, or extreme breathlessness after mild exertion.
- Blood pressure that is too high and not under control.
- Heart disease that has been diagnosed, a heart murmur, or you have suffered a heart attack.
- Arthritis.
- A medical condition that might need special attention, such as insulin-dependent diabetes mellitus.

 ## LONG-TERM EFFECTS OF AEROBIC EXERCISE

The long-term effect of aerobic exercise—also referred to as *chronic adaptations*—are those physiological and psychological changes that result from training. These changes represent the training effect gradually developed after repeated bouts of exercise.

● Heart Rate

A few months of participation in an aerobic exercise program will decrease the resting heart rate (RHR) by 10 to 25 beats per minute (bpm). This can drop the RHR below 60 bpm. The decline in RHR is accompanied by a decline in exercise heart rate for a given workload. For example, a bout of exercise that elicits a heart rate of 150 beats per minute prior to training may produce a heart rate of 125 beats per minute after a few months of training. Five to six months of training will realistically lower the submaximum exercise heart rate by 20 to 40 beats per minute. Also, the exercise heart rate returns to resting level more rapidly as physical fitness improves.

The importance of lowered resting and exercise heart rates is that it allows more time for filling the ventricles with blood to be pumped to all of the body's tissues and more time for the delivery of oxygen and nutrients to the heart muscle. The delivery of these substances occurs during diastole (resting phase of the heart cycle) because relaxation of the heart muscle allows the coronary vessels to open up and receive the blood that it needs. Training substantially prolongs the heart's diastolic phase. The net result is that the heart operates more efficiently and with longer periods of rest.

Table 6.3 illustrates the differences between the trained and untrained heart. The efficiency of the trained heart at rest is readily apparent because it can pump the same amount of blood with fewer beats, thereby reducing its energy requirements. During maximum exercise, even though the maximal heart rate is the same for the trained and untrained heart, the stroke volume is considerably higher for

TABLE 6.3	Comparison of Cardiac Effciency—Trained Versus Untrained			
EFFICIENCY MEASUREMENT	**REST**		**MAXIMUM EXERCISE**	
	Untrained	*Trained*	*Untrained*	*Trained*
Cardiac Output (ml)	5,200	5,200	22,000	34,000
Heart Rate (bpm)	74	52	200	200
Stroke Volume	70	100	110	170

the former. The result is that more blood can be pumped per heart beat, which increases the level at which one can exercise.

Stroke Volume

Stroke volume and heart rate are inversely related. The heart rate at rest and for a given workload is lower because of the heart's enhanced ability to pump more blood per beat. This is accomplished because of more complete filling of the left ventricle, combined with an increase in the contractile strength of the left ventricle's muscular walls. Together these produce a more forceful contraction and greater emptying of the blood in the chamber. This stronger, more efficient heart is capable of meeting circulatory challenges with fewer beats both at rest and during submaximum exercise.

Cardiac Output

Posttraining cardiac output is increased considerably during maximum exercise. However, there is little change during rest or submaximum work, primarily because the trained individual is able to extract more oxygen from arterial blood. Cardiac output improves with training, primarily because of the increase in stroke volume. The training effect is apparent during maximum exercise.

Blood Pressure

Some controversy exists regarding the effect of exercise in reducing essential hypertension (high blood pressure, the causes of which are unknown). Essential hypertension comprises 90 percent to 95 percent of all cases of high blood pressure. Most of the evidence suggests that aerobic forms of exercise seem to be the most effective in reducing blood pressure.[6] The evidence is not as strong regarding the effectiveness of progressive resistance exercise as a moderating influence on hypertension. However, several studies have suggested that this type of exercise can also lower blood pressure.[7]

At this point, at least three generalizations about the relationship between exercise and blood pressure are supported by research: (1) very sedentary people tend to get the most benefit from exercise with regard to lowering the blood pressure, (2) exercise seems to be slightly more effective in lowering the blood pressure of women, and (3) heavier people tend to have smaller reductions in systolic blood pressure than lighter people unless they lose weight simultaneously.[8]

The mechanisms by which exercise may lower blood pressure involve the hormones epinephrine and norepinephrine and their effect on resistance to blood flow in the arteries. Both hormones are vasoconstrictors that decrease the diameters of the arterioles (the smallest arteries). Sixteen weeks of aerobic exercise reduced the blood level of norepinephrine and also reduced the blood pressure.[9]

The resistance to blood flow—or peripheral resistance—is another major contributor to blood pressure. The diameter of the arterioles is largely responsible for peripheral resistance. The relationship between the two is inverse, so that the larger the diameter of the arterioles, the less the peripheral resistance, and the smaller the diameter, the greater the resistance. Three days of aerobic exercise per week decreased peripheral resistance by 18 percent, while daily exercise resulted in a decrease of 24 percent.[10] Plasma norepinephrine levels, peripheral resistance, and blood pressure decreased as exercise frequency increased.

Blood Volume

Blood volume increases with endurance training. The volume change occurs from a significant increase in the amount of plasma (the liquid portion of the blood) and a lesser increase in blood solids (primarily the number of red blood cells). The increase in plasma volume versus red blood cells is disproportionate. The greater increase in plasma volume results in less viscous blood that is thinner (more watery). This is an important adaptation to training because thinner blood can be circulated more efficiently and with less resistance.

A trained person's red cell count is usually below average, causing the individual to appear to be anemic. In reality, trained people have a higher absolute number of red blood cells than untrained people, but on a relative basis, because of the expanded plasma volume, the numbers appear to be low. The average hematocrit (the ratio of red blood cells to plasma volume) of the general public is 40 percent to 50 percent, with males having slightly higher values (more red blood cells per unit of blood) than females. The lower hematocrit of trained people not only is an important adaptation for endurance performance but also represents a healthy change. The ideal hematocrit for running a marathon is about 50 percent, but for health it is probably closer to 40 percent for men and 35 percent for women.[11]

Heart Volume

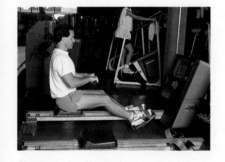

Rowing

The heart responds to regular exercise in a similar manner as the other muscles of the body; it becomes stronger and oftentimes larger. The volume and the weight of the heart are increased with endurance training. The effects of bed rest and training upon heart volume have been determined. Prior to bed rest, the mean heart volume of five young male subjects was 867 ml.[12] Twenty days of bed rest reduced the volume to 778 ml. Bed rest was followed by 50 days of training that increased the volume to 900 ml. Many other studies have confirmed the change in heart volume with aerobic training.

In the not-so-distant past, exercise-induced changes in the heart were considered to be pathological. The term "athlete's heart" was assigned to describe the cardiac hypertrophy (heart enlargement) seen in many athletes, and the connotation was that such a heart was harmful to health and longevity. Today, the medical community accepts these changes as normal responses to endurance training that have no long-term detrimental effects. In fact, it would be beneficial to maintain such a heart for as long as possible. Six months of inactivity following a training program will reduce heart weight and size to pretraining levels. The atrophy associated with inactivity is unavoidable.

Respiratory Responses

Some training-induced adaptations also occur in the respiratory system. The muscles that support breathing improve in both strength and endurance. This increases the amount of air that can be expired after a maximum inhalation (**vital capacity**) and decreases the amount of air remaining in the lungs (**residual volume**). Ventilation decreases slightly for a given workload and increases signficantly during maximum exercise as a result of training, indicating an improvement in the efficiency of the system. The depth of each breath (tidal volume) also increases during vigorous exercise.

Training increases blood flow in the lungs. In the sitting or standing position, many of the pulmonary capillaries in the upper regions of the lungs close down because gravity pulls blood down to the lower portions of the lungs. Exercise forces blood into the upper lobes and creates a greater surface area for the diffusion of oxygen from the **alveoli** (air sacs) to the pulmonary blood. Perfusion of the upper lobes of the lungs is improved with training. See Figure 6.4 for an illustration of the respiratory system.

Metabolic Responses

Improving the Aerobic System   Endurance training improves aerobic capacity (VO_2 max) by 5 percent to 25 percent. The magnitude of the increase is dependent primarily upon the initial level of fitness. Those who are the least fit make the most improvement simply because they are furtherst away from their genetic potential.

Fitness gains come rather quickly during the first few months of training, with further increases occurring in smaller increments as fitness improves until VO_2 max reaches its peak. VO_2 max is reached with six months to two years of training.[13]

The improvement in VO_2 max is caused by a combination of physiological adaptations. First, the number and size of mitochondria increase. The **mitochondria** (often referred to as the cells' powerhouse) are organelles within the cells that utilize oxygen to produce the ATP needed by the muscles. ATP (adenosine triphosphate) is a high-energy compound that provides the fuel that the body

---

| **FIGURE 6.4** | **The Human Respiratory System**   On the left is the structure of the interior of the lungs. The insert on the right magnifies the alveoli and their blood and oxygen supply. Oxygen and carbon dioxide are exchanged in the alveoli. |

Reprinted by permission. D. D. Chiras, *Biology the Web of Life*, St. Paul: West, 1993. Art rendered by Cyndie Wooley.

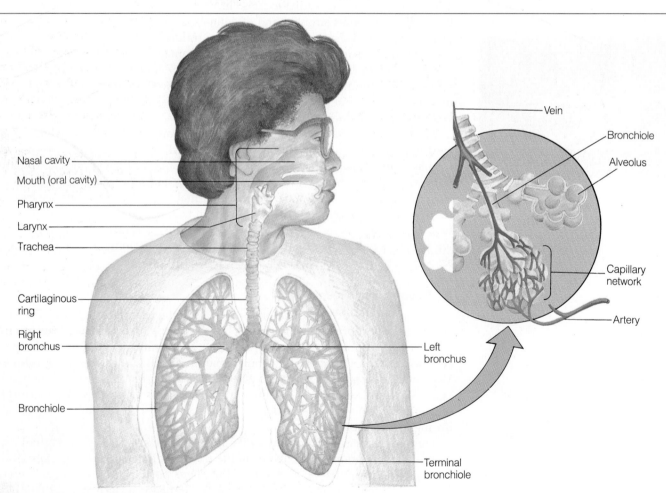

uses. Second, enzymes located within the mitochondria that accelerate the chemical reactions needed for the production of ATP are increased. These increases in the mitochondria and their enzymes produce greater amounts of energy and an improvement in physical fitness. Third, there is an increase in maximal cardiac output and local blood supply in the exercising muscles. Fourth, more oxygen is extracted from the blood by the exercising muscles. At rest, the arteries carry approximately 20 ml O_2 per 100 ml of blood. The veins carry about 14 ml O_2 per 100 ml of blood. When the oxygen value in the veins is subtracted from the oxygen values in the arteries, it yields the amount of oxygen used by the body. This value is termed the **arterial-venous oxygen difference (a-vO$_2$diff),** and at rest it is equal to 6 ml O_2/100 ml blood. Since exercise increases the body's need for oxygen, the extraction rate increases and the a-vO$_2$ difference widens. Training increases the a-vO$_2$ difference during maximum exercise but may not increase it at rest or during submaximum exercise (see Table 6.4).

The Genetic Factor   Aerobic capacity is finite. Each of us is endowed with an aerobic potential limited by our heredity. A small percentage of people inherit the potential to achieve amazing feats of endurance, as exemplified by performances in marathons, ultramarathons, Iron Man Triathalons, cross-country runs lasting weeks or months, and long-distance bike races. Most of us are in the average category for aerobic capacity, but all of us can achieve our potential with endurance training.

Researchers have attempted to quantify the influence of heredity as a component of VO$_2$ max. In other words, how much of the variability seen among people in VO$_2$ max is due to inherited factors? Although this line of inquiry is yet to be fully resolved, the differences observed among identical twins, fraternal twins, and other siblings have provided some clues.[14] The best available evidence suggests that the genetic component represents 40 percent of the known factors regarding the achievable VO$_2$ max for any individual. Those who have inherited a superior cardiorespiratory endowment have the physical structure to benefit maximally from training and may become national or world-class performers. Those who are endowed to a lesser extent (the majority of people) also benefit from training. They may not have the foundation to become high-level competitors, but they can train to their potential and enjoy their own accomplishments.

The Anaerobic Threshold (Onset of Blood Lactic Acid)   Even though VO$_2$ max reaches a peak early in the training program, aerobic performance continues to improve for many years with harder and continued training. The question, then, is, How can physical performance continue to improve after VO$_2$ max has leveled off? This question can be answered with an example. Let us assume that a female jogger has achieved her aerobic potential of 54 ml/kg/min with two years of regular training. At this point, she is abel to jog a five-mile course at 38 ml/kg/min, or 70 percent of her aerobic capacity. After two more years of vigorous training (VO$_2$ max still at 54 ml/kg/min), she is now able to sustain a 47 ml/kg/min pace

TABLE 6.4	Comparison of A-VO$_2$ Difference—Rest Versus Maximum Exercise*		
Rest		Arterial blood	20 ml O_2/100 ml blood
		Venous blood	– 14 ml O_2/100 ml blood
			6 ml O_2/100 ml blood
Maximum Exercise		Arterial blood	20 ml O_2/100 ml blood
		Venous blood	– 4 ml O_2/100 ml blood
			16 ml O_2/100 ml blood

*Note that the venous blood values of oxygen change from rest to severe exercise because the body is extracting and using more of the oxygen in arterial blood.

for the same distance, or 88 percent of her aerobic capacity. The past two years of training have permitted her to use more oxygen, thereby sustaining a faster pace for the course without dipping materially into the anaerobic fuel systems that produce lactic acid and oxygen debt.

The point during exercise where blood lactate sudenly begins to increase is defined as the anaerobic threshold and is also known as "the onset of blood lactate accumulation."[15] Training moves the anaerobic threshold closer to the VO_2 max, allowing people to exercise at a higher percentage of their capacity before lactic acid accumulates to the point where it begins to interfere with muscle contraction and physical performance. Two people with the same VO_2 max will perform differently in an endurance event if one has an anaerobic threshold substantially higher than the other.

The Effect of Aging on Aerobic Capacity   Aerobic capacity decreases with age, but it decreases more slowly for people who are physically fit. Researchers at San Diego State University studied the effect of exercise on 15 men who walked, jogged, swam, and cycled 3 to 4 days per week for 23 years.[16] The men averaged 45 years of age at the start of the study and 68 years at the 23-year mark. Their VO_2 max declined 13 percent during 23 years, compared to an amazing 41 percent decline for a nonexercising group of men of similar age. The average loss in VO_2 max as people age is a gradual but systematic 1 percent per year. The researchers concluded that the 13 percent loss in VO_2 max for the exercise group represented a true effect of aging. If the aging effect (13 percent decline) is factored out of the decline experienced by the nonexercisers, two thirds of their decrease in VO_2 max is due to inactivity rather than aging.

This important long-term study has provided evidence to support what many exercisers and researchers by logical deduction and anecdotal evidence already knew—that physcial training delays the deterioration of aerobic capacity at least until people reach their sixties.

Estimating the Oxygen Demand of the Heart   The oxygen demand of the heart during aerobic exercise can be estimated by multiplying the heart rate by the systolic blood pressure. This is referred to as the **double product,** or the **rate pressure product (RPP),** and represents the volume of oxygen required by the heart muscle per minute. Training reduces the double product for a given amount of work. For example, an untrained individual may respond to a specific submaximal workload with a heart rate of 150 beats per minute and a systolic blood pressure of 160 mmHg, for a double product of 240 (150 × 160 = 24000). The last two zeros are dropped to produce a three-digit, more manageable figure. After training, the same workload may provoke a heart rate of 130 beats per minute with a systolic blood pressure of 140 mmHg, for a double product of 182. This represents (1) a reduced myocardial oxygen requirement for the same level of work, (2) an objective indication that aerobic conditioning has occurred, and (3) a response that implies the development of some degree of protection against ischemia (diminished blood flow).

DECONDITIONING—LOSS OF TRAINING EFFECT

Deconditioning takes place when training is discontinued or significantly reduced. E. F. Coyle investigated the physiological changes that accompany detraining as well as the approximate timetable of their occurrence.[17] The subjects in this study had been actively training for ten years. They abandoned training for 84 days so that Coyle could observe and measure the changes that took place. Coyle noted that some systems of the body showed the effects of detraining rapidly, while others reacted more slowly. Stroke volume declined substantially in the first 12 days. As expected, the decline was accompanied by a significant reduction

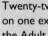
Twenty-two years of continuous data on one exercising population makes the Adult Fitness Study a treasure chest of information on the effects of exercise.

—Lan Barnes

in aerobic capacity, which declined 16 percent by the fifty-sixth day of the deconditioning period. The oxidative enzyme level in the muscles dropped 40 percent at the end of eight weeks. However, the capillary density of the muscles declined by only 7 percent below the trained state by the end of the detraining period, and mitochondrial enzymes remained 50 percent higher than those of sedentary control subjects.[18]

EXERCISE AND INFECTION: HELP OR HYPE?

People who have exercised for years claim that they have fewer viral infections and colds than they did in their sedentary days. Although this response is prevalent among exercisers, research evidence remains equivocal on this point. That physically active people are less susceptible to these infections is probably true. However, is it because of natural buildup of antibodies as we age, or is it because of the effect of exercise in boosting the immune system, or is it that people who exercise are more aware and take better care of their health than nonexercisers?

Support for enhancement of the immune system through exercise comes from increased production of lymphocytes, interleukin-1, and interferon, which has been observed in some studies. The lymphocytes are the primariy cells involved in the immune response. Most studies have shown an increase in the number of circulating lymphocytes with strenuous exercise, but the effects may be short-lived.[19] Moderate exercise has increased circulating levels of interleukin-1,[20] which stimulates the immune system by increasing the activity of both T- and B-lymphocytes. Interleukin-1 also exerts a pyrogenic effect (produces a fever), which is part of the body's natural defense in combatting infections.

Moderate exercise also stimulates the production of interferons,[21] a group of naturally occurring proteins that have antiviral properties. The response of interferons to viral infections is initiated only a matter of hours after an infection develops. Exercise-induced increases in interferons last for approximately two hours. First, the effectiveness of this transient response is debatable, and second, the amount of interferons produced by exercise is less than that which naturally occurs to the virus alone.

Persistent, very strenuous exercise that produces chronic fatigue may have the opposite effect by reducing the activity of the immune system, lowering one's resistance to disease. High-intensity exercise performed frequently tends to increase the likelihood of respiratory infection by suppressing some components of the immune system for up to two hours after exercise.[22]

Is exercise a help or a hindrance with regard to infections? The research shows that exercise of moderate intensity may enhance the immune system and that exhaustive exercise might suppress it. The suggestion for those who exercise for reasons other than competition is quite clear: exercise moderately and frequently.

Lymphocytes are the most important link in the relationship between exercise and immune function.
—Harvey Simon

ACTIVITIES FOR IMPROVING CARDIORESPIRATORY ENDURANCE

Cardiorespiratory endurance can be developed through participation in rhythmic and continuous activities that elevate the heart rate to desired levels at least three times a week for at least 20 to 60 minutes at a time. Any activity meeting these criteria will suffice. Remember, since fitness cannot be developed or maintained without effort and consistent participation, it is very important that you select activities that are enjoyable and satisfying.

Many activities—some more than others—have the potential for developing cardiorespiratory fitness. Many of them are more amenable to regulation in terms of exercise intensity and require neither an opponent nor a companion. The frequency, duration, and intensity of these activities are under your control. Some

1. People perspire to a greater extent immediately after exercise than during exercise.

   There are several reasons for this phenomenon. Exercising muscles always receive the lion's share of blood, but the skin receives more than its normal share to remove the heat produced by exercising muscles. When exercise stops, more blood is diverted to the skin as the muscles' demand for oxygen diminishes. This stimulates the production of sweat, accelerating heat removal from the body. We notice less sweat during exercise because sweat evaporates more efficiently while we are in motion. The evaporative process is augmented by convective heat loss. Sweat production does not reduce during exercise; sweat simply evaporates more efficiently.

2. Should people exercise when they are sick? A few guidelines are in order:

   a. People should not exercise if they have a fever above 100 degrees F.

   b. People may exercise with a fever of 100 degress F or less, but they should reduce the intensity and duration of the workout.

   c. A resting heart rate 10 beats/minute above normal would indicate that exercise should be postponed.

3. Breathing becomes much easier and exercise becomes more comfortable two to three minutes after exercise begins.

   The phenomenon known as second wind appears to be the result of greater circulatory efficiency coupled with more appropriate metabolic responses. After a couple of minutes, a steady exercise state, or equilibrium between oxygen demand and oxygen supply, is achieved. The oxygen deficit incurred during the first couple of minutes of exercise abates, resulting in greater comfort.

4. Exercise develops an enlarged heart, which may be harmful to health.

   An enlarged heart is a normal response to those forms of exercise that stimulate enlargement. Jogging, rowing, cycling, cross-country skiing, and other endurance events do produce heart enlargement because of the circulatory demands by the muscles involved in exercise. The cardiac response to these demands leads to heart muscle hypertrophy. This is not a pathological adaptation. In fact, the athlete's heart is a very efficient, powerful, healthy organ capable of meeting the body's blood and oxygen needs with fewer beats. Hearts that are pathologically enlarged are the result of disease processes. Such hearts are weak and inefficient.

5. Runner's anemia is harmful to health.

   Runner's anemia is an adaptation to strenuous exercise. It is not harmful to health, because the body's ability to produce healthy red blood cells is not compromised. Actually, runners experience an increase in the number of red blood cells. The reason that runners appear to be anemic is that the plasma portion of their blood increases more rapidly and to a greater extent than the number of red blood cells. The change in ratio between the two gives the appearance of a decrease in the number of red blood cells.

events that fall into this category include fast walking, jogging, biking, swimming, rope jumping, fitness trails, cross-country skiing, stair climbing, rowing, and skating (ice and roller). Competition in these activities is not precluded, but their nature is such that they allow for individual participation and latitude in scheduling plus control of the criteria that must be met to develop and maintain cardiorespiratory endurance.

Many sports and games also have the capacity to develop and maintain cardiorespiratory endurance, but some flexibility and control is lost. For example, the intensity of a game is dependent upon the skill level and motivation of the players as well as the degree to which the action is continuous. Court games such as squash, racquetball, handball, badminton, and tennis are noncontinuous activities. Optimal fitness benefits from these games are attained when two highly skilled players of equal ability oppose each other in singles competition.

Team sports such as basketball, ice and roller hockey, lacrosse, rugby, soccer, and water polo have the potential to develop aerobic fitness. The action in these sports is also intermittent, and they pose the additional obstacle of rounding up more people to play as well as gaining access to an appropriate facility. It becomes more difficult to schedule these activities three or more days per week.

A more serious problem associated with court games and team sports is that they may be too strenuous for sedentary beginners. A sensible approach for those who want to maintain fitness through sports and games is to first develop a fit-

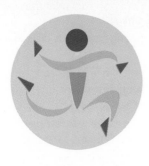

INTRODUCTION

This chapter will introduce you to how and why the death and disease patterns in the United States have changed. Infectious diseases have given way to the chronic diseases. **Cardiovascular disease,** the foremost of the chronic diseases, is the number one killer of Americans. This chapter focuses upon (1) the basics of circulation, (2) pediatric origins of cardiovascular disease, (3) the signs and symptoms of heart disease, and (4) the risk factors for heart disease and strokes.

In the American Heart Association's (AHA's) publication *1992 Heart and Stroke Facts*, the risk factors for heart disease are categorized as follows:[1]

1. Major risk factors that can't be changed (heredity, male sex, and increasing age).

2. Major risk factors that can be changed (cigarette smoking, high blood pressure, blood cholesterol level, and physical inactivity).

3. Other contributing risk factors (diabetes, obesity, and stress).

The major risk factors are those that, based upon medical research, are significantly related to the development of cardiovascular disease. The contributing risk factors are related to the development of cardiovascular disease, but research has yet to document their importance.

The risk factors for strokes also include controllable and noncontrollable factors. The controllable or treatable factors include (1) high blood pressure, (2) heart disease, (3) cigarette smoking, (4) high red blood cell count, and (5) transient ischemic attacks (ministrokes). According to the AHA, the following risk factors

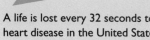

A life is lost every 32 seconds to heart disease in the United States.
—American Heart Association

Miniglossary

Aorta   Largest artery in the body.

a-vO$_2$ Difference   The amount of oxygen in the venous blood subtracted from the oxygen in arterial blood. This represents the extraction rate of oxygen by the tissues of the body.

Atherosclerosis   A progressive disease that results in the narrowing of arterial channels caused by the buildup of plaque.

Blood Platelets   Blood cells involved in preventing blood loss. Platelets are important components in clot formation.

Blood Pressure   The force that the blood exerts against the walls of the blood vessels.

Carbon Monoxide   A colorless, odorless gas formed by the incomplete oxidation of carbon and highly poisonous when inhaled.

Cardiovascular Diseases   Diseases of the heart and blood vessels.

Cerebrovascular Accidents   Diseases of the blood vessels to the brain or in the brain that result in a stroke.

Cholesterol   An organic substance—the most abundant steroid in animal tissues, especially in bile and gallstones. Elevated blood cholesterol is a primary risk factor for heart disease.

Chylomicrons   Large, buoyant particles that are the primary transporters of triglycerides in the fasting state.

Congential Heart Disease   Heart defects that exist at birth and occur when the heart or its structures or the blood vessels near the heart fail to develop normally before birth.

Diabetes Mellitus   A metabolic disorder in which the ability to oxidize carbohydrates is more or less completely lost because of faulty pancreatic activity

Continued

—Continued

and consequent disturbance of normal insulin mechanisms. It is often accompanied by resistance of receptor cells to insulin.

Diastolic Blood Pressure   The lowest pressure of arterial blood against the walls of the vessels or heart during diastole.

Endogenous Cholesterol   Cholesterol manufactured within the body.

Erythrocytes   The red blood cells that transport oxygen from the lungs to the various tissues of the body and carbon dioxide from the tissues to the lungs.

Exogenous Cholesterol   Cholesterol received through the diet.

HDL   A lipoprotein that transports cholesterol from the blood to the liver for degradation and removal (good cholesterol).

Hemoglobin   The protein molecule to which oxygen and carbon dioxide attach for transport by the erythrocytes.

Hypertension   Medical term for high blood pressure.

Hypokinesis   Lack of physical activity.

LDL   A lipoprotein that transports cholesterol to the tissues. It is involved in the atherosclerotic process (bad cholesterol).

Leukocytes   White blood cells that protect the body against invading microorganisms and remove dead cells and debris from the body.

Myocardial Infarction   A heart attack. The term literally means "death of heart muscle tissue."

Myocardium   Heart muscle.

Nicotine   A stimulant and poisonous drug found in tobacco products.

Obesity   Excessive body fat—23 percent to 24 percent or greater for males; 30 percent or greater for females.

Systolic Blood Pressure   The greatest pressure in the blood vessels or heart during a cardiac cycle as the result of systole.

Triglycerides   Glycerol with three attached fatty acids.

VLDL   Lipoproteins that are the primary transporters of endogenous triglycerides in the fasting state.

indirectly increase the risk of stroke: (1) elevated blood cholesterol and lipids (fats), (2) excessive alcohol intake, (3) physical inactivity, and (4) obesity. Risks that can't be changed include (1) age, (2) sex, (3) race, (4) diabetes mellitus, (5) prior stroke, (6) heredity, and (7) asymptomatic carotid bruit (the sound created by turbulent blood flow as it passes through a partially blocked artery).

Four Self-Assessment activities appear in Appendix C that apply directly to the contents of this chapter:

7.1 Cardiac Risk Assessment

7.2 Case Study—Robert S.

7.3 Distribution of Body Fat

7.4 Diabetes Check

 PREVALENCE OF CARDIOVASCULAR DISEASES

Cardiovascular diseases (diseases of the heart and blood vessels) were responsible for 43.8 percent of all deaths in the United States in 1989[2] (the most recent year that statistics are available). The total number of such deaths was 944,688. Approximately 69,000,000 Americans have one or more forms of cardiovascular disease. The leading form of cardiovascular death—claiming 497,850 victims in 1989—is coronary heart disease. The 1989 projections indicated that coronary heart disease would cause 1.5 million heart attacks and approximately 500,000 deaths in 1992.

These data are ominous, and much remains to be accomplished in the battle against all forms of cardiovascular disease. However, substantial headway has been made. The death rate from cardiovascular disease has declined by 51 percent since 1950.[3] Coronary heart disease declined by 30 percent between 1979 and 1989.

Stroke or cerebrovascular disease (disease of the brain and the blood vessels supplying it) is the third leading cause of death. Strokes were responsible for 147,470 deaths in 1989. Strokes and cardiovascular diseases share similar etiologies. When blood flow to the heart or brain is interrupted or stopped for a few minutes, the affected organ suffers damage and/or death. The death rate from strokes has declined by 31.5 percent between 1979 and 1989.

The decline in the death rates from cardiovascular and cerebrovascular diseases is due to many factors, but certainly the lifestyle behavioral changes made by many Americans have exerted considerable influence. Some of those behavior changes include (1) more people exercising, (2) healthy changes in nutritional habits, (3) reduction in the number of people who smoke cigarettes, (4) awareness of the importance of blood pressure screening and control, (5) awareness of the importance of blood lipids (fats) control, (6) stress management awareness, and (7) weight management.

THE BASICS OF CIRCULATION

The Heart and Blood Vessels

The basic anatomy and function of the heart must be grasped—at least in an elementary way—to understand circulation and the consequences of the interruption of the circulatory system's natural order. The circulatory system consists of the heart and blood vessels. The heart, a muscular organ made up of specialized cardiac muscle, weighs between eight and ten ounces. About the size of a fist, it lies slightly to the left of center in the chest. The heart is a four-chambered hollow organ whose muscular wall or **myocardium** (*myo:* muscle; *cardium:* heart) is surrounded by a fiberlike bag, the pericardium (*peri:* around) and lined by a strong, thin membrane, the endocardium (*endo:* inner). Figure 7.1 shows the various structures of the heart.

The heart is divided into two halves by a wall (the septum), and each half is divided into an upper chamber (the atrium) and a lower chamber (the ventricle). The flow of blood entering and exiting the heart is regulated by valves located between the chambers, the aorta, and the pulmonary artery. See Figure 7.2 for the various structures of the heart.

FIGURE 7.1

Pericardial Sac

Source: L. Sherwood, *Human Psysiology,* St. Paul: West, 1993. Reprinted with permission. Art rendered by Rolin Graphics.

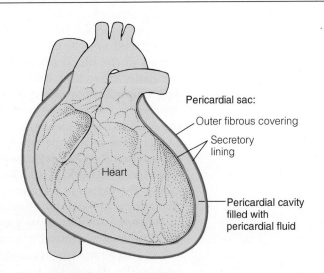

Pericardial sac:

Outer fibrous covering

Secretory lining

Heart

Pericardial cavity filled with pericardial fluid

FIGURE 7.2

Gross Anatomy of the Interior of the Heart

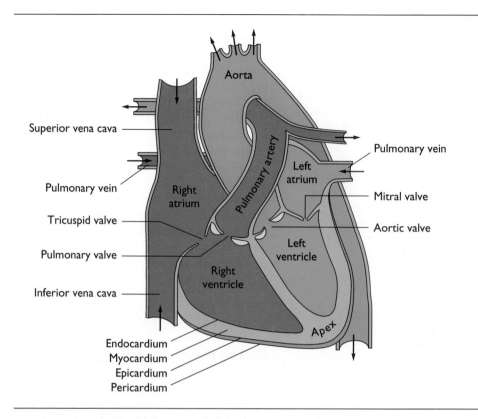

The heart is a double pump. The right heart, or "pulmonary pump" (*pulmonary:* lungs), has the singular task of transporting deoxygenated blood to the lungs where it can exchange carbon dioxide for a fresh supply of oxygen. From the lungs, the oxygen-rich blood is circulated to the left heart, or "systemic pump" (*systemic:* system or body), so that it can be sent to all of the tissues of the body (see Figure 7.3).

The tissues extract their oxygen requirements and, in exchange, give up their waste products (principally carbon dioxide) to the blood. The blood, now carrying a reduced oxygen load and an increased amount of carbon dioxide, returns to the right heart, where the cycle begins again. Both pumps work simultaneously and continuously. The left pump, which circulates blood throughout the entire body and therefore carries the heavier workload, has a thicker and stronger ventricular wall.

Blood leaves the left heart via the **aorta**—the largest artery in the body. It then travels through conduits of muscular vessels called arteries. The arteries subdivide into arterioles (the smallest arteries), which eventually empty into the smallest of blood vessels, the capillaries. In the capillaries, oxygen, nutrients, and hormones in the blood are exchanged for waste products from the tissues. The capillaries are so tiny that blood cells pass through them in single file. The arterial and venous systems are joined together by the capillary network. The venules (smallest veins) emanate from these tiny vessels and empty into the veins, allowing the removal of metabolic wastes from the tissues. Providing a constant supply of fuel to the cells while removing their wastes is the principal job of the circulatory system. When red oxygenated blood leaves the left ventricle and courses down the arterial network, it contains 20 milliliters of oxygen (ml O_2) in each 100 ml of blood. The tissues at rest extract about 6 ml of O_2 so that the bluish venous blood that returns to the right atrium contains 14 ml of oxygen per 100 ml of blood.

When the amount of oxygen in the veins is subtracted from that in the arteries, the difference is referred to as the arterio-venous oxygen difference (**a-vO_2 difference**). This represents the amount of oxygen that is extracted by the body's tissues and organs. At rest, the a-vO_2 is about 6 mlO_2 per 100 ml of blood. The extraction

FIGURE 7.3

Circulation of the Pulmonary and Systemic Pumps

Deoxygenated (carbon dioxide-enriched) blood (blue) flows into the right atrium from the systemic circulation, then is pumped into the right ventricle. The right ventricle, in turn, pumps the blood into the pulmonary artery, which delivers it to the lungs, where carbon dioxide is released and oxygen is picked up. Reoxygenated blood (red) is returned to the left atrium, then flows into the left ventricle, which pumps it to the rest of the body through the systemic circuit.

Source: Chiras, *Biology: The Web of Life,* 1993, West Publishing Company. Reproduced with Permission. Layout by Darwin and Vally Hennings and modification by Cyndie Wooley.

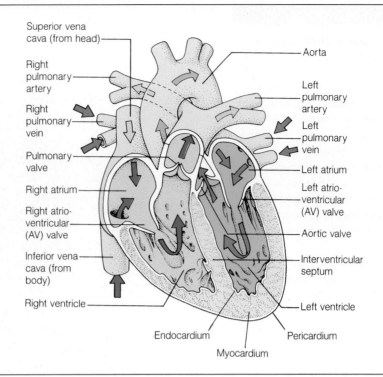

rate increases when one goes from a resting state to an exercising state. The more vigorous the exercise, the greater the extraction rate, up to a maximum value of about 16 to 17 ml of oxygen per 100 ml of blood.

Arteries carry oxygenated blood to all of the body's tissues. The pulmonary artery is the lone exception in that its cargo is deoxygenated blood. It transports its oxygen-poor blood from the right half of the heart to the lungs, where it gives up carbon dioxide in exchange for a supply of oxygen. The veins carry deoxygenated blood back to the right half of the heart. The pulmonary vein is the lone exception in that it transports fully oxygenated blood from the lungs to the left half of the heart for distribution to all parts of the body.

The heart's failure to pump blood for a few minutes can be catastrophic. Under usual circumstances, oxygen deprivation for as little as four minutes can destroy the ability of the brain to function normally, and it can lead to death. The heart is so vital that nature has attempted to protect it by locating it behind the breastbone, encircling it with ribs, and surrounding it with a tough multiple membrane, the pericardium. Fluid between the membranes cushions the heart from trauma and reduces friction as the heart beats against the breastbone and the diaphragm.

At rest, the heart's pumping rate averages between 70 and 80 beats per minute. Some variance from the average occurs, however, such as among endurance athletes, who often have resting rates in the 30s and 40s on the one hand, and among some overweight, sedentary smokers, with resting rates in the 90s on the other. Physicians consider 50 to 100 beats per minute normal, but they have recognized in the past few years the the low heart rates of endurance athletes are adaptations to training and represent normal values for this group.

The heart's beating rate is established by the heart's pacemaker—the sinoatrial node (SA node), shown in Figure 7.4. The electrical stimulus that causes the heart to contract originates in this node. The atria contract and force blood into the ventricles while the impulse travels to the atrioventricular node (AV node). A split second later, the ventricles contract, sending blood through the body as the impulse travels down the Bundle of His and spreads throughout the ventricular walls.

Blood that enters the chambers of the heart does not directly nourish heart muscle. Heart muscle receives its nourishment when the heart contracts and ejects

FIGURE 7.4

The Electrical Conduction System of the Heart The heart beat originates in the SA node causing the atria to contract. The electrical impulse travels downward to the AV node where it stops for a fraction of a second allowing the ventricles to fill with blood. From here it continues downward through the bundle branches and spreads upward through the periphery causing the ventricles to contract. The cycle is repeated for every heartbeat.

Source: Chiras *Biology: The Web of Life*, 1993, West Publishing Company. Reproduced with Permission. Layout by Darwin and Vally Hennings and modification by Cyndie Wooley.

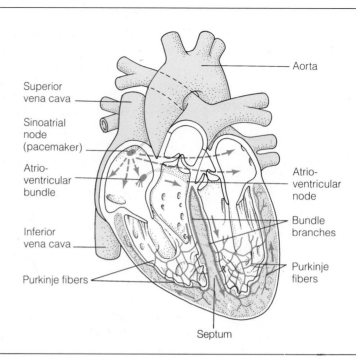

blood out of the chambers and into an elaborate network of coronary blood vessels (see Figure 7.5). Originating at the aorta, the coronary arteries lie around the surface of the heart like a crown and supply the heart muscle with its nutrient needs. The left coronary artery carries the larger volume of blood, supplying the cells of the left atrium and ventricle as well as a portion of the right ventricle. The right coronary artery supplies the right atrium and the remainder of the right ventricle. These major vessels divide downstream and eventually culminate in a very dense network of capillaries structured precisely so that at least one capillary services each of the heart's muscle fibers. The coronary veins return deoxygenated blood to the right atrium.

FIGURE 7.5

Coronary Circulation

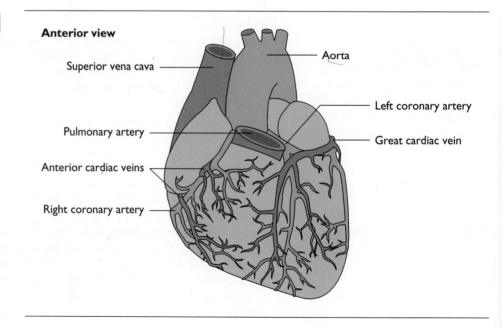

The Blood

Plasma, a clear yellowish fluid that carries approximately 100 chemicals, constitutes about 55 percent of the blood. The other 45 percent is made up of several types of cells that are suspended in the plasma. These include the **erythrocytes** (red cells), **leukocytes** (white cells), and **blood platelets.** The red cells, which represent the majority of blood cells, carry oxygen and carbon dioxide to and from the tissues of the body. **Hemoglobin**—the iron-containing protein of the red cells—combines with and transports oxygen to the tissues. The white cells are the body's defense mechanism against invading microorganisms and are actively engaged in combatting bacterial infections and other foreign substances that invade the body. The blood platelets are involved in the process of clotting and repair of damaged blood vessels. See Figure 7.6 for the composition of blood.

CARDIOVASCULAR DISEASES: THE TWENTIETH-CENTURY EPIDEMIC

Cardiovascular disease is a phenomenon of this century. The reasons advanced for this unfortunate occurrence relate to the living habits discussed in Chapter 1. There are several types of cardiovascular disease.

Congenital Heart Diseases

Congenital heart diseases—more accurately labeled as congenital heart defects— exist at birth and occur when the heart or its structures or the blood vessels near the heart fail to develop normally before birth. Approximately 30,000 infants are affected annually, and 5,800 of them die from heart defects. Medical scientists are not sure of the causes, but it appears that maternal alcohol and other drug abuse are implicated. Viral infections may also interfere with the normal development of the heart during uterine life. Many congenital defects can be identified and corrected as a result of new diagnostic methods and sophisticated surgical techniques. Undiagnosed congenital heart defects are usually the cause of death when a young, seemingly healthy athlete collapses and dies during athletic competition.

Rheumatic Heart Disease

Rheumatic heart disease affects youngsters between the ages of 5 and 15. This form of heart disease is virtually 100 percent preventable because it progresses through a series of stages initiated by a streptococcal infection. The first phase is usually a

---

FIGURE 7.6

Blood Composition Blood removed from a person can be centrifuged to separate plasma from the cellular component. Red blood cells constitute about 45% of the blood volume, except at higher altitudes where they make up about 50% of the volume to compensate for the lower oxygen levels.

Source: Adapted from Chiras, *Biology: The Web of Life,* 1993, West Publishing Company. Reproduced with Permission. Art rendered by John and Judy Waller.

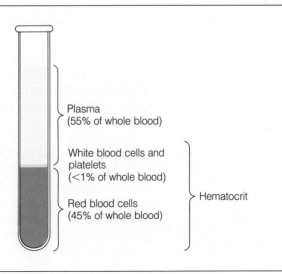

Plasma
(55% of whole blood)

White blood cells and platelets
(<1% of whole blood)

Red blood cells
(45% of whole blood)

Hematocrit

strep throat and sometimes a strep ear. Antibiotic treatment at this stage will arrest the infection and prevent it from developing into rheumatic heart disease.

Congestive Heart Failure

Congestive heart failure occurs when the heart muscle is unable to contract with sufficient force to effectively pump blood throughout the body. The major causes are high blood pressure, atherosclerosis, heart attack, rheumatic fever, and birth defects. Treatment centers upon drug therapy, including diuretics to remove excess fluid and medication to increase the heart's contractile power. Exercise does not contribute to the prevention of congential or rheumatic heart disease, but it exerts a preventive or delaying effect upon some of the processes that produce congestive heart failure.

Coronary Heart Disease

Coronary heart disease is the leading cause of death in the United States.[4] In 1989, this lethal form of cardiovascular disease, was responsible for 497, 850 deaths and 1.5 million heart attacks. Coronary heart disease is actually a disease of the coronary blood vessels that supply the heart with oxygen and nutrients. A heart attack, or **myocardial infarction** (death of heart muscle tissue), occurs when obstructions or spasms disrupt the flow of blood to a portion of the heart muscle. The location of the obstruction or spasm determines the extent of muscle damage. Heart attacks of any magnitude result in irreversible injury and myocardial tissue death. The dead tissue forms a scar, contributes no further to the function of the heart, and results in a less efficient pump. If the heart attack causes extensive muscle damage, the heart will die and, of course, so will its host.

Although most heart attack deaths occur late in life (55 percent after age 65), the processes that cause them begin quite early—often before adolescence. These processes are insidious and often undetected until, without warning, a heart attack occurs. The attack is sudden, but the processes are long-standing. The medical community accepts moderate exercise as an important strategy in the prevention of and rehabilitation from coronary heart disease.

Strokes

Cerebrovascular (*cerebro:* brain; *vascular:* blood vessels) **accidents,** or strokes, in many instances follow the same course as coronary heart disease. The problem takes years to develop, strokes are essentially a disease of the blood vessels that supply the brain, they share the same risk factors as coronary heart disease, and they respond to exercise. Strokes are caused by a thrombus (a clot that forms and enlarges in an artery leading to the brain) or an embolus (a clot that forms elsewhere, dislodges or fractures, and circulates to one of the cerebral arteries that is too small for its passage). Cerebral hemorrhage—the bursting of a blood vessel in the brain—is a third cause of stroke. This can result from head trauma or an aneurysm (a weak spot in an artery that forms a blood-filled pouch similar to a balloon that may burst and bleed into the brain). Another type of hemorrhage (subarachnoid) occurs when a blood vessel on the surface of the brain bursts and bleeds into the space between the brain and the skull, but not the brain itself.

The amount of bleeding determines the severity of the stroke. Fifty percent of the strokes caused by a cerebral hemorrhage lead to death because of increased pressure on the brain. Those who survive are apt to recover more fully than stroke victims whose stroke was caused by a blood clot. The reason for this is that blood clots result in oxygen deprivation to a portion of the brain. That portion dies and never regenerates. The prognosis is better for a survivor of a stroke caused by a cerebral hemorrhage because the pressure will gradually diminish and the brain will possibly return to its former state as the dried blood is absorbed by the body.

Heart Attacks

Some heart attacks are silent and imperceptible to the victim. These attacks, which are quite common, involve small areas of heart muscle and may go unnoticed or undetected unless discovered by an electrocardiogram (ECG or EKG). But if a clot occurs in a large vessel supplying a substantial amount of heart muscle, the individual will experience some or all of the various symptoms of a heart attack (see Figure 7.7), and a larger portion of the heart will die. If the attack is of massive proportions, the victim will die.

POINTS TO PONDER

1. The causes of death in the United States have changed since 1990. How have they changed, and why have they changed?
2. Discuss the function of the heart as a double pump. What are the functions of the pulmonary and systemic pump?
3. What is coronary heart disease?
4. What are the signs and symptoms of a heart attack? A stroke?
5. Describe the electrical conduction system of the heart.
6. What is an aneurysm?
7. Why is rheumatic heart disease preventable?

◤ CARDIOVASCULAR RISK FACTORS

There are certain characteristics that increase the likelihood of developing cardiovascular disease. These characteristics are referred to as risk factors. Some of these can be changed while others cannot, but a healthy lifestyle can affect both categories of risk factors in a positive way. The risk factors that cannot be changed will be discussed first.

FIGURE 7.7

Signs of Heart Attack

Source: The American Heart Association.

1. Uncomfortable pressure, fullness, squeezing, or pain in the center of the chest that lasts longer than two minutes.
2. Pain that spreads to the shoulders, arms, or neck.
3. Severe pain, dizziness, fainting, sweating, nausea, or shortness of breath can occur.

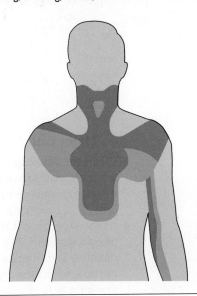

Major Risk Factors That Can't Be Changed

Heredity According to the American Heart Association, "A tendency toward heart disease or atherosclerosis appears to be hereditary, so children of parents with cardiovascular diseases are more likely to develop it themselves."[5] Separating genetic factors from a learned lifestyle is a complex problem. An overweight individual with elevated blood pressure and cholesterol may be the product not of heredity but of an overindulgent and underactive lifestyle. First-degree relatives (parents, grandparents, siblings) who have died of coronary diseases before the age of 55 would strongly indicate the possibility of familial tendencies toward cardiovascular disease. If your family history reads this way, it is imperative that you make an effort to keep the modifiable risk factors in check.

Male Sex Men are and have been the primary candidates for cardiovascular disease. As a result, research studies have used males as subjects when attempting to discover the causes, risks, and treatments of cardiovascular disease. Until recently, many physicians regarded cardiovascular disease as a minor threat to premenopausal women. Also, physicians have historically treated heart disease in women less aggressively than they do for men.

This unintentional neglect is rapidly disappearing because the statistics clearly indicate a high incidence of cardiovascular disease, death and disability among women.[6] In 1989, all cardiovascular diseases combined resulted in the death of 503,000 women. Coronary heart disease alone accounted for 240,000 deaths among women, and more than 90,000 women died of stroke.[7] By comparison, all forms of cancer kill less than half the number of women who die of cardiovascular disease.

The realization that women are almost as susceptible to cardiovascular disease as men has prompted the National Institutes of Health to initiate a 500-million-dollar, 10-year, community-based research project to study the effects of health maintenance strategies and therapies on the cardiovascular health of women.

The risk factors associated with the onset of heart disease impact both males and females.[8] Premenopausal women are unlikely candidates for heart disease if they have no risk factors. But women with a family history and one or more of the other risk factors are at a significant risk. Before menopause, women are at less risk than men because estrogen (the female sex hormone) and generally favorable blood/fat ratios protect the coronary arteries from premature damage. After menopause (permanent cessation of the menstrual cycle), women's vulnerability to heart disease increases. A post-menopausal 60-year-old woman runs the same risk of heart attack as a 50-year-old man. By her late seventies, the woman's risk will be equal to that of a man her own age.

Increasing Age Although Americans 65 years of age and older represent about 12 percent of the total population, their health care expenditure is approximately one-third of the U.S. total.[9] Cardiovascular diseases, primarily coronary heart disease, are responsible for 55 percent of the total number of heart attacks that occur and 80 percent of all fatalities from heart attacks. The statistical probability that death will occur from heart disease increases with advancing age.

Major Risk Factors That Can Be Changed

Cigarette Smoking Cigarette smoking is considered the most potent of the preventable risk factors associated with chronic illness and premature death. It is directly responsible for 21 percent of all mortality from heart disease[10] and 35 percent of all cancer mortality.[11] Smoking is involved in 390,000 deaths annually.

Forty percent of the population smoked cigarettes in 1965, but by 1987, this figure dropped to 29 percent.[12] The decline has been much greater for males than females. The number of women smokers declined by about 5 percent, but the proportion of deaths from coronary heart disease attributable directly to cigarette smoking actually increased from 26 percent in 1965 to 41 percent in 1985. This

Of all people alive today, fully 500 million will die from tobacco-related diseases according to estimates by the World Health Organization.
—University of California, Berkeley, *Wellness Letter* October 1992

apparent anomaly is explained by the fact that there is a dose-response relationship between the number of cigarettes smoked and the risk of heart disease.[13] Women who continue to smoke are smoking more heavily, and the percentage of those who smoke more than 25 cigarettes a day has risen in the past decade.

Smoking accounts for almost half of all heart attacks that occur in women before the age of 55. In a mistaken effort to lower the risk of heart disease, a number of women have switched to "low-yield" cigarettes (low in tars and nicotine). But the evidence indicates that this practice does not materially reduce the excess risk.[14]

The risk of heart disease decreases rapidly in both men and women who quit smoking.[15] The heart attack risk is similar to that of nonsmokers after one quits for two to three years. This time period was found to be constant regardless of how long or how much a person smoked. The cancer risk takes longer to normalize—7 to 10 years.

Ninety percent of former smokers report quitting on their own.[16] A number of stop-smoking programs and techniques are available, including professional counseling, nicotine chewing gum, nicotine skin patches, artificial cigarettes, hypnosis, acupuncture, aversive conditioning, and behavioral self-management. The one-year success rate for these programs and techniques ranges from 10 percent to 40 percent.[17]

Exercise offers another option for cigarette smokers who have inclinations to become nonsmokers. The bottom line may be that if one is truly committed to quitting, one will succeed in spite of the method, but if the resolve is weak, one will fail regardless of the method. Exercise is a viable and valid option because the benefits received from physical activity cannot be maximized while continuing to smoke. Many smokers who become hooked on the exercise and fitness habit become unhooked from the smoking habit.

Complicating the effort to quit smoking for young adults is the fear of gaining weight. Of course, exercise is an effective weight-management technique and can play a significant role in this regard. In addition, exercise is so good at producing relaxation that it may lessen the anxiety that often accompanies quitting. Women are more likely than men to continue smoking as a means of weight control.[18] Approximately 65 percent of those who quit smoking do gain weight. The mechanisms involved are not well understood but the most likely candidates include metabolism that slows down (fewer calories being burned) and a slower advancement of food through the digestive tract so that more of the calories are absorbed by the body. These mechanisms may be responsible for a 7- to 8-pound weight gain. Additional weight gain is due to altered eating patterns and sedentary habits. When a person no longer smokes, food smells and tastes better, it can act as a substitute for a cigarette, especially during social activities or periods of anxiety or tension, and it can provide some of the oral gratification once obtained from cigarettes. Weight gain can be avoided by appropriate exercise coupled with sensible eating.

Smokers often light up reflexively—they aren't aware of it. Various cues stimulate this automatic behavior. Smokers light up after a meal, with a cup of coffee or an alcoholic drink, while talking on the telephone, at social gatherings, at parties, when they feel anxious or tense, and when they get into the car to drive anywhere. These smoking triggers have reinforced smoking behavior for many years. The ties between these social cues and smoking are extremely difficult to break and can last for years, constantly tempting the ex-smoker.

As a group, cigarette smokers are 7 percent lighter than a matched group of nonsmokers.[19] This apparent benefit appears to be better than it actually is, since smoking encourages the body to deposit fat in the abdomen and upper body, and fat distributed in this manner is associated with and increases the risk of heart disease, stroke, diabetes, and some forms of cancer.[20] Even a few extra pounds deposited in this manner increases the risk. Fat that accumulates in the lower half of the body (hips, buttocks, and thighs) does not appear to carry the same degree of risk.

Iowa became the first state to make it illegal for anyone under the age of 18 to smoke a cigarette. The sale of cigarettes to minors is illegal in 44 states (it is rarely enforced) but it is not against the law for minors to smoke cigarettes.
—University of California, Berkeley, *Wellness Letter* November 1991

Cigarettes contain many hazardous products, including **carbon monoxide** and other poisonous gases, **nicotine,** tars, and chemical additives for flavor and taste. Carbon monoxide is a noxious gas that is the by-product of combustible tobacco products (cigarettes, cigars, pipe). Hemoglobin, the protein pigment that carries oxygen in the blood stream, has a much greater affinity for carbon monoxide. When both are present in the air, carbon monoxide displaces oxygen by attaching to hemoglobin. Carbon monoxide does not disassociate rapidly from hemoglobin. It has a half-life of about 5 ½ hours. As a result, the oxygen-carrying capacity of the blood is reduced. Carbon monoxide is absorbed with every puff of tobacco smoke that is inhaled and probably accounts for the shortness of breath experienced by smokers during moderate physical exertion such as climbing a couple of flights of stairs or walking up a hill.

Nicotine is a powerful stimulant that has a profound effect on the cardiovascular system. The following are some of its major consequences:

1. It has a negative effect on serum cholesterol, which increases the risk for heart disease and stroke.

2. It contributes to spasms of the coronary blood vessels that may cause chest pain or heart attack.

3. It increases the oxygen requirements of the heart at rest and during physical exertion.

4. It constricts small blood vessels, increasing peripheral resistance to blood flow.

5. It contributes to irregular heartbeats.

The tobacco industry has not divulged the sources of the chemical additives in cigarettes. It is not regulated by the Food and Drug Administration, and no other governmental agency has the power to force such disclosure. These chemicals may or may not be carcinogenic (cancer-producing). The best guess at this time is that cigarettes contain 2,000 to 4,000 chemicals at least 30 of which are carcinogenic.

Cigarette sales have declined because the "quitters" are outnumbering those who take up smoking for the first time. To partly compensate for the loss, tobacco companies are aggressively pursuing the export of their products to other countries. They are also marketing "smokeless" tobacco products in the United States. Young males are the primary users of these products, but a few teenage females are also regular users. The typical smokeless tobacco user begins to experiment with these products by the age of 10.[21]

Nicotine is an addictive drug regardless of the method of delivery. The effects are the same whether it is inhaled, as in cigarette smoking, or absorbed through the tissues of the oral cavity, as in chewing or dipping. When the users of either of these products stop using them, they suffer an array of withdrawal symptoms—restlessness, anxiety, irritability, and sleep disturbances.

The American Cancer Society estimates that there were 30,600 new cases of oral cancer in 1989. When tobacco is held in the mouth, nicotine and other substances, some of which are carcinogenic, are absorbed through the oral tissues. The prevalence of oral cancer may be 50 times higher among long-term users of smokeless tobacco than for nonusers. The incidence of tooth decay and gum diseases is also significantly higher in users of these products. The data indicate that smokeless tobacco is both addictive and deadly.

Involuntary or passive smoking is associated with premature disease and death. Estimates indicate that 53,000 nonsmokers who are regularly exposed to the smoke of others (environmental smoke) die annually.[22] The vast majority of these—37,000—succumb to heart disease, another 4,000 die of lung cancer, and the remaining 12,000 die of other forms of cancer.

The risk of heart disease for a nonsmoker who is married to a smoker increases by 30 percent. Once again, there is a dose-response effect—the more the smoker smokes, the greater the risk to the nonsmoker. If the nonsmoking spouse works in a smoking environment, the risk increases according to the total exposure.

Inhaling the smoke of others is a serious cause of atherosclerosis and heart attacks. Cigarette smoke, either direct or environmental, damages the walls of the coronary arteries. The damage is believed to result from the action of smoke particles called "polycyclic aromatic hydrocarbons." Additionally, cigarette smoke activates the blood platelets which can cause a spasm or blood clot to occur in a diseased artery. All of the compounds that damage the blood vessels of active smokers are also present in environmental smoke.

Children of smoking parents are more likely to experience higher ratios of respiratory illness, including colds, influenza, bronchitis, asthma, and pneumonia. The lung capacity of young male children was decreased by 7 percent when their mothers were smokers, and when teenage boys of smoking mothers also smoked, their lung capacity was reduced by 25 percent. The impact of passive smoking on children can last a lifetime, and it may include delayed physical and intellectual development as well as the hazards associated with prolonged exposure to carcinogenic substances.

The price tag due to smoking is shared by all Americans—smokers and nonsmokers alike. Premature death, medical treatment for smoking-related illnesses, and lost productivity run approximately $65 billion annually. This translates to $2.17 expended for every pack of cigarettes sold. The financial cost to the smoker just to purchase tobacco products for a lifetime of use is staggering, and smokers lose in other financial ways as well. Nonsmoking men and women collect more of their retirement benefits than do smokers, simply because they live longer. Nonsmoking men collect $21,000 and nonsmoking women collect $9,000 more than smokers in Social Security benefits.

The medical profession measures smoking danger in pack-years. For example, smoking one pack per day for 20 years results in 20 pack years (20 years × 1 pack per day = 20 pack-years). One and one-half packs per day for 20 years equals 30 pack-years (20 × 1 ½ = 30). Twenty to twenty-five pack years represent a point beyond which medical problems associated with smoking become evident. Cigarette smoking is such a serious threat to public health the the Surgeon General has set a goal of a smoke-free society by the year 2000.

Blood Pressure Blood Pressure—recorded in millimeters of mercury (mm Hg)—is the force exerted against the walls of the arteries as blood courses through the circulatory system. A certain level of pressure, created by contractions of the heart muscle, is needed to circulate blood throughout the body. Blood pressures that exceed normal limits are referred to as **hypertension.**

Blood pressure is routinely measured by an indirect method using a sphygmomanometer (see Figure 7.8). The measurement consists of two readings. The larger number, or **systolic pressure,** represents the pressure of blood flow in the vessels when the heart beats. The second, and smaller measure of the two, is the **diastolic pressure,** which represents the pressure between heart beats. An average adult blood pressure is 120/80 (read as 120 over 80). Normality covers a range of blood pressure from low normal (100/60) to high normal (140/90). The standards developed for classifying blood pressures in adults are found in Table 7.1.

The heart is adversely affected by long-standing hypertension. Pumping blood against high resistance in the arteries increases the workload of the heart. As a result, the heart enlarges much as any other muscle that is stimulated over a period of time. The problem for the heart is that since the resistance is consistently high, the heart receives inadequate rest. Years of pumping against such a resistance produces muscle fibers that become overly extended or stretched. The muscle fibers progressively lose their ability to snap back, and the end result is a less forceful contraction. The heart becomes inefficient and weak. The blood vessels are affected when blood pressure is high because hypertension may lead to tears of the interior lining of the arteries accelerating the process of atherosclerosis.

Children whose mothers smoke at least half a pack of cigarettes a day are twice as likely to have asthma as children of nonsmoking mothers.
—University of California, Berkeley, *Wellness Letter* November 1990

The number of premature deaths due to smoking in the U.S. is the equivalent of 920 fully loaded 747 jumbo jets crashing every year—350,000 people each year.
—American Lung Association

FIGURE 7.8

Using a Sphygmomanometer to Measure Blood Pressure

Source: Chiras *Biology: The Web of Life*, 1993, West Publishing Company. Reproduced with Permission. Art rendered by John and Judy Waller.

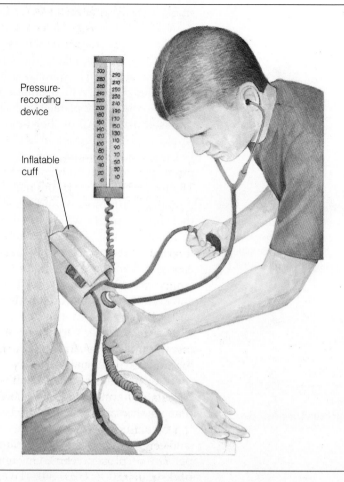

Pressure-recording device

Inflatable cuff

62,770,000 American adults and children have high blood pressure.
—American Heart Association

Hypertension can usually be controlled with medication, salt restriction, weight loss, and exercise. Since medications for controlling blood pressure can produce undesirable side effects, a better strategy might concentrate upon salt restriction, weight control, and exercise supplemented with such stress-reduction techniques as progressive muscle relaxation, Benson's relaxation response, transcendental meditation, yoga, biofeedback, and hypnotherapy. Explaining, defining, and demonstrating these techniques is beyond the scope of this text, and the interested reader is encouraged to learn from instructors of these methods or possibly from self-help books. However, the following guidelines might provide some insight for budding practitioners of these techniques. First, find a quiet place that is free of interruptions. Sit in a comfortable position, close your eyes, and repeat a phrase, such as "I am relaxed," with each exhalation. Do this daily for five minutes for about two weeks, and you should be able to determine whether this type of exercise is appropriate for you. Next, select one of the relaxation techniques mentioned above. You may need to experiment with more than one of them to find the one most effective for you. Then, you need to practice the technique every day; most techniques require that you participate twice a day. Practice will improve your ability to relax. There is no guarantee that blood pressure can be normalized without medication, but many people have experienced success utilizing these approaches, and control without drugs is highly desirable.

Essential hypertension constitutes 90 percent to 95 percent of all blood pressure problems. In medical terms, *essential* means "of unknown cause." This type of hypertension is incurable, but it is treatable by those behaviors and techniques previously mentioned. If the lifestyle behaviors are not effective in normalizing the blood pressure, medication must be added to the mix.

Salt restriction is an important strategy in the control of blood pressure. Salt consists of 40 percent sodium and 60 percent chloride. Sodium is the component

TABLE 7.1	Standards for Classification of Blood Pressure for Adults Age 18 Years and Older

CATEGORY	SYSTOLIC (mm Hg)	DIASTOLIC (mm Hg)
Normal	< 130	< 85
High Normal	130–139	85–89
Hypertension		
Stage 1 (Mild)	140–159	90–99
Stage 2 (Moderate)	160–179	100–109
Stage 3 (Severe)	180–209	110–119
Stage 4 (Very Severe)	≥210	≥120

Source: National Institutes of Health, *The Fifth Report of the Joint National Committee on Detection, Evaluation and Treatment of High Blood Pressure*, U.S. Dept. of Health and Human Services: NIH Publication No. 93-1088, January, 1993.

that raises the blood pressure. The average American consumes 7.5 to 18 grams of salt per day which translates to 3 to 7 grams of sodium. (A teaspoon of salt is equivalent to 5 grams of salt, 2 of which are sodium.) Nutritional guidelines suggest that adults limit their sodium intake to 2.4 to 3.0 grams per day to limit the risk of hypertension.[23]

Approximately 10 percent of the U.S. population is salt sensitive, and these people must carefully monitor their salt intake. Salt increases the blood pressure because it encourages the body to retain water, which distributes itself in all fluid compartments, including the blood stream. The expanded plasma volume in the circulatory system requires more force to transport it through the blood vessels. People who are not salt sensitive would do well to restrict their intake just to be on the safe side.

Weight loss is another component in the management of blood pressure. Excess fat places a strain or greater workload upon the heart, which must meet the circulatory demands of the extra tissue. Weight loss usually results in a lowered blood pressure.

Daily drinking of alcoholic beverages will raise the blood pressure of some people. More than two ounces of alcohol a day seems to be a threshold for raising blood pressure. Two ounces of alcohol can be obtained by drinking two four-ounce glasses of wine, two eight-ounce glasses of beer, or two shots or jiggers of hard liquor. Alcohol should be eliminated from the diet or at least consumed in moderation.

Exercise is another contributor to blood pressure control. A number of investigations have found that aerobic exercise can lower the blood pressure of hypertensive and borderline hypertensive people. The studies found that people who had exercised had systolic blood pressures that were 5 to 25 mm Hg lower than nonexercisers and diastolic pressures that were 3 to 15 mm Hg lower.[24] Aerobic exercises seem to have the greatest effect in lowering the blood pressure, but there is evidence that weight training can also have a lowering effect.

The Harvard Alumni study was a major epidemiological investigation that followed thousands of subjects for many years. The results indicated that those who did not engage in vigorous sports or physical activities had a 35 percent greater risk of developing hypertension than those who were regularly active, and this relationship held for all ages from 35 to 74.

There are several possibilities regarding the mechanisms through which exercise lowers blood pressure. Adrenaline (epinephrine) and noradrenaline (norepinephrine) are important hormones that regulate blood pressure. Both decrease the diameters of the arterioles (the smallest arteries). Training reduces the circulating level of noradrenaline, allowing the arterioles to relax and thus lowering the diastolic pressure. Furthermore, this effect is independent of weight loss. Also, there is usually a post-exercise reduction in blood pressure that lasts for an average of 12.7 hours for hypertensive men. This effect is independent of the intensity of exercise,[25] probably because of the vasodilation of the arterioles and a reduction in resistance to blood flow that may persist if exercise is continued on a regular basis. Additionally, cells become more sensitive to insulin. As a result, the insulin level in the blood decreases, leading to sodium excretion by the kidneys and a lower blood pressure.[26] Finally, exercise contributes to weight loss. This is considered a secondary rather than a direct effect. Reducing the body weight is almost guaranteed to reduce the blood pressure to some extent.

High blood pressure is found in 2.8 million children and adolescents ages 6 to 17. The roots of much adult hypertension can be traced back to childhood. In fact, most childhood hypertension tracks into adulthood.[27] Most cases of pediatric and adolescent hypertension are classified essential and can be treated with exercise and diet.[28] Average blood pressures and categories of hypertension for children and adolescents are presented by age and gender in Table 7.2.

Cholesterol   Chemically, **cholesterol** is an organic substance classified as a crystalline or solid alcohol. It is a steroid required for the manufacture of hormones as well as bile (for the digestion and absorption of fats), it serves as one of the structural components of neural tissue, and it is used in the construction of cell walls.[29] A certain amount of cholesterol is essential for good health, but high levels in the blood are associated with heart attack and stroke. Since the liver produces enough cholesterol to meet the body's needs, cholesterol does not have to be consumed to maintain health.[30]

Although Americans consume 400 to 500 mg of cholesterol daily, the amount suggested by the American Heart Association is less than 300 mg. Additionally, 37 percent to 38 percent of the total calories consumed by the typical American comes from fat, almost half of which is saturated. Dietary cholesterol, or **exogenous cholesterol,** contributes to the level of serum cholesterol (that which circulates in the blood). (Table 7.3 lists selected foods and their cholesterol and saturated fat content.) An even greater source of serum cholesterol comes from that which is manufactured **(endogenous cholesterol)** by the liver from saturated fats. The liver manages to produce 1,000 to 2,000 mg of cholesterol per day. Most authorities suggest that it may be more important to limit one's intake of saturated fat than to be overly restrictive of dietary cholesterol, although it is prudent to limit both.

TABLE 7.2   **Standards Defining Upper Blood Pressure Ranges (Systolic/Diastolic) for Children and Adolescents**

	MALES				FEMALES			
Age	Average	Upper Normal	Hypertension	Severe Hypertension	Average	Upper Normal	Hypertension	Severe Hypertension
6	95/57	111/70	115/74	121/80	96/57	111/70	115/73	122/82
7	97/58	112/71	116/75	124/84	97/58	112/71	116/75	124/84
8	99/60	113/72	117/76	124/84	99/59	113/72	118/76	126/84
9	101/61	115/74	119/77	128/86	100/61	115/74	119/77	126/84
10	102/62	117/75	122/78	130/86	102/62	117/75	121/79	130/86
11	105/63	119/76	123/80	132/88	105/64	119/77	123/81	134/86
12	107/64	122/77	126/81	134/88	107/65	122/78	126/82	134/88
13	109/66	124/77	128/81	140/84	109/67	124/78	128/83	138/86
14	112/64	126/78	130/82	144/87	111/67	125/81	129/85	138/90
15	114/65	129/79	133/83	146/88	111/68	126/82	130/86	138/86
16	117/67	132/81	136/85	149/90	112/67	127/81	131/85	140/88
17	119/69	133/83	138/87	150/90	112/66	127/81	132/84	138/88
18	121/70	136/84	140/88	153/94	113/66	127/80	132/84	139/89

Adapted from the National Heart, Blood, and Lung Institute's Task Force on Blood Pressure Control in Children—1987, *Pediatrics*, 79, no. 1 (1987): 1.

TABLE 7.3   Dietary Cholesterol and Saturated Fat

ITEM	CHOLESTEROL (IN MILLIGRAMS)*	SATURATED FAT (IN MILLIGRAMS)*
Meats (3 oz)		
Beef liver	372	2500
Veal	86	4000
Pork	80	3200
Lean beef	56	2400
Chicken (dark meat)	82	2700
Chicken (white meat)	76	1300
One egg	215	1700
Dairy Products (1 cup; cheese, 1 oz)		
Ice cream	59	8900
Whole milk	33	5100
Butter (1 tbsp)	31	7100
Yogurt (low fat)	11	1800
Cheddar cheese	30	6000
American cheese	27	5600
Camembert cheese	20	4300
Parmesan cheese	8	2000
Oils (1 tbsp)		
Coconut	0	11,800
Palm	0	6700
Olive	0	1800
Corn	0	1700
Safflower	0	1200
Fish (3 oz)		
Squid	153	200
Oily fish	59	1200
Lean fish	59	300
Shrimp (6 large)	48	200
Clams (6 large)	36	300
Lobster	46.5	75
Other Foods		
Pork brains	2169	1800
Beef kidney	683	3800
Beef hot dog	75	9900
Prime rib of beef	66.5	5300
Doughnut	36	4000
Milk chocolate (1 oz.)	18	16,300
Green or yellow vegetable or fruit	0	trace
Peanut butter (1 tbsp)	0	1500
Angel food cake	0	1960
Skim milk (1 cup)	4	300
Cheese pizza (3 oz)	6	800
Buttermilk (1 cup)	9	1300
Ice milk, soft (1 cup)	13	2900
Turkey, white meat (3 oz)	59	900

*1000 mg = 1 gram; 454 grams = 1 lb.

Ideally, plasma cholesterol levels should be below 200 mg/dL (read as milligrams of cholesterol per deciliter of blood). Table 7.4 illustrates and quantifies the risk of cardiac disease associated with various cholesterol levels. Actually, the ideal cholesterol level for adults is found between 130 and 190 mg/dL.

Some observational studies have demonstrated an inverse relationship between cholesterol and certain types of cancer; that is, people with very low cholesterol levels had a higher than normal death rate from cancer, particularly cancer of the colon. Of course, this was very unsettling news, considering that low cholesterol levels, which decrease the risk of cardiovascular disease, seemed to increase the risk of cancer. However, later studies indicated that the decrease in cholesterol occurred secondarily to the onset of cancer or other disease processes associated with an increased risk of cancer. In other words, the cancer was in its incipient or preclinical stage and had not yet been detected. Cancerous cells consume more cholesterol than healthy cells, and this gives credence to the concept that cancer significantly reduces the level of cholesterol rather than that low cholesterol causes cancer. If your cholesterol level drops substantially without reason (diet modification, weight loss, exercise, etc.), you should schedule a medical checkup.

After reviewing the research, the National Heart, Lung, and Blood Institute has concluded that the relationship between high serum cholesterol and heart disease is a causal one.[31] Several of the studies in that review indicated that every 1 percent reduction in serum cholesterol resulted in a 2 percent to 3 percent reduction in the risk of heart disease.

Strategies for lowering total cholesterol include (1) reduction in dietary cholesterol and saturated fat, (2) increase in the consumption of soluble fiber (found in oats, beans, fruits, and vegetables), (3) weight loss, and (4) cessation of cigarette smoking.

> We are persuaded that the blood cholesterol levels of most Americans are undesirably high, in large part because of our high dietary intake of calories, saturated fat, and cholesterol.
> —National Heart, Lung, and Blood Institute

REDUCE THE CHOLESTEROL RISK— EAT WALNUTS

Can eating walnuts really lower one's blood cholesterol level? The answer, according to a recent *New England Journal of Medicine* study, is yes. The results of the study suggested that substituting walnuts, which are high in monounsaturated fat, for an equal amount of fat in a cholesterol-lowering diet was more effective in lowering serum cholesterol than the standard diet. In other words, the effect of the diet containing walnuts on the lipoprotein risk profile was more favorable than that of the standard cholesterol-lowering diet. This occurred in spite of the fact that the subjects had relatively low serum cholesterol levels at the start of the study. The walnut eaters (the diet lasted only four weeks) reduced their total cholesterol level 12.4% and LDL cholesterol 16.3% more than the subjects on the standard diet.

A prior study found that people who ate nuts five or more times per week had only one half the risk of suffering a heart attack compared to those who never eat nuts. The protective effect of nuts was independent of other risk factors, including a number of other foods, and was consistent across several population subgroups.

The investigators suggest that one ounce of walnuts per day will provide substantial protection against heart attacks. Remember, however, that walnuts are high in calories, with about 81% of their total calories being derived from fat.

Sources: J. Sabate et al., "Effect of Walnuts on Serum Lipid Levels and Blood Pressure in Normal Men," *New England Journal of Medicine*, March 4, 1993, p. 603. G. E. Fraser et al., "A Possible Protective Effect of Nut Consumption on Risk of Coronary Heart Disease: The Adventist Health Study," *Archives of Internal Medicine* 152 (1992): 1416.

TABLE 7.4

Cholesterol Level and Cardiac Risk

CHOLESTEROL (MG/DL)	RISK
Less than 200	Desirable level
200–239	Borderline
240 or greater	High level

Adapted from "Report of the National Cholesterol Education Program Expert Panel on Detection, Evaluation, and Treatment of High Blood Cholesterol in Adults," *Archives of Internal Medicine*, 148, (January, 1988): 36.

The amount of circulating cholesterol in the blood accounts for only a part of the story. To gain greater insight into cholesterol as a risk factor, one must understand how cholesterol is packaged and transported in the circulatory system. To begin, the mechanisms of cholesterol distribution are very complex and not completely known at this time, but researchers are continuing to unravel the mystery. The following paragraphs are a brief synopsis of the synthesis, transport, and function of cholesterol.

Cholesterol does not dissolve in the blood in a manner similar to sugar and salt. It is transported through the circulatory system attached to protein packages that facilitate its solubility. These transporters, the lipoproteins (fats bound to a protein) include (1) the chylomicrons, (2) very low density lipoprotein **(VLDL),** (3) intermediate density lipoprotein (IDL), (4) low-density lipoprotein **(LDL),** and high-density lipoprotein **(HDL).** Each of the lipoproteins carries different concentrations of fats (lipids) and protein (see Figure 7.9 for the concentrations). Note in Figure 7.9 the size relationship between the lipoproteins. Note also that each of the lipoproteins carries triglycerides, phospholipids, and cholesterol. The greater the concentration of lipids, the less dense the lipoprotein.

The **chylomicrons** are fatty particles produced in the intestinal wall that are the major carriers of triglycerides. The chylomicrons circulate through the blood stream until eventually coming in contact with binding sites on the capillaries where they release most of their triglyceride load to the muscles and adipose tissues (fat cells). They are essentially stripped of their cargo approximately 12 to 14 hours after leaving the digestive system. The liver contains receptor sites that recognize, remove, and dismantle these chylomicron remnants, from which the liver manufactures VLDL (the largest of the lipoproteins).

The VLDLs transport triglycerides that are made in the liver from fats, carbohydrates, alcohol, and cholesterol. VLDLs exit the liver and circulate to the capillaries, where their triglycerides are removed, broken down, and used for energy or storage by the muscles and adipose cells. The remnants are referred to as intermediate density lipoproteins (IDLs). Some of the IDLs are removed from circulation by the liver, but the remainder are transformed into low-density lipoproteins (LDLs). Sixty to eighty percent of all of the cholesterol circulating through the blood stream is carried by the LDLs.

The evidence linking LDL to coronary heart disease has been accumulating rapidly in the past decade. It appears that LDL is the most atherogenic (capable of producing atherosclerosis) of the lipoproteins. Our understanding of the role of LDL transport was substantially increased by the Nobel Prize winning research of Brown and Goldstein, who discovered that the cells have receptor sites that bind LDLs, thus removing them from the blood stream. Binding allows cholesterol to enter the cell, where it can be stored or used to synthesize plasma membranes, bile acids, and steroid hormones. By removing LDL from the blood for cellular use, the receptors contribute to the prevention of atherosclerosis. However, when the diet is high in animal fat (the typical American diet), the receptors become sat-

We now have strong evidence that lowering LDL concentrations will reduce the risk of coronary heart disease.

—Scott M. Grundy

FIGURE 7.9

Schematic of the Lipid Carriers

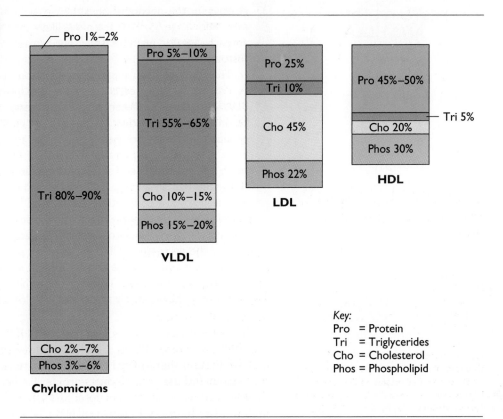

Chylomicrons

Key:
Pro = Protein
Tri = Triglycerides
Cho = Cholesterol
Phos = Phospholipid

urated and removal of LDL from the blood is significantly reduced. The excess LDLs are then oxidized in the cells of the artery walls. This is the beginning of atherosclerosis and the formation of plaques that eventually clog the arteries supplying the heart and brain.

LDLs are programmed to carry cholesterol to the cells of the body; they become harmful only when there are too many of them so that some are oxidized. Animal species who typically do not develop atherosclerosis have plasma LDL levels lower than 80 mg/dL. Human infants have LDL levels that are approximately 70 mg/dL, but this value increases with age. If a low-fat diet is maintained during growth and adulthood, LDL will generally remain below 80 mg/dL. The typical American diet usually results in an LDL value that exceeds 100 mg/dL. Heart attacks are rare when the LDL level is below 100 mg/dL. A national panel of experts has developed guidelines for LDL levels (see Table 7.5). While the panel stated that an LDL level below 130 mg/dL is desirable, it acknowledges that the lower the better. An LDL of 160 mg/dL is roughly equivalent to a total cholesterol (TC) of 240 mg/dL, and an LDL of 130 mg/dL is equivalent to a TC of 200 mg/dL to 239 mg/dL.

Low-density lipoprotein cholesterol may be lowered by reducing saturated fat and cholesterol in the diet.[32] Schafer concluded after a literature review that the optimal diet for the prevention of coronary artery disease consists of 10 percent to 15 percent of the total calories coming from protein, 65 percent from carbohydrate (mainly complex carbohydrate), 20 percent to 25 percent from fat (less than 10 percent saturated), and no more than 200 mg of cholesterol per day.[33] The results of at least two studies have shown that LDL levels respond to exercise, and people whose fitness has improved the most experience the greatest reduction. Conversely, excessive caloric intake produces an overproduction of VLDL. You will recall that LDLs are made from VLDL remnants; therefore, an increase in the latter will result in an accompanying increase in the former.

TABLE 7.5

Guidelines for LDL Levels

LDL CHOLESTEROL (MG/DL)	RISK
Less than 130	Desirable level
130–159	Borderline–high risk
160 or greater	High risk

Adapted from "Report of the National Cholesterol Education Program Expert Panel on Detection, Evaluation, and Treatment of High Blood Cholesterol in Adults," *Archives of Internal Medicine*, 148, (1988): 36.

TESTOSTERONE AND HDL

Women live approximately eight years longer than men. One of the primary reasons for this phenomenon is the higher incident of heart attack deaths among men before age 55. Men are more likely than women to have a heart attack at an early age for many reasons, but a major factor is the male sex hormone testosterone.

Testosterone has a suppressant effect on the production of HDL cholesterol. A 1987 study by researchers at Baylor University College of Medicine of 57 boys who were at different stages of puberty indicated that increases in testosterone production affected the level of circulating HDL. The subjects were grouped according to their position on the puberty continuum. Those who were prepubertal had an average HDL of 66.6 mg/dL and were producing one tenth the testosterone of subjects who were at or nearing postpuberty. This latter group had an average HDL level of 54.4 mg/dL. As the stages of puberty advanced toward completion, the level of HDL decreased. Some of the prepubertal subjects were given injections of testosterone, and the HDL level was significantly reduced in two weeks. The larger the dose of testosterone, the greater the decrease of HDL. Adult males produce 10 to 20 times more testosterone than adult females and have HDL level that are typically below that of females of the same age. Testosterone, which is positively associated with virility, seems to be negatively associated with longevity.

An inverse relationship exists between HDL and heart disease. A low circulating level of serum HDL is a powerful independent predictor of coronary heart disease. Factors that lower HDL are cigarette smoking, diabetes, elevated triglycerides, and the use of anabolic steroids. Factors that increase HDL are moderate alcohol consumption, weight loss, and physical exercise. The most potent factor for stimulating the production of HDL is aerobic exercise. People who regularly participate in endurance exercises are leaner and more physically fit and have higher HDL, lower total cholesterol, and lower LDL than sedentary people. This profile is associated with a relatively lower risk for coronary heart disease and conversely reflects high-level wellness.

How much and what kind of exercise is needed, and how often should one exercise to change the pattern of cholesterol into a healthier one? Reducing the risk of heart disease begins with as little as 20 minutes of moderate intensity exercise just three days a week. Up to a point, more vigorous exercise performed more frequently and for a longer duration produces even greater results. A minimum of 1,000 calories per week expended in exercise and physical activity will significantly increase HDLs. This is translated into 10 miles of walking or its equivalent in a week's time. This is certainly an attainable goal within the reach of almost everyone. Middle-age mail carriers who are involved in daily low-level walking have higher HDLs than normally expected for this age group.[34] The implications of the results from various studies for public health are enormous. The suggestion is that one need not be a marathon runner to attain the health benefits of exercise. Instead, consistent low- to moderate-intensity exercise for at least 30 minutes a day, three to five days per week will suffice for health enhancement.

The effect of alcohol on HDL might prompt a few people to substitute a couple of drinks for exercise to produce the same effect. But HDL consists of subfractions, two of which are HDL2 and HDL3. HDL3 appears to be neutral in that it is not involved in the processes of arterial protection or disease. However, HDL2 is established as a protective element actively involved in the removal of cholesterol from the arteries. Alcohol appears to raise the neutral HDL3, while exercise increases the protective HDL2. However, raising total HDL by increasing either or both fractions seems to be protective. Based on that, alcohol does make a contribution, but it contributes only if used in moderation. Heavy alcohol consumption significantly increases the risk for heart disease, stroke, and cancer. Also, heavy drinking may lead to full-blown active alcoholism, which adds other life-threatening risks and the risk of premature death. It is definitely better to raise HDLs through exercise than through increased alcohol consumption. In addition, weight loss whether through exercise and/or diet also raises HDL cholesterol. This effect has been observed consistently.[35]

Researchers have examined the ratio between total cholesterol (TC) and HDL as a predictor of heart disease. Dividing TC by HDL yields a number that can be interpreted in terms of the risk for heart disease. Ratios of 5 and 4.5 represent the average risk for males and females, respectively. Table 7.6 elucidates the risk for values above and below the average.

Atherosclerosis is the major cause of cardiovascular and cerebrovascular disease. It is a slow progressive disease of large and medium size arteries in which fatty substances, cholesterol, calcium, fibrin, and cellular debris collect to obstruct the flow of blood. These elements are deposited in the arterial lining and bulge out to form fibrous lesions called plaques. Two catastrophic events occur when plaque grows to the point that it significantly narrows an arterial channel: (1) a hemorrhage or bleeding into the plaque can occur, and (2) a clot (thrombus) can

TABLE 7.6 Ratio of Total Cholesterol to HDL Cholesterol

RISK	MALE	FEMALE
Very low (½ average)	Under 3.4	Under 3.3
Low risk	4.0	3.8
Average risk	5.0	4.5
Moderate risk (2 × average)	9.5	7.0
High risk (3 × average)	Over 23	Over 11

Adapted from the "National Institutes of Health Consensus Development Conference Statement: Lowering Blood Cholesterol," *Journal of the American Medical Association* 253 (1985): 2080.

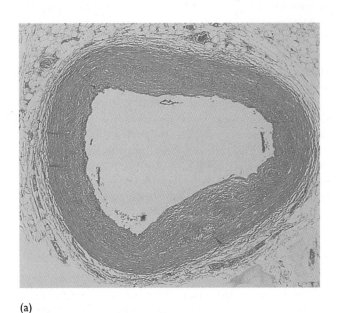

(a)

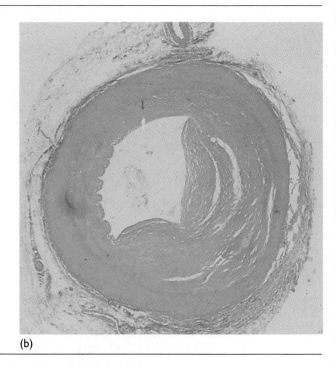

(b)

FIGURE 7.10

An Artery Undergoing Atherosclerosis Degeneration (a) Normal artery in cross-section. (b) Atheroslerotic artery that is significantly narrowed.

Source: Chiras *Biology: The Web of Life*, 1993, West Publishing Company. Reproduced with Permission.

form on the plaque's surface. If either of these events stops the flow of blood completely, a heart attack or stroke is the result (see figure 7.10).

Medical scientists are not sure how atherosclerosis begins, but the latest and most plausible explanation is the oxidized LDL theory.[36] When there is a high circulating level of LDL in the blood (refer to Table 7.5), some of the excess becomes trapped in the artery wall, where it is oxidized, engulfed, and neutralized by cells attempting to protect the arteries. LDL levels that are consistently high for years overwhelm the defense system and damage the arteries, ultimately resulting in plaque that chokes off blood supply to heart or brain tissues.

Physical Inactivity Physical inactivity **(hypokinesis)** has finally been recognized by the American Heart Association (AHA) as a major modifiable risk factor for coronary heart disease. This change in position occurred during the AHA's 1992 annual scientific meeting. It reflects the AHA's recognition that regular exercise is beneficial and is an important lifestyle factor within the grasp of most Americans. The AHA does not make such changes lightly. The impact of a physically inactive life on cardiovascular disease has been documented by several significant long-term studies. The weight of the evidence caused the AHA to take its current position.

If carried to an extreme, physical inactivity it is very debilitating to the human body. For example, the changes brought about by the aging process can be simulated in young healthy adults by a few weeks of bed rest. Muscles atrophy (get smaller and weaker), bones demineralize and weaken, and maximum respiratory capacity and cardiovascular endurance decrease. As people grow older, they tend to become less active. Inactivity leads to further inactivity, so that physical decline follows a predictable course.

Aerobic exercise pursued on a regular basis is protective in that it favorably influences most of the modifiable risk factors for heart disease. The evidence generated from recent studies indicates that the effectiveness of habitual exercise in producing good health and longevity is no longer moot. What remains to be

Leisure-time activity can be an effective way of physically and mentally separating oneself from stress-producing situations at home or work.

—William Haskell

Facts, Fallacies, and Timely Tidbits

In November 1992, a well-known television news program ran a piece proclaiming that the French consume 30% more fat than American do and have 40% less heart disease. Additionally, the French exercise less, smoke more, and live longer than Americans. If this is so, how can the French avoid or delay atherosclerosis and heart disease? The answer from the Wine Institute in San Francisco is that the French drink more red wine than Americans do.

Now let us examine this objectively. The assertion is that the French are doing all of the wrong things for cardiovascular health but seem to be getting a great deal of protection from heart disease by drinking red wine. Actually, heart disease is the number one killer of French people, but because of their high alcohol consumption, cirrhosis of the liver causes twice as many deaths among the French as Americans. Also, their heavy cigarette consumption is the cause of the rising death rate from lung cancer.

Does wine consumption actually confer some degree of immunity to heart disease? There are no mysterious ingredients in wine that could lead to such a conclusion. The reason the French have fewer heart attacks than Americans is related to the French lifestyle. We get our perception of French eating habits from the rich cuisine that is served in swanky French restaurants. The rich sauces and fatty foods served in these establishments is not reflective of the way the average French person eats. Records have been kept since 1961 regarding the food supply in France. In 1961, fat supplied 28% of the calories in the average French diet, while that same year, fat supplied more than 40% of the calories in the typical American diet. In 1975, fat supplied 34% of the calories in the French diet; it eased up to 35% by 1980, to 37% in 1985, and to 39% by 1988. Today, the French consume as much fat as we do, but we have been consuming this amount for many more years than the French. We have been consuming a minimum of 39% of our calories from fat since 1923, while the French have been consuming this amount only since the late 1980s.

The previous low fat consumption in France, rather than the drinking of red wine, has been responsible for the French people's lower incidence of heart disease. If the French continue to eat fat at the present rate, however, the incidence of heart disease will increase in the near future. Wine can raise HDL cholesterol, but even this cannot nullify the effect of a high-fat diet as a causative agent for heart disease.

There's no doubt whatever that insufficient activity will shorten your life.
—Robert Hyde

determined is the quantity, the intensity, the duration, and the type of activity that is required to achieve these ends. The majority of exercise scientists do agree that one does not need to become a marathon runner to achieve the health benefits of physical activity. Somewhere between couch potato status and marathon running lies a threshold of exercise where the health benefits begin to accumulate.

Considerable agreement exists among researchers that consistent, moderate amounts of exercise or physical activity will promote health and longevity. But for those who have hypertension or elevated cholesterol, the evidence indicates that the more physically fit such people become, the less likely they are to die prematurely from heart disease.[37] The MR FIT (Multiple Risk Factor Intervention Trial) study utilized as subjects high-risk middle-aged males. The results showed that moderately active subjects (burning 224 calories/day in physical activity) had only 63 percent of the fatal heart attacks of the light activity group (burning 74 calories/day in physical activity).[38] A third group—the heavy activity group (burning 638 calories/day in physical activity)—had as many fatal heart attacks of the moderately active group but 20 percent fewer nonfatal heart attacks. These data suggest that moderate activity provides substantial protection from heart attacks, while heavy activity produces a bit more protection but at a significantly greater commitment of time and energy. To put physical activity levels in perspective for this study: (1) burning 74 calories a day is equal to walking approximately three quarters of a mile or its equivalent; (2) burning 224 calories a day is equal to walking approximately 2 ¼ miles or its equivalent, and (3) burning 638 calories a day is equal to walking approximately 6 ½ miles or its equivalent. These values are based on the assumption that a mile walked or jogged results in 100 Kcals of expended energy.

A consensus of many studies is that 150 calories a day expended in physical activity (equal to walking 1 ½ miles) represents a threshold above which the risks of coronary heart disease decreases. There appears to be an upper level effect as well, so that the protection afforded by exercise plateaus when energy expenditures reach 400 calories a day.

Subjects who walked, climbed stairs, and participated in sports activities lived longer, had less heart disease, and suffered fewer deaths from all causes than sedentary subjects.[39] Two thousand calories (20 miles of walking or its equivalent) of energy expended in a week was optimal with regard to longevity and health enhancement. For those whose energy expenditure was more, the benefits increase, but at a markedly slower rate, so that the health return was not proportional to the energy and time invested. See Figure 7.11.

An eight-year followup of 10,224 men and 3,120 women showed that those subjects who were in the lowest fitness category regardless of gender had the highest mortality rates.[40] The difference in all-cause mortality was greatest between low-fit subjects and moderately fit subjects, but there was little difference between the moderately fit and the high-fit subjects. This well-chronicled study reconfirmed the emerging trend in exercise for health that indicates that moderate levels of physical activity are about as protective against morbidity as heavy levels of exercise. In a 1989, speech, Steve Blair, the lead author of this study, discussed the development of physical fitness as a deterrent to the consequences of existing risk factors. He and his research team found that physically fit people with high cholesterol levels (≥280 mg/dL) were three times less likely to die prematurely of heart disease than unfit people with desirable levels of cholesterol. In the same study, physically fit hypertensives had less chance of dying from coronary heart disease than physically unfit normotensives (normal blood pressure). In other words, it is better to be fit and hypercholesteremic or hypertensive than to be unfit with normal levels of both. Blair stated that the amount of activity required to obtain this degree of protection could be acquired by walking. He further stated that lack of exercise is a potent risk for coronary heart disease, and official agencies such as the American Heart Association need to recognize this fact and reflect it in their guidelines. Three years and much evidence later have convinced the AHA to make this change.

While moderate levels of physical activity can lead to only moderate levels of physical fitness, the effort is sufficient to produce healthful changes in the risk factors for coronary heart disease and other chronic diseases. Researchers at the Centers for Disease Control in Atlanta critiqued 43 studies that investigated the relationship between physical inactivity and coronary heart disease and found a causal relationship between the two.[41] Furthermore, the strength of the relationship was similar in magnitude to the relationship between coronary heart disease and each of the primary risk factors—cigarette smoking, high blood pressure, and elevated cholesterol. This relationship is even more meaningful because the most active subjects in these studies exercised only 20 minutes per day three times per week. The researchers concluded that the one lifestyle change that would have the

FIGURE 7.11

Weekly Energy Expenditure and Longevity

Chart drawn using data from R. S. Paffenbarger et al., "Physical Activity All-Cause Mortality, and Longevity of College Alumni," *New England Journal of Medicine* 314 (1986): 605.

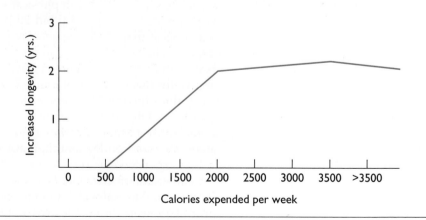

most impact on the health of the nation would be for everyone to participate consistently in some form of physical activity. The rationale is quite simple: approximately 30 percent of Americans have blood pressures that are greater than 140/90; approximately 32 percent have cholesterol levels in excess of 200 mg/dL; and 29 percent smoke cigarettes. Compare those percentages individually to the 80 percent of Americans who either are completely sedentary or exercise infrequently and you can readily see that sheer numbers alone make physical inactivity a risk worth changing.

A study completed using only women as subjects investigated the physical fitness benefits versus the health benefits of three levels of walking intensity.[42] One group walked at 5 mph, a second group walked at 4 mph, and a third group walked at 3 mph. The results showed that physical fitness improved on a predictable does-response basis. The fastest walkers improved the most, the slowest walkers improved the least. But the cardiovascular risk reduced equally among the three groups. Low-level exercise was equally as effective as the highest level in promoting cardiovascular health. This is important for the public to understand.

The problem is that most sedentary people don't like to exercise. To them, the word *exercise* conjures up sweating and pain, neither of which is appealing. The approach to motivating such people should focus upon everyday activities rather than on such fitness activities as jogging, swimming, and cycling. Everyday activities such as walking, climbing stairs, carrying packages from the store, mopping floors, vacuuming and doing other household chores with enthusiasm, mowing the lawn (without a riding mower), gardening, and substituting some physical activity for coffee and doughnuts at the break will minimally contribute to physical fitness, but they can have a profound effect upon health status. The protective effects of exercise are independent of the other known risk factors; that is, exercise produces changes in the cardiovascular system that tend to lower the risk.

> It doesn't take an enormous amount of activity to obtain considerable health benefits.
> —Steve N. Blair

THE COSTS OF A SEDENTARY LIFESTYLE

Many studies have shown that exercise may lessen the severity of chronic disease and it may also delay or prevent the onset of these diseases. Health enhancement as a result of exercise translates into decreased use of health services and increased occupational productivity, which in turn are economically beneficial to society at large. Conversely, those who choose to lead essentially sedentary lives actually impose costs on others.

The cost that others pay for those who lead inactive lives are termed "external costs." These costs are incurred from additional payments received by sedentary individuals from collectively financed programs such as health insurance, sick-leave payments, disability insurance, and group life insurance. The premiums and payroll taxes that finance these programs are the same for sedentary and active individuals. As such, these social welfare programs have an undesirable side effect: they subsidize unhealthy behavior.

All people benefit when those who are sedentary switch to an active life. Each minute that people spend walking will increase their life expectancy by a similar amount; joggers who burn their calories twice as fast as walkers can expect to get double their exercise time back in increased life expectancy.

The costs associated with a sedentary lifestyle can be summed up this way: the external costs of a sedentary life are almost twice the external costs of smoking.

E. B. Keeler et al., "The External Costs of a Sedentary Lifestyle," *American Journal of Public Health* 79 (1989): 975.

A benefit versus risk relationship is associated with exercise. The potential risk of sudden cardiac death during vigorous exercise and the potential benefit of participating in habitual exercise in the same population has been examined. The results indicated that sedentary men who engaged in vigorous exercise less than 20 minutes per week are three times more likely to die suddenly than men who exercise vigorously more than two hours and twenty minutes per week.[43]

Although the active men have a slightly elevated risk of sudden death during exercise, the long-term health benefits clearly outweigh the mortality risk when compared to the sedentary men. The risk of sudden death during exercise for sedentary men was 56 times greater than their risk at other times. Active men have a mortality advantage at rest and during exercise when compared to sedentary men.

Actually, the occurrence of sudden death during exercise is relatively rare.[44] The precise number of these deaths is not known, but newspaper reports place the incidence between 10 and 25 per year. This is a small number when one considers the millions of competitive and recreational athletes in the United States. The results of a study of U.S. Air Force recruits who participated in 42 days of basic training over a 20-year period reinforced the low prevalence of sudden death among young people (17 to 28 years of age). There were 21 deaths during this time, 19 of them sudden, caused by heart attack that occurred while engaged in or immediately after exercise.[45] During the 20-year period, 1,606,167 recruits went through basic training, accumulating millions of hours of exercise time. There was one death for each three million hours of exercise. Only one of the 21 deaths was caused by the buildup of fatty cholesterol deposits in the coronary arteries. The majority of the deaths were attributed to myocarditis (inflammation of heart muscle) and birth defects. Exercise-related cardiac deaths that occur among young people are usually the result of cardiac anomalies,[46] while cardiac deaths in older participants are usually the result of severe atherosclerotic coronary artery disease.

Jim Fixx is an example of severe coronary artery disease. On the other hand, Pete Maravich, former basketball great, died suddenly at the age of 40 while playing a leisurely pickup basketball game with friends. An autopsy revealed that his left coronary artery (the major blood vessel supplying a large portion of heart muscle) and its branches were missing. This was a congential defect that had gone undetected. Flo Hyman, U.S. Olympic volleyball star in her mid-thirties, collapsed and died during a match. She had Marfan's syndrome, an inherited disorder of the connective tissues common in very tall people. Her death was caused by a rupture of the aorta (largest artery in the body) which was a consequence of Marfan's disease. The infrequent deaths that do occur to young people during exercise are usually due to congential problems.

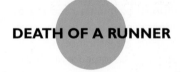

DEATH OF A RUNNER

Jim Fixx, jogging guru and author of the best-selling text *The Complete Book of Running*, died of a massive heart attack while on a training run in July 1984 at the age of 52. Since Fixx had been jogging 80 miles per week, his abrupt death sent shock waves through the running community. It also raised questions about the protective effect of vigorous exercise against heart disease. Also, many pointed to his death as further evidence that vigorous exercise is a risk for precipitating a heart attack.

An autopsy revealed that Fixx had significant coronary artery disease. That he was able to jog 80 miles per week with severely narrowed coronary arteries attests to the trainability and adaptability of the human body. But did jogging contribute to this death or prolong his life? Before becoming a jogger, Fixx was a sedentary, two-pack-a-day cigarette smoker who was approximately 60 lbs. overweight and who worked in a high-stress job. He had a family history of heart disease (his father died of a heart attack at the age of 43). This was definitely not a wellness profile. At 35 years of age, Fixx turned his life around by starting a jogging program. He lost 60 lbs. and gave up smoking. Many authorities are convinced that these changes in living habits helped to prolong his life—he outlived his father by 9 years. But for some unknown reason, Fixx refused to heed the advice he offered millions of others through his writings, that is, to submit to a medical examination that would include an EKG stress test. Ironically, his last refusal to take such a test came just three weeks before his

Continued

death. After his death, it was learned that he had been suffering from angina (chest pain) for at least six weeks and would probably have had an abnormal stress test. Medical intervention at that point might have substantially delayed his death.

Whether jogging increased Fixx's life or caused an early death cannot be answered, but the lifestyle changes that he instituted at age 35 were certainly consistent with longer life. Regardless, the quality of his life improved as a result of those changes.

What can we learn from Fixx's death? One, he had a combination of factors that most runners don't have: he had severe heart disease that probably began before his change to a healthier lifestyle, he had the risk factors associated with heart disease, and he had a warning (angina) of its occurrence. Two, heart disease is a killer that not even jogging can cure. Three, making positive lifestyle changes should be accompanied by medical feedback before initiating vigorous exercise and should continue periodically during the life of the individual. This is particularly appropriate for those who manifest more than one risk factor.

POINTS TO PONDER

1. In relation to men, what is the risk of cardiovascular disease for pre-menopausal and postmenopausal women?
2. Most people who quit smoking cigarettes gain weight. What are the physiological mechanisms that are involved? In addition to these mechanisms, what other factors are involved in weight gain?
3. What advice would you give to a smoker who is reluctant to quit the habit because of the fear of gaining weight.
4. Identify and describe the noxious products in cigarette smoke.
5. Describe the effects of environmental smoke on nonsmokers.
6. What is essential hypertension?
7. What lifestyle behaviors have the capacity to modify the blood pressure?
8. What is the role of exercise in blood pressure control?
9. Define endogenous and exogenous sources of cholesterol.
10. Describe the lipoproteins and their role in heart disease.
11. Explain how HDL can be increased. Explain how TC and LDL can be decreased.
12. What is atherosclerosis, and how does it begin?
13. Cite the evidence that caused the AHA to move physical inactivity from other risk factors to major risk factors that can be changed?
14. Discuss the role of moderate exercise versus heavy exercise for physical fitness and for health.

Other Contributing Risk Factors

Obesity   In 1985, the NIH Consensus Development Conference formally declared obesity a disease.[47] Obesity is highly correlated with coronary heart disease, stroke, atherosclerosis, and diabetes—four of the top ten killers of Americans. **Obesity** is defined by the National Institutes of Health as 20 percent above desirable weight. The American Heart Association states that those who are 30 percent above desirable weight are more likely to develop cardiovascular disease even in the absence of other risk factors. Severely obese people are at three times the risk of having coronary heart disease.[48] Even mild to moderate overweight was associated with an 80 percent increase in the risk. Forty percent of the coronary events that occurred in this study were attributable to being overweight. The risk doubled for people who gained 22 pounds between early and mid-adulthood, which refutes the idea that weight gain during this time period is expected and harmless. Excess weight puts a strain on the heart, and it usually coexists with high blood pressure, elevated cholesterol, and diabetes.

The manner in which fat is distributed in the body (touched upon in the section on cigarette smoking) may intensify the risk. If the waist measurement of a male exceeds his hip measurement and if the waist measurement of a female is more than 80 percent of her hip measurement, both are at increased risk for heart attack, stroke, diabetes, and some forms of cancer.

Exercise plus sensible eating can produce weight loss for most people. Exercise uniquely contributes to weight loss and weight management by burning calories, speeding up muscle metabolism, building muscle tissue, and balancing appetite with energy expenditure.

Diabetes Mellitus   **Diabetes mellitus** (honey-urine disease) is a metabolic disorder in which the body is unable to regulate the level of glucose (sugar) in the blood. It is one of the ten leading causes of death in the United States, affecting as many as 10 million Americans. Most cases of diabetes occur in middle age to overweight people.

Diabetes produces severe consequences, including cardiovascular disease, kidney disease, blindness, and nerve and blood vessel damage. More than 80 percent of all diabetics die of some form of cardiovascular disease.[49] The mortality rate from coronary heart disease for diabetic men is two to three times greater than for nondiabetic men, and for diabetic women the rate is three to seven times greater than for nondiabetic women.[50]

Diabetes is an independent risk for coronary heart disease because of the increased tendency for diabetics to form blood clots and because there is a greater than normal risk of developing heart muscle pathology.[51] Also, diabetes appears to accelerate the onset of some of the coronary risk factors, particularly circulating levels of cholesterol and triglycerides.

Diabetics must live well-regulated lives that include attention to a low-fat, high-complex carbohydrate diet, weight loss and maintenance, and exercise. These factors must be balanced to achieve control of the amount of sugar (glucose) in the blood. Some diabetics must include medication in addition to the lifestyle measures to achieve control.

Exercise plays an important role by increasing the sensitivity of body cells to insulin—a hormone that is needed to move sugar from the blood to the cells so that it can fuel the functions of the cells. Diabetics who either produce little or no insulin or have few cell receptor sites for insulin are markedly helped by exercise, which increases sensitivity of the cells to insulin. Blood platelet adhesiveness is reduced for about 24 hours following exercise. Exercise also moderates many of the risk factors for coronary heart disease.

Stress It is estimated that 50 percent to 75 percent of all people who visit a physician do so for psychosomatic disorders (illnesses that originate in the mind and manifest themselves in physical ailments). Animal experiments have shown that the higher centers of the brain can influence the physical state. Human studies are far from conclusive, but certain mental states such as grief over the loss of a loved one increase the risk of contracting infectious diseases on the one hand to dying of a cardiovascular event on the other. In the near future, researchers will be able to delineate the role of emotions in the genesis of health and disease.

Stress can be acute or chronic. Acute stress is situational; that is, an event triggers the stress response, but the effect of that response is short-lived. For example, a mid-term exam, a speech before a group, or the emergency evasive maneuvers require to avoid a traffic accident provoke the physiologic stress response. The hormone epinephrine initiates a series of responses that readies the body for action. Heart rate, blood pressure, and oxygen consumption increase, the heart pumps with greater force, muscles respond more forcefully and rapidly, metabolism increases, and pupils dilate in response to acute stress. These altered states are temporary and usually return to normal within the first hour after the emergency or event is perceived to have ended.

Chronic stress, on the other hand, is long-term, permeates the very fabric of our lives, and has a negative effect on the body. It provokes the stress response at lower levels than acute stress but lasts for a much longer period of time. Constantly rushing to meet deadlines and quotas, losing control of one's life, feeling helpless, and perceiving that there is too much to do and not enough time to do it result in chronic stress.

The response to stress cannot be measured as precisely as blood pressure or cholesterol, but most authorities consider it to be a factor in the development and acceleration of cardiovascular disease. Exposure to stress is inescapable, but it can be controlled by voluntary relaxation techniques, development of time-management skills, and exercise. Stress and its management will be covered in greater detail in Chapter 8.

Triglycerides **Triglycerides** are found in food, can be synthesized by the liver and intestines, and constitute the most space-efficient form of energy storage in the body. Most of the fat in the body is stored in the form of triglycerides, composed of fatty acids of varying lengths that are attached to a molecule of glycerol.

The relationship between hypertriglyceridemia (elevated plasma triglycerides) and coronary heart disease remains controversial. The National Institutes of Health (NIH) has reported that elevated plasma triglycerides may be associated with heart disease under certain circumstances,[52] including coexistence with diabetes, kidney disease, obesity elevated total cholesterol, low concentrations of HDL cholesterol, high concentrations of LDL cholesterol, hypertension, and cigarette smoking.[53] Elevated triglyceride levels do not seem to be independently predictive of coronary risk. Values up to 250 mg/dL are considered to be normal; values between 250 and 500 mg/dL are borderline; and values above 500 mg/dL are excessive. Values below 250 mg/dL do not increase the risk for heart disease unless accompanied by elevated LDL and low HDL cholesterol. People whose values are between 250 and 500 mg/dL may be at higher risk, particularly if the elevation is caused by familial or genetic factors. Intervention should be established for these people as well as for those whose levels are above 500 mg/dL.

Intervention programs designed to lower plasma triglycerides include smoking cessation, alcohol restriction, low-fat, low-cholesterol diet, exercise, and medication. A single bout of aerobic exercise will decrease the concentration of plasma triglycerides. Aerobic exercise performed on consecutive days lowers the level further and keeps it suppressed for 48 to 72 hours. But if several days are allowed

Rules for Handling Stress
- Don't sweat the small stuff.
- Everything is small stuff.
- If you can't "fight" or "flee," then flow.

—Robert Eliot, M.D.,
Time, June 6, 1983

to pass without exercise, triglyceride values return to pre-exercise levels. The optimal intensity and duration of exercise for the purpose of reducing plasma triglycerides are not known at this time. It is probably a safe bet if one follows the American College of Sports Medicine guidelines for exercise (discussed in Chapter 3), triglyceride values will drop.

HEART DISEASE AND THE IRON CONNECTION

A recent study of 1,900 men in Finland showed that those with high levels of iron (ferritin) in the bloodstream were twice as likely to have a heart attack as men whose iron concentration was in the low-normal range.[54] The link between iron and heart disease is that iron promotes the oxidation of LDLs. (Only LDLs that are oxidized are involved in the development and promotion of atherosclerosis.)

Of course, this one study, provocative though it is, can only be considered preliminary. However, if valid, it adds credence to some observed phenomena regarding heart disease. First, premenopausal women have less heart disease than men and have less iron than men, primarily because of monthly blood loss during menstruation. Second, societies that consume red meat are at greater risk because red meat is rich in iron. This would add to the saturated fat risk present in red meat. Third, aspirin and fish oil protect against heart disease—aspirin induces minor bleeding, and fish oil prolongs bleeding, so that both contribute to iron loss. Fourth, oral contraception reduces menstrual blood loss so that more iron is retained. Fifth, the incidence of cardiovascular disease increases substantially after menopause because menstruation ceases and iron is no longer lost each month. The researchers suggested that it is a good idea for all people to donate blood once a month to periodically reduce iron stores.

The idea that excessive iron might cause heart disease is not new, although it has been largely ignored for the past decade. Since other investigators are studying the possible connection between the two, we should see some answers in the next five to ten years.

J. T. Salonen et al. "High Stored Iron Levels Are Associated with Excess Risk of Myocardial Infarction in Eastern Finnish Men,: *Circulation* 86, no. 3 (September, 1992): 803.

CAN LIFESTYLE CHANGES REVERSE CORONARY HEART DISEASE?

Forty-eight heart patients participated in a study to determine whether comprehensive lifestyle changes could affect coronary atherosclerosis.[55] Approximately half of the group (the experimentals) were put on a low-fat vegetarian diet and a moderate aerobic exercise program, were given training in stress management, and stopped smoking. The other half (the controls) followed the usual care procedures for heart patients. All subjects were followed for one year.

The vegetarian diet contained only 10 percent of the total calories as fat and only 5 mg of cholesterol per day. The exercise program consisted primarily of walking for at least 30 minutes three times per week. Control-group patients were not asked to make lifestyle changes, but they were free to do so.

At the end of one year, persons in the experimental group showed significant regression of coronary atherosclerosis, while atherosclerosis continued to progress in the usual care control group. This study indicated that small changes in lifestyle can only slow the progression of atherosclerosis. Comprehensive lifestyle changes are required to halt or reverse coronary atherosclerosis. While it takes some effort to make substantial lifestyle changes, the results are very worthwhile.

POINTS TO PONDER

1. What evidence can you cite that supports the proposition that moderate-intensity exercise produces health-related benefits?
2. What seems to be the optimal level of weekly caloric expenditure for improvement in longevity?
3. Can physical fitness nullify the effect of some of the risk factors for heart disease?
4. Comment on the following: If Americans could make only one lifestyle behavioral change, it should be that all would engage in exercise and a physically active way of life. This would significantly enhance the health of the nation.
5. What is the likelihood of sudden death during exercise?
6. Why is diabetes a risk for cardiovascular disease?
7. Discuss the relationship between high iron levels in the blood and heart disease.

CHAPTER HIGHLIGHTS

- Although cardiovascular disease is the number one killer of Americans, the death rate from this disease has declined by 51% since 1950.
- The heart is a double pump: the pulmonary pump sends deoxygenated blood to the lungs; the systemic pump sends oxygenated blood to all of the tissues.
- The heart is autoregulatory: it has its own pacemaker and electrical conduction system.
- Strokes are caused by a thrombus, an embolus, or a hemorrhage.
- Cigarette smoking is considered the most potent preventable risk factor associated with chronic illness and premature death.
- Smoking accounts for almost half of all heart attacks that occur in women before the age of 55.
- Nonsmokers who live or work with smokers are at increased risk for heart disease and cancer.
- The typical user of smokeless tobacco products begins experimenting with them at about 10 years of age.
- The incidence of oral cancer is as much as 50 times higher for long-term users of smokeless tobacco products than for nonusers.
- Essential hypertension cannot be cured, but it can be treated.
- Exercise lowers blood pressure because it decreases the resistance to blood flow, results in weight loss, and promotes sodium excretion by the kidneys.
- We get cholesterol in two ways: (1) through the diet (exogenous) and (2) manufactured by the liver (endogenous).
- To accurately assess cholesterol as a risk factor, one must know the total amount of cholesterol and the LDL and HDL fractions.
- Reducing cholesterol by 1% in the blood reduces the risk of cardiovascular disease by 2% to 3%.
- Exercise raises HDL.
- Moderate exercises performed regularly produce many health benefits.
- Diabetes produces severe consequences, including cardiovascular disease, kidney disease, blindness, and nerve and blood vessel damage.
- Chronic stress is long-term, permeates the very fabric of our lives, and has a negative effect on the body.
- Some evidence exists that supports the link between high iron levels in the blood and heart disease.

1. American Heart Association, *1992 Heart and Stroke Facts*, Dallas: American Heart Association, 1991.

2. Ibid.

3. Ibid.

4. Ibid.

5. Ibid.

6. Ibid.

7. T. L. Bush, "Influence on Cholesterol and Lipoprotein Levels in Women," *Cholesterol and Coronary Disease—Reducing the Risk* 2, no. 6 (February 1990): 1.

8. S. Wichmann and D. R. Martin, "Heart Disease: Not for Men Only," *The Physician and Sportsmedicine* 20, no. 8, (August 1992): 138.

9. S. P. Van Camp and J. L. Boyer, "Cardiovascular Aspects of Aging," *The Physician and Sportsmedicine* 17, no. 4 (April 1989): 121.

10. J. E. Manson et al., "The Primary Prevention of Myocardial Infarction," *New England Journal of Medicine*, May 21, 1992, p. 1406.

11. American Cancer Society, *Cancer Facts and Figure—1992*, Atlanta, Ga.: American Cancer Society, 1992.

12. Department of Health and Human Services, *Reducing the Health Consequences of Smoking: 25 Years of Progress: A Report of the Surgeon General*, Washington, D.C.: U.S. Government Printing Office, 1989. (DHHS publication number (CDC) 89–8411)

13. W. C. Willett et al., "Relative and Absolute Excess Risks of Coronary Heart Disease Among Women Who Smoke Cigarettes," *New England Journal of Medicine* 317 (1987): 1303.

14. J. R. Plamer, L. Rosenberg, and S. Shapiro, "Low Yield Cigarettes and the Risk of Nonfatal Myocardial Infarction in Women," *New England Journal of Medicine* 320 (1989): 1569.

15. L. Rosenberg, J. R. Palmer, and S. Shapiro, "Decline in the Risk of Myocardial Infarction Among Women Who Stopped Smoking," *New England Journal of Medicine* 322 (1990): 322.

16. M. Fiore et al., "Smoking Cessation: Data from the 1986 Adult Use of Tobacco Survey," in M. Aoki, S. Hisamichi, and S. Tominaga (Eds.), *Smoking and Health 1987: Proceeding of the Sixth World Conference on Smoking and Health*, Amsterdam: Excerpta Medica, 1988.

17. Department of Health and Human Services, *Reducing the Health Consequences*, 1989.

18. P. L. Pirie, D. M. Murray, and R. V. Luepker, "Gender Differences in Cigarette Smoking and Quitting in a Cohort of Young Adults," *American Journal of Public Health* 81, no. 3 (1991): 324.

19. *The Health Consequences of Smoking—Nicotine Addiction*, A report of the Surgeon General, Rockville, Md.: Department of Health and Human Services, 1988.

20. J. L. Christopher, B. Lees, and J. C. Stevenson, "Sex and Menopause—Associated Changes in Body-Fat Distribution," *American Journal of Clinical Nutrition* 55 (1992): 950.

21. Office of the Inspector General, *Youth Use of Smokeless Tobacco: More Than a Pinch of Trouble*, Washington, D.C.: U.S. Dept. of Health and Human Services, 1986.

22. "Passive Smoking: A Threat to the Heart?" *Harvard Heart Letter* 1, no. 12 (August 1991): 1.

23. G. M. Wardlaw and P. M. Insel, *Perspectives in Nutrition*, St. Louis: Times Mirror/Mosby, 1990.

24. C. M. Tipton, "Exercise, Training, and Hypertension," in J. D. Hollozsy (Ed.), *Exercise Sport Science Reviews*, Baltimore: Williams and Wilkins, 1991.

25. L. S. Pescatello et al., "Short-term Effect of Dynamic Exercise on Arterial Blood Pressure," *Circulation* 83 no. 5 (1991): 1557.

26. S. R. Daniels and J. M. H. Loggie, "Hypertension in Children and Adolescents," *The Physician and Sportsmedicine* 20, no. 3 (March 1992): 120.

27. "Report of the Second Task Force on Blood Pressure Control in Children—1987," *Pediatrics* 79, no. 1 (1987): 3.

28. S. R. Daniels, and J. M. H. Loggie, "Hypertension," March 1992; p. 125.

29. L. Rosenberg, J. R. Plamer, and S. Shapiro, "Decline in the Risk," 1990.

30. AHA, *1992 Heart and Stroke Facts*, 1991, p. 8.

31. J. C. La Rosa et al., "The Cholesterol Facts: A Summary of the Evidence Relating Dietary Fats, Serum Cholesterol, and Coronary Heart Disease: A Joint Statement by the American Heart Association and the National Heart, Lung, and Blood Institute," *Circulation* 81 (1990): 1721.

32. U.S. Department of Health and Human Services. *Healthy People 2000*, Washington D.C.: U.S. Government Printing Office, DHHS Publication No. (PHS) 91–50212, 1990.

33. T. C. Cook et al., "Chronic Low Level Physical Activity as Determinant of High Density Lipoprotein Cholesterol and Subfractions" *Medicine and Science in Sports and Exercise* 18 (1986): 653.

34. E. J. Schaefer et al. "Nutrition, Lipoproteins, and Atherosclerosis" *Clinical Nutrition*, 5 (1986): 99.

35. P. D. Wood et al., "Changes in Plasma Lipids and Lipoproteins in Overweight Men During Weight Loss Through Dieting as Compared with Exercise," *New England Journal of Medicine* 319 (1988): 1173.

36. D. Steinberg and J. L. Witztum, "Lipoprotein and Atherogenesis—Current Concepts," *Journal of the American Medical Association*, December 19, 1990, p. 3047.

37. S. N. Blair et al., "Physical Fitness and All-Cause Mortality—A Prospective Study of Healthy Men and Women," *Journal of the American Medical Association*, November 3, 1989, p. 2395.

38. A. S. Leon et al., "Leisure-time Physical Activity Levels and Risk of Coronary Heart Disease and Death," *Journal of the American Medical Association* 258 (1987): 2388.

39. R. S. Paffenbarger et al., "Physical Activity, All-Cause Mortality, and Longevity of College Alumni," *New England Journal of Medicine* 314 (1986): 605.

40. S. N. Blair et al., "Physical Fitness," November 3, 1989, p. 2400.

41. K. E. Powell, "Physical Activity and the Incidence of Coronary Heart Disease," *Annual Reviews of Public Health* 8 (1987): 253.

42. J. J. Duncan et al., "Women Walking for Health and Fitness," *Journal of the American Medical Association* 266 (1991): 3295.

43. D. S. Siscovick et al., "The Incidence of Primary Cardiac Arrest During Vigorous Exercise," *New England Journal of Medicine* 311 (1984): 874.

44. S. P. Van Camp, "Exercise-Related Sudden Death: Risks and Causes," *The Physician and Sportsmedicine* 16 (1988): 96.

45. L. Lamb (Ed.), "Sudden Cardiac Death in Young Men," *The Health Letter,* June 12, 1987, p. 1.

46. S. P. Van Camp, "Exercise-Related Sudden Death," 1988, p. 99.

47. W. R. Foster and B. T. Burton (Eds.), "Health Implications of Obesity: National Institutes of Health Development Conference," *Annals of Internal Medicine* 103 (1985, Supp. 6, Part 2): 977.

48. S. P. Van Camp and J. L. Boyer, "Cardiovascular Aspects," April 1989, p. 122.

49. AHA, *1992 Heart and Stroke Facts,* 1991, p. 22.

50. J. E. Manson et al., "The Primary Prevention," May 21, 1992, p. 1411.

51. Ibid. p. 1411.

52. E. L. Bierman, "The Treatment of Hypertriglyceridemia: Views from the National Institutes of Health Consensus Conference," *Cholesterol and Coronary Disease—Reducing the Risk* 2 (1988): 6.

53. "More on Triglycerides," *Harvard Heart Letter* 2, no. 10 (June 1992): 7.

54. J. T. Salonen and others. "High Stored Iron Levels are Associated With Excess Risk of Myocardial Infarction In Eastern Finnish Men," *Circulation,* 86, No. 3 (Sept. 1992): 803.

55. D. Ornish and others. "Can Lifestyle Changes Reverse Coronary Heart Disease?" *The Lancet,* 336 (July 21, 1990): 129.

Other Chronic Conditions

CHAPTER OUTLINE

INTRODUCTION

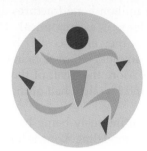

This chapter focuses on osteoporosis, low-back problems, osteoarthritis, asthma, cancer, and stress. These prevalent chronic disorders are covered because most Americans are affected by one or more, and a relationship exists between them and exercise. For instance, many people do not exercise because they fear that exercise contributes to the wear and tear of joints, thus resulting in osteoarthritis. We explore that possibility by presenting samples of the available evidence and then arrive at some conclusions. Many asthmatics do not exercise because exercise generally induces an asthma attack. While this certainly does occur, should asthmatics deny themselves the health benefits of exercise? Can asthmatics exercise in safety? How do osteoporosis, low-back problems, and cancer respond to exercise? How can stress be relieved through exercise? These and other questions and concerns are discussed in this chapter.

Four self-assessment activities appear in Appendix C that apply directly to the contents of this chapter:

8.1 Cancer Awareness

8.2 Years of Life Lost From Smoking

8.3 Life Events Scale—Student Version

8.4 Manifestations of Stress—Mind, Body, Combination of Both

Miniglossary

Asthma Widespread narrowing of the airways of the lungs because of varying degrees of contraction or spasm of smooth muscle, edema of the mucosa, and mucus in the bronchi and bronchioles.

Cancer A large group of disorders characterized by abnormal cellular growth.

Cortical Bone The dense, hard outer layer of bone such as that which appears in the shafts of the long bones of the arms and legs.

Depression Prolonged sadness that persists beyond a reasonable length of time.

Distressor Negative or bad stress.

Eustressor Positive or good stress.

Homeostasis A state of equilibrium in the body with respect to the body's various functions as well as chemical composition of the body's fluids and tissues.

Kyphosis Abnormal curvature of the thoracic region of the spine.

Lordosis Abnormal curvature of the lumbar region of the spine.

Metastasis The spread of cancer from the original site to other sites in the body.

Neoplasm Growth of new tissue (tumor).

Oncogene A cancer-causing gene.

Osteoarthritis Degenerative joint disease characterized by the deterioration of articular cartilage, particularly in the weight-bearing joints. Often referred to as the wear-and-tear disease.

Osteoblast Bone-forming cells.

Osteoclasts Cells that break down and absorb bone.

Osteoporosis Reduction in the quantity of bone as a result of demineralization and atrophy of skeletal tissue.

Scoliosis Abnormal lateral curvature of the spine.

Stressor Any event, condition, or situation that results in change, threat, or loss.

Trabecular Bone Spongy bone; not as dense as cortical bone.

Osteoporosis is Latin for "porous bone." It is a silent condition with no overt symptoms. There is a gradual loss of bone mass, so that the bones weaken and become susceptible to fractures. Twenty-five million Americans—80 percent of whom are elderly women—have osteoporosis. The incidence of osteoporosis has been on the increase and will continue to rise as more Americans live longer.

The critical period for the development of bone mass occurs from 11 to 15 years of age.[1] The greater the accumulation of bone mass during these early years, the more bone that can be lost before incurring an osteoporatic-related fracture during the later years.

Osteoporosis is responsible for more than a million bone fractures annually. The medical cost to the nation for these incidents is astronomical. There are approximately 300,000 hip fractures per year, and they alone cost $7 billion.[2] Up to 20 percent of these victims will die from pneumonia, blood clots in the lungs, and heart failure in the first year after surgery.[3] More than half of the survivors will require a walking aid (a cane or a walker), and less than half of the survivors will return to their former level of activity.

Bone is not inert; it is living tissue that is continuously being broken down (resorbed) and rebuilt by a process referred to as remodeling. Bone is formed from a protein framework into which calcium is deposited. Approximately 99 percent of the body's calcium is stored in the skeletal system and teeth. Calcium significantly contributes to bone strength.

Osteoclasts are specialized cells that break down and absorb bone. **Osteoblasts** are bone-forming cells. It takes about 90 days for old bone to be resorbed and replaced by new bone, and then the cycle begins anew. During childhood and adolescence, the activity of the osteoblasts is greater than that of the osteoclasts, so that new bone is added to the skeleton faster than old bone is removed. By early adulthood, the processes of resorption and growth begin to equalize until about age 35, when bone removal overtakes bone replacement. Women experience the greatest bone loss during the first five years following menopause. After this period, bone loss continues, but at a slower rate. On the average, women with established osteoporosis have lost about one-third of the bone mass that they had earlier in life. Since males do not experience a comparable period where bone loss is accelerated, they lose bone at a relatively constant rate.

Cortical bone is the dense, hard outer layer of bone, such as the shafts of the long bones of the arms and legs. **Trabecular bone** is spongy and less dense and is surrounded by cortical bone. The vertebrae consist primarily of trabecular bone. The trabecular bone is weaker than cortical bone and breaks more easily because of its spongy consistency. This accounts for the high incidence of fractures of the vertebrae and ball of the femur (thigh bone). Women with advanced osteoporosis will lose 35 percent of their cortical and 50 percent of their trabecular bone.

Two types of osteoporosis—each caused by different pathogenic mechanisms—have been identified.[4] Type I affects eight times more women than men, and it occurs after menopause (age 50 to 65).[5] The fracture sites in their order of prevalence in type I osteoporosis are vertebral crush fractures and fractures of the arm above the wrist (see Figure 8.1). These fractures are caused by accelerated bone loss because of estrogen deficiency after menopause. Type II osteoporosis affects twice as many women as men and usually occurs to both sexes in the 70 years of age group. Hip fractures are the most frequent events, and estrogen deficiency is only one of many possible contributing factors in this type of osteoporosis.

● Osteoporosis—The Risk Factors

The cause or causes of osteoporosis are not known, but many factors contribute to its development. Having the risk factors does not necessarily mean that one will

FIGURE 8.1

Effects of Osteoporosis

Source: Whitney and Rolfes, *Understanding Nutrition, 6/e,* 1993, West Publishing Company Reproduced with permission. Art rendered by J/B Woolsey Associates.

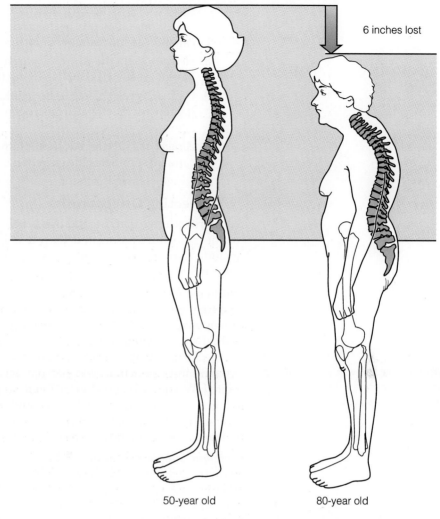

6 inches lost

50-year old   80-year old

Effects of osteoporosis on a woman's height. On the left is a woman at menopause and on the right, the same woman 30 years later. Notice the collapse of her vertebrae has shortened her back; the length of her legs has not changed.

definitely develop the disease, but it does increase the probability. The following are the risk factors for osteoporosis:

1. *Gender.* Women are about four times as likely to develop osteoporosis as men.

2. *Age.* Since this disease takes many years to evolve, the longer one lives, the higher the likelihood of developing osteoporosis.

3. *Thin, small-framed body.* People with slight skeletal systems (ectomorphic body type) are more susceptible because they have less bone to lose. Petite women are particularly at risk.

4. *Early menopause.* Early menopause that occurs naturally or is surgically induced (hysterectomy that includes the removal of the ovaries) increases the probability of developing osteoporosis because the protective effect of estrogen is lost prematurely.

5. *Lack of calcium in the diet.* Calcium deficiency contributes to the development of osteoporosis.

6. *Race.* Caucasian and Asian people are at a greater risk than black people.

7. *Lack of physical activity.* Inactivity—voluntary or enforced—increases the risk. Consistent physical activity, particularly the weight-bearing type, can increase or maintain bone mass.

8. *Heredity.* The offspring of parents and grandparents with osteoporosis have a greater risk of developing the condition.

9. *Cigarette smoking.* Cigarette smoking suppresses the estrogen level, leading to early menopause. Estrogen protects the skeletal system from mineral loss.

10. *Alcohol and caffeine.* Alcohol interferes with the absorption of calcium, and caffeine stimulates the excretion of calcium through the urine.

● Preventing Osteoporosis

Authorities agree that osteoporosis is better prevented than treated, because much of the deformity associated with it is irreversible. Prevention and treatment include hormone (estrogen) replacement therapy (ERT), calcium supplementation, and exercise.

Hormone Replacement Therapy   Women who are deficient in endogenous estrogen (that which they manufacture in the body) are at a greater risk of developing osteoporosis. Estrogen can be replaced with a commercial preparation that slows bone loss. However, the longer a postmenopausal woman stays on estrogen replacement therapy (ERT), the greater the risk of developing breast cancer.[6] A woman, in conjunction with her physician, should decide whether ERT is warranted. Women who do elect ERT can expect to have less than half of the hip fractures and substantially fewer spine and wrist fractures than women who do not take estrogen. It must be pointed out that estrogen is combined with progesterone to lessen the risk of breast cancer.

Calcium Supplementation   Calcium is an important mineral essential for the growth and maintenance of the teeth and skeletal system. In 1989, the U.S. National Academy of Sciences recommended that females 11 to 24 years of age should consume 1,200 mg of calcium daily. It recommended a reduction to 800 mg after the age of 24. By 1990, evidence emerged suggesting that optimal bone density in females was achieved with a daily intake of 800 to 1,000 mg. Calcium levels in excess of this amount did not appear to confer additional benefit. However, it was suggested that older women might need more because the ability to absorb calcium diminishes with age. Men need about 800 mg/day. Table 8.1 lists some selected food sources of calcium.

> Estrogen would prevent at least 90 percent of the vertebral fractures among postmenopausal women.
> —Robert Lindsay

BONE LOSS IN WOMEN—THE CALCIUM CONTROVERSY

A recent review of the medical literature indicated that calcium supplementation could arrest bone loss in women. Women are particularly susceptible to bone loss during the first five years after menopause. The loss at this time is attributed to estrogen deficiencies rather than insufficient calcium.

The amount of calcium required to maintain calcium balance to reduce bone loss is not known, but several studies have shown that at least 900mg/day are required for younger women, while 1,500 mg/day may be required for post-menopausal women. Estrogen deficiency accounts for the majority of bone loss for post-menopausal women, but calcium deficiency is responsible for a portion of the loss for women in Europe and North America.

At what stage of life should women become concerned about their calcium intake? The earlier the better, but a number of studies have shown that it is never too late to begin increasing one's calcium intake and that reductions in fracture rates from bone loss can occur in as little as 18 months.

Source: R.P. Heaney. "Talking Straight About Calcium," *New England Journal of Medicine,* February 18, 1993, p. 503.

TABLE 8.1 — Selected Food Sources of Calcium

ITEM	PORTION SIZE NEEDED TO PROVIDE 400 MG CALCIUM (½ SUGGESTED REQUIREMENT DAILY)*	KCALS NEEDED TO PROVIDE 400 MG OF CALCIUM
Milk		
Whole	11 oz.	206
Skim	10.6 oz.	112.6
Cheese		
Cheddar	2 oz.	230
Cottage—low fat (2%)	20.5 oz.	528
Mozzarella	2 oz.	160
Swiss	1.5 oz.	160.2
Fish		
Sardines (with bones)	4 oz.	250.2
Shrimp (boiled)	4.5 oz.	136
Vegetables		
Broccoli (cooked)	2 ¼ cups	103
Collards (fresh)	1.1 cups	73
Spinach (cooked)	1.6 cups	66
Turnip greens (cooked)	2 cups	60
Tofu	15.5 oz.	330
Wheat bread	13.3 slices	867
Oatmeal (fortified, instant)	2.5 pkgs	262.5
Almonds	5.3 oz	880

*RDA for adults is 800 mg

Source: Adapted from G. M. Wardlaw and P. M. Insel. *Perspectives in Nutrition,* St. Louis: Mosby, 1993, p. 445, and "U.S.D.A. Nutritive Value of Foods" *Home and Garden Bulletin,* no. 72, p. 8.

The earlier a person starts a regular exercise program, the greater the likelihood of meaningful osteogeneses (bone growth).

—Morris Notelovitz

Physical Activity   Bone responds to the downward force of gravity and the lateral forces generated by muscle contraction. The stimulus produced by exercise is important in treatment and prevention of osteoporosis.[7] Enforced bed rest (4 to 36 weeks) occurring to healthy people results in significant bone loss. Inactivity and the absence of gravitational force (weightlessness) produce the same deleterious effect upon the skeletal system. Some degree of stress must be periodically imposed upon the skeletal system for bone to maintain its integrity. Disuse osteoporosis results from prolonged periods of inactivity. Physical activity forces bone to adapt and respond to the stresses imposed upon it, and as with other body tissues, bone hypertrophies (grows larger and stronger). When unstressed, bone atrophies. The development of muscle tissue is important to the development and maintenance of bone mass. A direct relationship exists between the size of the muscles and the thickness of the bones.

Athletes have greater bone density than age-matched sedentary persons (controls), probably because of their greater muscle mass.[8] Strong muscles capable of exerting strong forces upon the bones, result in thicker, stronger bones. In addition, athletes participating in different sports show different skeletal adaptations based upon the load to which bone is subjected. When the thigh bones of athletes competing in different sports were compared, the greatest bone density was found in the weightlifters, followed by the weight throwers, runners, soccer players, and swimmers, in that order. "Swimmers were not significantly different than age-matched sedentary controls in bone density. Weight-bearing activities are more effective in maintaining skeletal integrity than nonweight-bearing activities such as swimming and cycling."[9]

Unilateral athletes are excellent candidates for studying the effects of physical activity upon selected sites in the skeletal system. Tennis players and baseball pitchers make extensive use of the dominant arm as they practice and perform in their sports. Because of muscle and bone hypertrophy, their dominant arm is larger than their nondominant arm. The bone density of the dominant arm of male tennis players was as much s 35 percent greater than the nondominant arm,[10] and female tennis players showed a 28 percent difference.[11]

Studies employing mild to moderate exercises for the elderly in the 60- to 95-year-old age group have shown increases in bone mineral content and/or cessation of mineral loss.[12] The subjects in the two studies were females whose average ages were 82 and 72 years.

LOW-BACK PROBLEMS

Basic knowledge of the major anatomical components of the back is important to understand the causes and treatment of low-back pain. The vertebral column, consisting of 33 bones, is the only bone connection between the upper and lower halves of the body (see Figure 8.2). It supports the weight of the torso and surrounds and protects the spinal cord. Its landmarks are sources of attachment for muscles and ligaments. The spinal cord extends downward from the base of the brain through most of the length of the vertebral column. Nerves exit from the spinal cord through openings between each of the vertebrae. Discs are cartilage located between each of the vertebrae, where they act as shock absorbers and keep the vertebrae from rubbing against each other. They have a ring of tough fibrous tissue with a white spongelike nucleus in the center. Discs are avascular; that is, they have no blood supply of their own and must rely on nearby tissues to provide their nutrient needs. This is one of the reasons that injured discs take so long to heal.

It is estimated that eight out of every ten Americans will suffer a back injury sometime in their life.[13] Low-back pain is the second leading cause of lost work time for people under the age of 45. It costs business and industry $250 million in workers' compensation and approximately one billion dollars in lost output annually. Twenty-five percent to thirty percent of all disability payments are paid for back injuries. Humans are particularly susceptible to back injury because of their upright posture. Since they do not have the structural advantage conferred by walking on all fours, the burden of supporting the weight of the torso falls upon the lower portion of the spine. The spinal column is not straight; it curves inward in the lower region (lumbar area), and when the curvature is accentuated, the likelihood of injury increases markedly.

The problem is concisely stated by L. Root, who remarks, "A simple law of physics states that when a force or weight is applied to a curved structure, the greatest stress is exerted on the concave or inner side of the curve. Therefore the more pronounced a curve in the spine is, the more uneven is the load of pressure over its surface, with the greatest loads concentrated at the apex of the curve. This in turn will cause excessive wear (a form of chronic trauma) on the intervertebral joints at the curve's apex so that degenerative changes and the wear and tear factor will occur earlier than normal in the spine's life."[14]

Abnormal Curvatures of the Spine

Three abnormal curves of the spine can lead to discomfort, pain and restricted motion. **Lordosis** is an abnormal curvature of the lumbar region (Figure 8.3). This type of curve increases one's susceptibility to low-back problems. **Kyphosis** is an abnormal curvature of the thoracic region of the spine. Referred to as "humpback," this condition is commonly seen in those with osteoporosis (Figure 8.1). **Scoliosis** is an abnormal lateral curvature of the spine (Figure 8.4). If this condi-

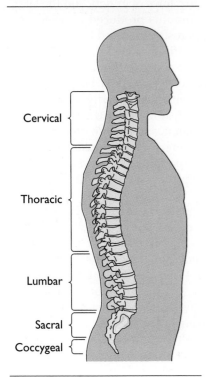

FIGURE 8.2

Normal Curvature of the Spine

Cervical

Thoracic

Lumbar

Sacral

Coccygeal

FIGURE 8.3

Lordosis

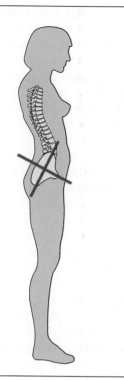

tion is diagnosed early in life—before age 16—it can be corrected with an appropriate brace. Bracing is not effective if scoliosis is allowed to continue unchecked into adulthood. If scoliosis continues to advance after growth has stopped, surgical insertion of steel rods in the spinal column may be necessary.

Patients with scoliosis should exercise to maintain strength and flexibility of the spinal column. This is particularly true for those who wear a brace part of the time. The brace holds the back and trunk in a static position, which can cause muscles to weaken and joints to lose flexibility. The exercises in Figure 8.6 are appropriate for scoliosis: the pelvic tilt, alternate knee to chest, double knee to chest, partial sit-up, and prone press-ups.

● Preventing Low-back Problems

Low-back pain can occur from a variety of causes, the majority of which can be classified as resulting from mechanical factors, including excess body weight, poor posture, and lack of physical fitness.[15] Most low-back pain involves muscle and ligament strain as well as inflamed joints along the vertebral column. Some injuries involve discs that herniate or tear, and the jell-like pulpy material that escapes exerts pressure on the spinal nerves. Back pain also occurs from injuries sustained from accidents, falls, lifting heavy objects, and athletic injuries. Arthritis and osteoporosis also cause low-back pain.

Strategies for preventing low-back problems include maintaining normal body weight; doing strength development exercises for the back and abdominals and flexibility exercises for the back, hips, and legs; and using correct lifting techniques. The muscles of the low back, the abdominals, and the hamstrings all attach to the vertebrae or the pelvis and can all be factors in low-back pain.

Excess weight carried in the abdominal region contributes to low-back problems. The further out front the weight protrudes, the greater the force exerted on the lower back. Paring down the waist and losing weight in general are important components of a healthy back program.

Proper standing, sitting, and lying-down postures are also important to a healthy lower back. Correct standing posture occurs when a vertical line can be drawn from the ear lobes to the anterior of the ankle bone. On the way down, the line should bisect the tip of the shoulder and the middle of the hip bone and continue on just behind the kneecap. To determine whether your posture conforms to

FIGURE 8.4

Scoliosis

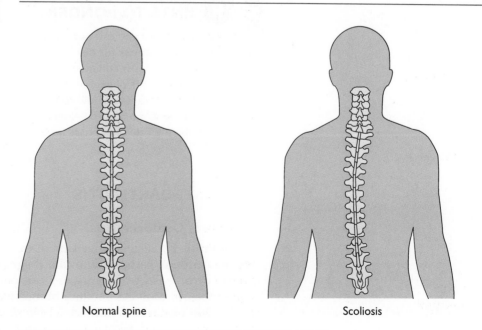

Normal spine

Scoliosis

this description, back up to a flat wall and press your shoulders against it. Press your lower back against the wall by contracting your abdominal muscles and walk away from the wall holding that position.

When sitting, avoid slumping, since this creates unusual stress on the shoulders and neck. See Figure 8.5 for some do's and don'ts for proper posture.

Exercises that develop strength of the lower back and the abdominal muscles as well as those that develop and maintain flexibility of the hamstrings and hip flexors can help prevent back injuries. Exercise also plays a significant role in rehabilitating the back after an injury. Strains and sprains respond well to exercise.[16] Many people with minimal disc herniation (tears) also respond well to exercise and may very well avoid surgery as a result. If surgery is necessary, exercise seems to accelerate the recovery process.

Today, one can choose exercises to treat the specific problem. Williams's flexion exercises (Figure 8.6) are used for low-back problems caused by extension movements. They involve the posterior elements of the spine—that is, those structures behind the body of the vertebrae. Extending the back in activities such as walking or others that involve arching the back usually increase the pain. Flexion activities such as forward bending, sitting, and driving usually reduce the pain. McKenzie's extension exercises (Figure 8.6) are more appropriate for disc problems. In these instances, flexion movements cause pain, while extension movements (arching the back and walking) provide some relief.

In addition to recommending either the Williams or the McKenzie exercises, we encourage patients at the appropriate time to participate in exercises that develop cardiorespiratory endurance and muscular strength. Cardiorespiratory endurance is important because it increases one's level of energy. Increased energy should help with the maintenance of good posture, since fatigue can cause people to slouch.

For beginners, light-weight resistance exercises should accompany the cardiorespiratory conditioning program. There should be a gradual progression of resistance as physical fitness improves. Exercises should work the major muscles of the back, hips, and legs as well as the abdominal muscles. The abdominal muscles may be developed by employing modified sit-ups or variations of abdominal crunches.[17] The majority of people can benefit from trunk curls where the trunk is flexed no more than 30 degrees, which is approximately that point when the shoulder blades clear the floor.

POINTS TO PONDER

1. Define and describe osteoporosis.
2. Who is most at risk for developing osteoporosis, and why?
3. What are the most common fracture sites in type I and type II osteoporosis?
4. Describe the role of exercises in preventing, delaying, and treating osteoporosis.
5. What are the causes of low-back problems?
6. What strategies might you employ in preventing low-back problems?
7. Describe the role of exercise in the treatment of low-back pain.

OSTEOARTHRITIS

What Is Osteoarthritis?

Osteoarthritis is a degenerative joint disease characterized by the deterioration of articular cartilage, particularly in the weight-bearing joints. It is called the wear-and-tear disease. Since the cartilage wears out, it is believed that the habitual participation in activities that produce trauma would accelerate the course of the disease. Weight-bearing activities have been studied to determine their impact upon the development or exacerbation of osteoarthritis.

FIGURE 8.5   Some Do's and Dont's for Proper Posture

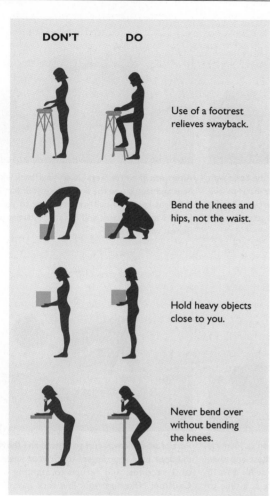

DON'T   **DO**

Use of a footrest relieves swayback.

Bend the knees and hips, not the waist.

Hold heavy objects close to you.

Never bend over without bending the knees.

Proper Bed Posture

For proper bed posture, a firm mattress is essential. Bedboards, sold commercially, or devised at home, may be used with soft mattresses. Bedboards should preferably be made of 3/4-inch plywood. Faulty sleeping positions intensify swayback and result not only in backache but also in numbness, tingling, and pain in arms and legs.

DON'T   **DO**

Lying flat on back makes swayback worse.

Lying on side with knees bent effectively flattens the back. Flat pillow may be used to support neck, especially when shoulders are broad.

Use of high pillow strains neck, arms, shoulders.

Sleeping on back is restful and correct when knees are properly supported.

Sleeping face down exaggerates swayback, strains neck and shoulders.

Raise the foot of the mattress eight inches to discourage sleeping on the abdomen.

Bending one hip and knee does not relieve swayback.

Proper arrangement of pillows for resting or reading in bed.

How To Sit Correctly

A back's best friend is a straight, hard chair. If you can't get the chair you prefer, learn to sit properly on whatever chair you get. To correct sitting position from forward slump, throw head well back, then bend it forward to pull in the chin. This will straighten the back. Now tighten abdominal muscles to raise the chest. Check position frequently.

Correct way to sit while driving, close to pedals. Use seat belt or hard backrest, available commercially.

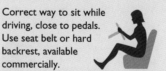

Keep neck and back in as straight a line as possible with the spine. Bend forward from hips.

Relieve strain by sitting well forward, flatten back by tightening abdominal muscles, and cross knees.

TV slump leads to "dowager's hump," strains neck and shoulders.

Driver's seat too far from pedals emphasizes curve in lower back.

Use of footrest relieves swayback. Aim is to have knees higher than hips.

If chair is too high, swayback is increased.

Strained reading position. Forward thrusting strains muscles of neck and head.

FIGURE 8.6

Exercises for Low-Back Pain

Certain exercises can help alleviate low-back pain and help prevent recurrence. The choice of exercises depends on your specific diagnosis. Extension exercises generally are best for persons with disk problems, while flexion exercises usually are best for persons with pain from other causes. Your physician can advise you as to which exercises are appropriate for you and may pre-scribe additional exercises to build strength and flexibility.

Flexion Exercises

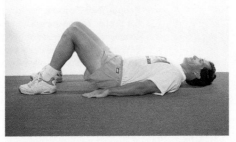

Pelvic tilt Lie on your back, feet flat on the floor with knees bent as shown. Press the lower back to the floor by contracting your stomach muscles. Do not push down with your legs. Hold 5 to 10 seconds.

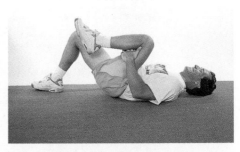

Alternate knee to chest Lie on your back with knees bent and feet flat on the floor. Place your hands under the right knee and pull your right leg to your chest. Hold 5 to 10 seconds and lower to starting position. Repeat with left leg.

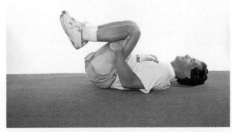

Double knee to chest Starting position is identical to the pelvic tilt. Pull right knee to chest and then pull left knee to chest. Hold both of these for 5 to 10 seconds and then slowly lower one leg at a time to starting position.

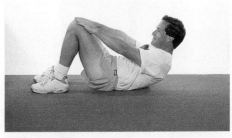

Partial sit-up Slowly curl your head and shoulders off the floor until your fingers touch your knees, hold 1 to 2 seconds, and return to starting position. **Caution:** Make sure your low back stays in contact with the floor.

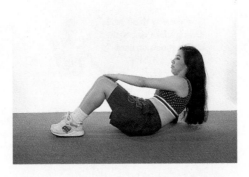

Partial sit-up with a twist Proceed as in the partial sit-up except that both hands touch the left knee. Return to the starting position and repeat with both hands touching the right knee.

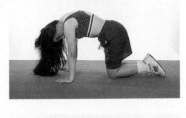
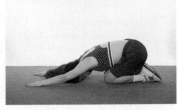

Trunk flexion Start on your hands and knees, tuck you chin to your chest, slowly sit back on your heels, and simultaneously lower your shoulders to the floor. Hold for 5 to 10 seconds and return to starting position.

Continued

FIGURE 8.6

**Exercises for Low-Back Pain—
*Continued***

Extension Exercises*

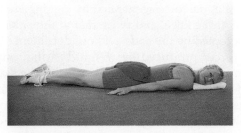

Lying prone Lie on your stomach, head turned to one side and arms at your sides. Lie in this position for 5 to 10 seconds.

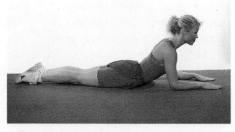

Lying prone propped on elbows Lie on your stomach with the weight supported on your elbows and forearms. Relax your back and allow hips to sag and contact the floor. Hold 5 to 10 minutes. If pain occurs, repeat the lying prone exercise and try it again.

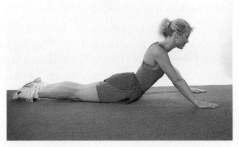

Prone press-ups Lie on your stomach, palms on the floor near the shoulders. Slowly push your shoulders up but keep your hips in contact with the floor by letting your back and stomach sag. Slowly return to starting position. Repeat 5 to 10 times.

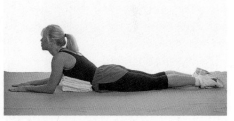

Progressive extension with pillows Lie on your stomach with one pillow under your chest. Add a pillow every two to three minutes until you are lying on three pillows. Stay in this position for 5 minutes and then remove the pillows one at a time over a period of two to three minutes.

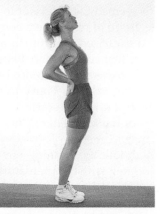

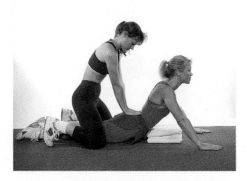

*Caution: It is acceptable to have mild back pain associated with these positions. But if a particular position causes pain to develop in a new location or increases existing hip or leg pain, it should be discontinued.

Standing back extension Stand with your feet approximately shoulder width apart with your hands against the back of the pelvis. Arch your back as far as is comfortable while pushing forward with your hands. Keep you head erect. Repeat 5 to 10 times.

Assisted prone press-ups Do the same prone press-ups but have a partner press down on your pelvis to stabilize it. This exercise can increase range of motion in the lumbar spine.

Currently, rheumatologists (physicians who specialize in the diagnosis and treatment of rheumatic conditions) believe that osteoarthritis has multiple causes and is probably the result of the interaction of genetic and mechanical factors.[18] Osteoarthritis runs in families, but scientists have yet to discover why.

Weight-bearing activities expose the joints to substantial forces. Compared to walking, the forces generated by jogging are twice as great at the hip, six times as great at the knee, and twice that at the ankle. Forces such as these, however, can be accepted by the body without detriment.[19] The joints are capable of dissipating the forces produced by weight-bearing, impact-loading activities. This occurs because the joints are supported by the voluntary muscles and movement is buffered by compressible shock-absorbing cartilage whose surfaces articulate in an essentially friction-free environment. The development of strong muscles surrounding the joints—particularly the knee—is imperative in the prevention of injury.

Osteoarthritis is the most common joint disease in the United States, and though its causes are not known, its prevalence is. Nearly 16 million Americans have osteoarthritis. Except for stroke, osteoarthritis causes as much disability as any cardiovascular disease.[20] Musculoskeletal disorders, including osteoarthritis, cost $35 billion per year in lost wages and productivity.

● Osteoarthritis and Physical Activity

Osteoarthritis is a progressive disease that worsens with age and ultimately affects most people to some extent. The degeneration of some joints begins before age 20 and continues throughout life. Thirty-five percent of 30-year-olds have clinically identifiable osteoarthritis of the knee. The weight-bearing joints of most 40- to 50-year-olds are affected, and 85 percent of 75-year-olds have diagnosable osteoarthritis.

Does jogging aggravate osteoarthritis? R.W. Moskowitz presents the majority opinion when he states, "It is my belief that jogging may aggravate osteoarthritis, especially when the hip or knee are [sic] already symptomatic."[21] Does jogging cause osteoarthritis in normal joints? The answer is no, and there is considerable evidence to support this position. In fact, there is evidence that suggests that jogging may slow the functional aspects of musculoskeletal aging. For several years, 498 runners and 365 nonrunners were followed.[22] The runners visited a physician less often and had less physical disability than age-matched nonrunners, and osteoarthritis seemed to be developing in them more slowly.

The same group of researchers compared 41 runners age 50 to 72 with matched controls who exercised one fourth as much and ran one tenth as much.[23] The results showed that runners had 40 percent more bone mineral content in the vertebrae and there was no difference between the two groups in the clinical manifestations of osteoarthritis. Thirty-five years of data collected in the Framingham study showed a strong relationship between obesity and development of osteoarthritis of the knee later in life.[24] The researchers concluded that obesity is probably a major cause of osteoarthritis of the knee and that running probably is not. Even high-mileage running (an average of 28 miles per week for 12 years) was not associated with the premature development of osteoarthritis.[25]

As long as a joint is not inflamed, people with osteoarthritis should exercise. Exercise increases strength, promotes flexibility, reduces pain, controls body weight, preserves mobility, and increases well-being.[26] The health of cartilage depends on regular use of the joints. When the joints move, fluid and waste products are squeezed out of cartilage. When the joint relaxes, fluid seeps back in, bringing oxygen and nutrients with it.

The osteoarthritic person may have to avoid weight-bearing or high-impact exercises. Pain that persists two hours after physical activity indicates that the osteoarthritic has exceeded his or her limits. Should this occur, a few days of rest are required before returning to physical activity. Activities such as swimming, water aerobics, walking, low-impact aerobics, riding stationary cycles, rowing and cross-country skiing are preferred forms of exercise.

 ## ASTHMA

Bronchial **asthma** is characterized by widespread narrowing of airways of the lungs because of contraction or spasm of smooth muscle and swelling of the mucous membranes in the pulmonary air passages. Breathing becomes very difficult during an asthma attack, which can be a frightening experience.

Nine million Americans are asthmatic, and nearly 5,000 die of asthma each year.[27] Allergies can trigger the asthmatic response. Ninety percent of the asthmatics under the age of 30 have allergies. Hay fever caused by allergies to specific substances such as ragweed, tree and grass pollen, cat dander, mold spores, mites, and other allergens can trigger an asthma attack. (Allergens are substances that cause allergic reactions in some people while producing no abnormal reaction in others.) Asthma can be caused by environmental factors (extrinsic) or intrinsic factors where no external factors can be identified. There is no cure for asthma, but there are effective medications to prevent or reduce the length and severity of an attack.

Exercise can precipitate an asthma attack. Seventy to eighty percent of all asthmatics develop bronchospasms during or following exercise. Bronchial narrowing peaks about 5 to 10 minutes after physical exertion, but recovery is spontaneous and complete within 30 to 90 minutes. Exercise-induced asthma is characterized by moderate airway obstruction and is usually not life-threatening. The severity of an attack depends upon the intensity of the exercise, or more specifically, on the level of ventilation required to meet the metabolic demands of the task. The environmental conditions in which the task is performed also influence the severity of the attack. Cold, dry air produces greater airway obstruction than warm, moist air. Most physicians are convinced that exercise-induced asthma is related to respiratory water loss and airway cooling from the volume and frequency of air that must be moved in and out of the lungs during vigorous exercise. Cold-weather masks or scarves worn over the mouth are useful in preventing cold-induced asthma.

The fear of exercise-induced asthma keeps many people sedentary. However, some asthma sufferers have participated in athletics at the national and international level as amateurs and professionals. The American Academy of Allergy and Immunology agree on the necessity of regular exercise for asthmatics. Regular exercise benefits the asthma sufferer in much the same way as it benefits other individuals. Improvements in aerobic endurance, muscular strength and flexibility, and general health status all occur to asthmatics who exercise. In addition, participation in fitness activities results in a decrease in the frequency and severity of exercise-induced asthma. Swimming and probably other water activities seem to be excellent because of the warm moist environment in which they take place and also because the high ventilation rates required to precipitate bronchospasms are difficult to achieve.[28] Swimming appears to be the least asthmogenic (asthma-producing) of the aerobic exercises, and running and cycling appear to be the most asthmogenic.

Even severely asthmatic hospitalized patients made significant grains in cardiopulmonary fitness after a conditioning program of stationary cycling. Their pulmonary function tests did not imporve significantly, but 92 percent of them improved their endurance and were able to increase their work capacity.[29]

Strange as it may sound, some people are allergic to exercise and experience annoying physiological reactions, including hives, itching, allergic shock (anaphylaxis), hypotension, bronchial spasms, irregular heartbeat, and gastrointestinal problems. Affected people may have one or more of these symptoms beginning about five minutes after the onset of exercise. The reactions usually subside spontaneously in 30 minutes to four hours, but persistent headaches may occur and last for several days. Some of these reactions are potentially life-threatening, but no fatalities have been reported thus far.

Several approaches can be taken to treating exercise-induced allergy. First, it may be possible to identify cocontributors without which the allergic reaction may not have occurred. For instance, a particular kind of food eaten before exercise may produce the allergic response when in fact neither the food nor the exercise alone would have. Avoiding that particular food would allow the individual to exercise safely. In addition, a host of medications are available—from inhalants to injections—that can be used to prevent or mitigate an attack. Exercising asthmatics should be following the treatment and advice of an allergist. It is probably a good idea for people who have allergic reactions to exercise with a friend or family member in case they need help.

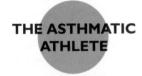

THE ASTHMATIC ATHLETE

Exercise-induced asthma (EIA) is very common among asthmatics. In fact, it affects more than 80% of those with ordinary asthma, 30% to 40% of those who suffer from hay fever, and 9% of people who have neither asthma nor allergies. Studies indicate that 3% to 11% of the world's elite athletes suffer from exercise-induced asthma.

In 1984, 67 athletes (11%) of the 597 members of the U.S. Olympic Team had asthma or exercise-induced asthma. But these 67 athletes collectively won 41 Olympic medals. Their successes were an eloquent testimony to the combination of the effectiveness of medical preventive treatment and the athlete's high level of physical fitness. The treatment applied to these athletes can be used by any asthmatic. First, airway-opening drugs should be used before exercise or competition. Second, a warmup period of 15 minutes should be followed by a 15-minute rest period. This reduces the likelihood of exercise-induced asthma for about two hours. Third, treatment must be individualized to find the optimal regimen for the exerciser. Asthmatics can exercise safely with proper treatment and instruction.

Source: D. Mahler, "Exercise-Induced Asthma," *Medicine and Science in Sports and Exercise* 25, no. 5 (May 1993): 554.

CANCER

● What Is Cancer?

Cancer involves a number of diseases (approximately 100) that are characterized by abnormal and uncontrolled cellular growth. Any cell can become cancerous if it is exposed under the right conditions to carcinogenic (cancer-producing) substances. These substances produce mutant cells that divide and grow uncontrollably. But carcinogens are not the only cancer-causing agents. Some cancerous tumors are probably caused by viral infections. Experimenters have shown that viruses could be isolated from certain tumors, and when implanted in members of the same species, they caused virus-containing tumors in the new hosts.

Normal cells follow an orderly pattern of division and growth which, in adulthood, is restricted to the replacement of lost cells. Cancerous cells lose their responsiveness to the body's signals to stop dividing, so that they and all of their offspring continue to grow wildly. The result is a mass of tissue growth called a tumor, or **neoplasm** (new tissue). A cancerous tumor is malignant. It grows rapidly and is not confined or localized. Cancerous tumors invade surrounding tissues and compete with normal cells for space and nutrients. Eventually, they interrupt the normal function of the tissues or organs in which they have grown.

As many as 2,000 industrial chemicals may pose a cancer risk.
—Jeffrey McKenna

Malignant tumors also shed their cells. These offspring ride the fluid pathways of the lymph and circulatory systems, where they invade and colonize other areas of the body. Metastasis is the medical term that defines the spread of cancer in this manner.

The processes that transform normal cells to malignant ones are complex and essentially unknown, but it appears that the cell's genetic material may be involved. **Oncogenes** are a part of that genetic material. Oncogenes probably start out as normal genes that undergo mutation. As the oncogenes mutate, they in turn change the character of the cells in which they reside, giving them their malignant characteristics. Because the oncogenes are part of the cell's genetic material, they are passed on from the parent cells to their progeny, which are malignant also. Researchers are attempting to identify and study the products produced by the oncogenes. If these can be identified, their analysis may yield information regarding who may have incipient cancer (cancer in its earliest stages). Since early detection is the key to curing cancer, early identification would significantly reduce mortality from the disease.

Surgery is the prescribed course of action as long as cancer is localized, but it is ineffective after metastasis. Cancer that has metastasized is treated with chemotherapy, radiation, or both. These modalities destroy cancerous cells or interfere with their division and growth. Unfortunately, normal cells respond to and are affected in the same manner, particularly those whose growth rate is rapid. Fast-growing blood cells and cells lining the digestive tract are susceptible to radiation and chemotherapy. Side effects associated with the cells' destruction cause substantial discomfort for patients who must be treated in this manner.

There were approximately 1,130,000 new cases of cancer in 1992. Another 600,000 had minor types of skin cancer. Cancer is the second leading cause of death among adults and the leading cause of death from disease among children 1 through 14 years of age.[30]

Cancer is considered cured when a patient shows no symptoms of the disease five years after treatment has stopped. Currently, 4 million cancer survivors have lived long enough to be considered cured.

Many persons in health-related professions and the medical profession agree that approximately 80 percent of all cancers could be avoided by intelligent lifestyle choices. About 35 percent of the total cancer death toll is associated with diet, and another 30 percent is attributed to cigarette smoking.[31] See Self-Assessement 8.1 in Appendix C for the symptoms of some of the common forms of cancer.

● Diagnosis and Treatment

Today, physicians have sophisticated, high-tech, diagnostic imaging techniques that can map the body.

1. Magnetic resonance imaging (MRI) and computerized tomography (CT scans) are painless noninvasive techniques used to detect and locate hidden tumors.

2. Genetic engineering may revolutionize the treatment of cancer. Scientists in the past 15 years have learned to manipulate the cells DNA (deoxyribonucleic acid—the basic storage vehicle or master plan of hereditary information). These techniques have allowed scientists to produce tumor-killing substances. It may be possible to correct impaired immune systems or to change hereditary susceptibility to disease as a result of this technology.

3. New and more effective drugs have been developed.

4. Immunotherapy is a method of enhancing the body's own disease-fighting systems to control or kill malignant cells.

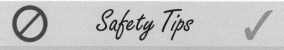

Safety Tips

PREVENTION OF CANCER

1. Avoid cigarette smoking and all other forms of tobacco. Cigarette smoking is responsible for 87 percent of all lung cancers and 30 percent of all cancer deaths.
2. Reduce exposure to sunlight. Almost all of the 600,000 cases each year of basal and squamous cell skin cancer are due to overexposure to the sun. Sun lamps and tanning booths are also hazardous.
3. Avoid overexposure to radiation. Ask physicians and dentists whether routine diagnostic x-rays are necessary.
4. Have your home checked for radon gas. Radon gas increases the risk of lung cancer, especially among cigarette smokers.

5. Drink alcohol sparingly or not at all.
6. Consume a diet high in fiber and low in fat. Eat a varied diet with plenty of fresh fruits and vegetables. Reduce consumption of salt-cured, smoked, and nitrite-cured foods.
7. Follow the American Cancer Society's recommendations for cancer screening.
8. Maintain normal body weight.
9. Exercise regularly.

5. Bone marrow transplants are currently employed in the battle against leukemia, and their use against other forms of cancer is under investigation.

6. Hyperthermic techniques, or methods of administering heat to the entire body or parts of the body, seem to have some promise. Cancerous cells are susceptible to heat. A temperature of 45 degrees C (113 degrees F) is necessary to kill malignant cells.

7. Treatments are being used in combination to enhance their effectiveness.

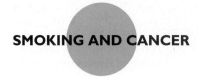

SMOKING AND CANCER

Lung cancer was a rare disease in the early part of this century for males and almost nonexistent for females. Figures 8.7 and 8.8 indicate that there is an approximate 20-year lag time between the advent of smoking behavior and the clinical manifestations of lung cancer. Notice in Figure 8.8 that very few women smoked before 1940; this was accompanied by a correspondingly low incidence of lung cancer. Notice also the acceleration of the lung cancer curve among women in the decade of the eighties and that it follows the curve of smoking incidence.

Smoking cigarettes is analogous to a variant of Russian Roulette. Imagine standing perfectly still in a large room. A blindfolded person with a gun is then ushered in. He cannot see you, nor does he know where you are. But he is instructed to shoot the gun one time in a random direction, after which he is escorted from the room, only to return every hour to fire one randomly aimed shot. Meanwhile, you assume the same position in the room.

Every time smokers light up, they are shooting mutagens (chemicals capable of damaging the cell's DNA) at their genes. But as with the blindfolded shooter, a hit is unlikely, and most shots will miss the target. But as one continues to shoot—or as the smoker continues to smoke—the chances of eventually scoring a hit get better.

Life insurance companies have statistically determined that smoking a single cigarette decreases life expectancy by 10.7 minutes.[32] That is more than the time it takes to smoke a cigarette. Three and one half hours of a smokers life are lost for every pack of cigarettes the person smokes. Self-Assessment 8.2 in Appendix C calculates the number of years of life lost based upon this statistic with regard to smoking.

FIGURE 8.7

Incidence of Smoking and Lung Cancer in Men

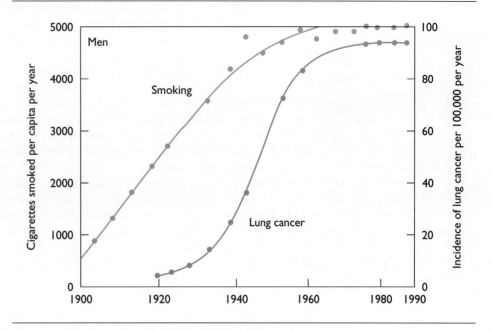

Role of Exercise in the Prevention of Cancer

The Harvard Alumni Study showed that cancer mortality was highest in those who exercised least, even after age and cigarette smoking were accounted for.[33] Women who participated in athletics for at least one year or who expended at least 1,000 calories per week in exercise and physical activity had a lower risk of developing breast cancer and cancers of the reproductive system than did sedentary women.[34] The risk of colon cancer in sedentary Swedish men was 1.3 times greater than for active men.[35] A low level of physical fitness was an important risk factor in both men and women at the Institute for Aerobic Research in Dallas.[36] The most fit of the 13,344 subjects had the lowest incidence of cancer, while the least fit had the highest.

FIGURE 8.8

Incidence of Smoking and Lung Cancer in Women

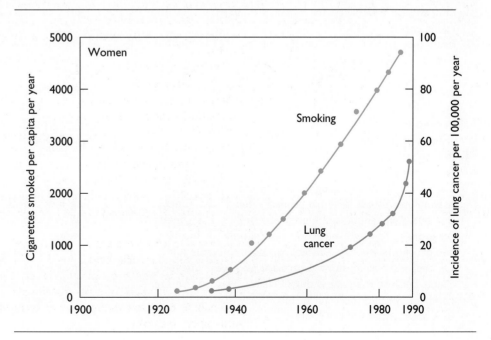

Just as exercise and a low-fat diet help prevent coronary heart disease, they may also help prevent cancer.
—Edward Eichner

The evidence of a relationship between physical fitness and cancer is mounting, but it falls short of establishing cause and effect. However, the results of the epidemiological studies that are investigating this relationship are encouraging, as they reveal a role for exercise and physical fitness in preventing cancer. Several hypotheses have been advanced to explain the mechanism through which exercise operates to prevent cancer. The first of these concerns the role of exercise in reducing body fat. The amount of body fat is positively correlated with the incidence of cancer.[37] R.E. Frisch suggested that the relative leanness of the female athletes in her study protected the women from cancer of the breast and uterus.[38] Fat in adipose tissue stimulates the production of estrogen, while slimness reduces the estrogen drive. The risk of cancers of the female reproductive system are positively associated with high estrogen levels.

Second, exercise may act as a stimulant to the body's immune system, which usually recognizes and destroys cancerous cells early in their development. Three types of immune cells function in an integrated manner to guard against the developing of cancer: (1) cytotoxic T cells, (2) natural killer cells, and (3) macrophages. All three types of cells directly attack and destroy cancer cells. All three also secrete interferon (a family of proteins that defend against viral infection), which enhances the killing capacity of the immune cells and inhibits the proliferation of cancer cells. However, the fact that cancer does occur indicates that the immune system is not infallible in recognizing and destroying malignant cells.

Several studies have shown that exercise may augment or boost the immune system. Plasma interferon levels doubled when eight untrained men exercised on

 Facts, Fallacies, and Timely Tidbits

1. Cancer causes more deaths among children ages 1 to 14 than any other disease in the U.S.

2. In terms of dollars, cancer costs the individual and the nation a substantial sum. The National Cancer Institute estimated that the total cost of cancer in 1990 was $104 billion. This was broken down as follows: (1) $35 billion for direct medical care, (2) $12 billion for lost production, and (3) $57 billion for mortality costs (the cost for taking care of burial).

3. Resistance training increases the thickness of bones for both sexes. Female bodybuilders have thicker bones than female endurance athletes, and research indicates that weight-training programs increase the bone mass of nonathletes. It also appears that weight training supplemented with an increase in calcium intake maximizes the gains in bone mass.

4. It is fallacious to view the cause of osteoarthritis as the result of normal wear and tear over the course of time. Today, most rheumatologists believe that osteoarthritis has multiple causes that are primarily due to the interaction between genetic and mechanical factors. The genetic component has evolved from observations of mothers and daughters who have osteoarthritis in the same joints. On the other hand, normal cartilage may wear unevenly simply because the joint is out of plumb. This may be the result of heredity or trauma, but it may lead to premature degeneration of the joint.

5. Asthmatics can benefit from exercise. Swimming and other water activities are best, but other forms of exercise can be beneficial when guidelines are followed:
   - Take medications as prescribed by your physician.
   - Perform a 5 to 10-minute warmup that includes moderate stretching.
   - Gradually increase the pace during the first 10 to 15 minutes of exercise, being careful to keep the heart rate below 140 beats per minute.
   - As your physical tolerance to exercise increases, you can gradually increase the intensity and/or duration of exercise.
   - Breathe slowly through your nose as much as possible, because nasal breathing reduces the likelihood of hyperventilation and humidifies and warms the air before it enters the lungs.
   - Breathe through a scarf or mask if you exercise outdoors during the winter.
   - Avoid exposure to allergens and air pollutants by exercising indoors during air pollution alerts. Exercise in areas with minimal auto traffic (public parks, golf courses).
   - Recognize that the pollen count is highest in the early morning hours.
   - Do a gradual cooldown to avoid rapid thermal changes in the airways.

a stationary cycle for 60 minutes at 70 percent of their aerobic capacity.[39] Plasma levels of interferon returned to normal two hours after exercise. Vigorous exercise stimulated the release of Interleukin-2 (IL-2), which enhances the activity of the cytotoxic T cells and natural killer cells.[40] Interleukin-2 is an antineoplastic agent that prevents the formation of tumors.

Strenuous exercise increases blood levels of natural killer cells and of B and T lymphocytes. The natural killer cells lyse (rupture) and destroy many kinds of virus-infected host and tumor cells. The B lymphocytes produce antibodies that attack substances that are recognized as foreign to their host, including viruses, bacteria, organ transplants, cancerous cells, and so on. The T cells defend the host against most viral and fungal infections and are involved in an important way with the regulatory control of the immune mechanisms. H.P. Simon stated, "Exercise is a known remedy for the weakness and low spirits that cancer patients experience during their recovery. It boosts energy and endurance, and also builds confidence and optimism. But, within the past five years, several medical investigations have revealed a surprising new fact: Exercise may also help prevent cancer." Recognition of the potential of exercise to prevent cancer came in 1985 when the American Cancer Society began recommending exercise to protect against cancer.[42]

STRESS AND ITS MANAGEMENT

Stress Defined

Stress is defined as the nonspecific response of the human organism to any demand, positive or negative, that it encounters. Stress is produced by any event, condition, or situation that results in change, threat, or loss. Such events are referred to as **stressors,** or stress triggers. The events themselves have stress-producing potential, but they cause stress only if the affected person allows it. In other words, it is the individual's response to a condition or event that empowers it as a stressor.

Those events or circumstances that are perceived to overload or exceed one's resources result in stress. The consequences are proportional to the response that stressors create in each person. Delivering a speech before a group might produce stress of crisis proportions for one individual, while the same event may be perceived by another as an exciting challenge. It is important for all of us to find constructive ways to cope with and manage stress so that it is not disruptive to bodily equilibrium.

Quantifying Stressors

Researchers have developed rating scales designed to measure the relative stressfulness of various life situations. The original scale, developed by Holmes and Rahe in 1967, itemized 43 life events ranging from those requiring the greatest personal adjustment to those requiring the least. Death of a spouse was evaluated as the most stressful of life's events, with the other 42 events tapering in value.

Research indicates that too many changes—good or bad—occurring during a one-year period increase the likelihood that the affected person will experience a health-related problem within the year or soon after. The higher the total score, the greater the possibility of a negative health change.

An examination of life event scales reveals that both negative and positive life changes produce stress. Death of a loved one and being fired from a job are significantly stressful events, but so too are positive life changes, such as marriage, job promotion, and retirement. Negative stressors are referred to as **distressors,** while positive stressors are classified as **eustressors.** While both are stress inducing, research suggests that eustressors may cause illness only in people with low self-

The real secret to a long healthy life is to enjoy what you are doing and be good at it. It's not to avoid stress.
—Paul Rosch

esteem. The reason advanced for this finding is that positive life events are perceived by those with low self-esteem as being inconsistent with their perception of self, and the conflict that arises between the two causes distress.

The life event scales quantify the potentially stressful changes in our lives that may lead to illness. But how do we know that these stress triggers are actually causing harmful stress responses? The warning signs indicative of excessive stress are presented in the following list:

1. Frequent illness—chronic fatigue, headaches, diarrhea, indigestion, sleep disturbance (difficulty with falling asleep or sleeping to excess).

2. Irritability, anxiety, and tension.

3. Apathy, pessimism, sarcasm, and humorlessness.

4. Denial that a problem exists.

5. Escapism, often in unhealthy ways, such as self-medication, including over-the-counter, prescription, and illicit drugs and alcohol.

6. Diminished ability to concentrate on tasks.

7. Avoidance of people—distancing, detachment, and despair.

8. Accident proneness.

9. Aberrant behavior—breaking rules, going to extremes.

10. Procrastination.

11. The perception that there is too much to do and not enough time to do it. Feeling overwhelmed.

12. Loss of objectivity, diminished insight, and impaired judgment.

It is important to understand that the predictability of life event scales is limited. Remember, the individual's response to a stressful event, rather than the event itself, is the primary determiner of its severity. Consequently, the ultimate effect of a life change event is dependent on one's reaction to the event as well as one's approach to coping with and constructively managing the event. Those with ineffective coping strategies who perceive the event to be very important in their lives are at greater risk. Table 8.2 presents selected coping strategies.

The original scale by Holmes and Rahe was modified for student use. Those items that typically do not affect college-age students were deleted in favor of more appropriate ones. This instrument, Self-Assessment 8.3, is presented in Appendix C. Turn to this self-assessment instrument and circle the point value for each life change that you have experienced in the past year, add the scores together for total, and then follow the interpretation guidelines.

THE GENERAL ADAPTATION SYNDROME

Homeostasis is a state of equilibrium in the body with respect to the body's various functions as well as the chemical composition of the body's fluids and tissues. These functions represent the processes through which bodily balance is maintained. The nervous system and the endocrine system are the two major vehicles for regulating homeostasis. Forces that disrupt this balanced state result in adaptive responses by the body. Hans Selye described the body's response to stressors and the ensuing adaptive processes as the general adaptation syndrome. Adaptation consists of three stages: alarm, resistance, and exhaustion.

The Alarm Stage

The alarm stage takes place when the body prepares for action. Adrenaline—the fight or flight hormone—is released, heart rate accelerates, blood pressure increas-

TABLE 8.2 Selected Strategies for Coping with Stress

Acceptance	Recognize a situation that cannot be changed and accepting it. No amount of grief can bring a dead loved one back.
Active thinking	Exploration of new ideas and alternative ways to lessen the stress in a given situation.
Avoidance	A temporary fix, such as staying busy to take one's mind off the stressor.
Catharsis	Expressing one's emotions (crying, anger, etc.) or channeling energy into vigorous physical activity or other pursuits.
Direct action	Taking an active rather than a passive approach to improve a stressful situation. Learn to say "no" more often.
Reappraisal	Assessing the situation and its possible impact on us. Attempting to perceive the stress inducer differently.
Re-examine priorities	Work to live—don't live to work.
Relaxation	Exploring one or two of the many methods of voluntary relaxation techniques or engaging in other relaxing and enjoyable activities for the purpose of experiencing inner peace and tranquility.
Religion	Attempting to obtain spiritual support and comfort from one's faith.
Social support	Talking about your problem with family and friends or, if needed, with a professional.

Adapted from E. Washing, and R. C. Kessler, "Situational Determinants of Aging and Coping Effectiveness," *Journal of Health and Social Behavior* 31 (1990): 103.

es, extra blood is sent to the muscles and less to the digestive system, pupils dilate to take in more information, blood coagulates more rapidly as a precaution against injury, blood sugar level rises, and the immune system slows down. These are some of the changes that occur that prepare the body to perform in a crisis. These changes represent a significant strain to the body and take a toll should they become numerous and persistent.

The Resistance Stage

In this stage, the body adapts to the continued presence of the stressor but at a significant cost in energy expenditure. If people cannot physically or psychologically remove themselves from the stressor, the adaptive mechanisms weaken, and the ability to resist deteriorates. Resistance may be a relatively long process, which is dependent upon the importance attached to the stressor by the affected person.

The Exhaustion Stage

The wear and tear upon the body and its organ systems is a substantial drain on energy reserves that leads to debilitation. Months or years of interaction with a stressor deplete the body's adaptive ability. At this point, professional help may be needed for guidance through the long rehabilitation process to return the individual to normal function.

THE EFFECT OF STRESS ON HEALTH AND WELLNESS

Distress that lasts for months or years prevents the body from repairing itself. Chronic stress produces unhealthy physical, mental, and emotional reactions whose underlying mechanisms are not well understood. Self-Assessment 8.4 in Appendix C will help you identify whether you manifest stress physically, mentally, or both. Regardless of how stress manifests itself, the reasons underlying its effect are theoretical.

We begin with the premise that stress probably does not cause disease but predisposes or increases one's vulnerability to illness and may also hasten the process of latent or subclinical disease. The question is, why? Previously, we saw how the mind can influence and change the body's physiology either positively or negatively. The body's immune system is somewhat depressed during the alarm stage of stress, but it returns to fully functioning status during the resistance stage. However, when stress is chronic, it may remain suppressed for a long period of time, thereby increasing susceptibility to illness.

The immune system responds to invading microorganisms and environmental assaults through a complex series of reactions designed to rid the body of these potentially harmful elements. This is accomplished through the development of specific antibodies and specialized blood cells (lymphocytes) that recognize and attack foreign substances inactivating and preparing them for removal. The immune response is the body's last but most effective line of defense against disease. Oftentimes, the immune response is long-lasting, conferring immunity for life from specific diseases, such as measles and chicken pox. If the immune system is temporarily impaired, as occurs in chronic stress, the individual becomes more vulnerable to disease. Paul Rosch, president of the American Institute of Stress, began research on this topic as a contemporary of Selye several decades ago. He states that cancer and other diseases invade the body when the immune system weakens. The lymphocytes have receptors in their walls that accept hormones such as ACTH (adrenocorticotropic hormone, which may assist in resisting stress) and endorphins (which reduce the perception of pain) and other brain hormones. This network provides a vehicle through which the brain and the immune system communicate. This is the rationale for supporting the connection between thoughts and feelings that cause changes in hormone levels and concomitantly produce responses from the immune system. Chronic stress changes hormone levels and depresses the immune system.

> In theory, stress could directly cause cancer by setting changes in the neuroendocrine system, causing a biochemical reaction that could transform normal cells into malignant ones.
> —Steven Locke

TECHNIQUES FOR MANAGING STRESS

Many techniques have been developed that may assist one to deal with and manage stress. Since not all techniques fit all personalities, it is wise to become familiar with at least a few of them. Examine those presented here and select one or two that appear to be most effective. For optimum effectiveness, these techniques must be practiced regularly.

● Aerobic and Anaerobic Exercise

Since this text approaches wellness through physical fitness, it emphasizes this vehicle for alleviating and controlling stress. Although this field of investigation is in its infancy, the preliminary data are encouraging. Three conclusions can be drawn from the literature regarding the relationship between physical fitness and stress: (1) physical fitness reduces the severity of the stress response, (2) it shortens the recovery time from stress, and (3) it reduces stress-related vulnerability to disease. The data leading to these conclusions were generated primarily from studies that employed aerobic exercise, which features continuous movement for at least 10 minutes at an intensity level that can be sustained without stopping to rest.

Thirty-four studies that examined the relationship between aerobic fitness and psychosocial stress were reviewed by Crews and Landers.[43] The subjects in these studies were exposed to laboratory-induced psychosocial stressors, which included solving math problems under a time deadline, observing films showing accidents or surgery, performing physical exercise of varying kinds, and immersing an extremity, usually an arm, in ice water. After statistical analysis, the researchers concluded that aerobically fit subjects displayed a reduced response to stress compared to unfit subjects, and this held regardless of the type of psychosocial stressor that was used. Fit subjects also recovered from stress sooner than the unfit. Some of these studies suggested that physically fit people have a more effective immune system and are better equipped to ward off disease. This may be possible through mechanisms that include an increase in body temperature during and immediately after exercise (discussed in Chapter 3), the production of endogenous opiates, and reduction in the levels of epinephrine and norepinephrine (catecholamines that prepare the individual for fight or flight).

The effect of anaerobic activity (high-intensity, short-burst activities such as weightlifting or sprinting 100 yards) on stress reduction is inconclusive. Researchers who support the notion that anaerobic training is effective in reducing the stress response accentuate the natural rhythm of these activities, which include periods of stress followed by periods of recovery.[44] Practice of this sort may facilitate one's ability to handle intermittent acute stress and may transfer to life situations, enabling one to more effectively handle such stress. Proponents suggest that anaerobically trained people show greater stress-response reduction than people who have had no physical training. It may be that any kind of exercise that leads to even minimal amounts of fitness may serve as a buffer against stress.[45] Opponents of anaerobic exercise as a stress reducer state that activities in this category do not produce the changes in the nervous system that are associated with stress reduction. They add that anaerobic exercise may be counterproductive in relieving stress, since it significantly raises the blood pressure.

Howard's longitudinal study has shown that exercise and fitness are beneficial for both mind and body in that they produce positive physiological and personality changes.[46] Improvements in body image and self-esteem result in satisfied individuals who genuinely like themselves. Exercise is a concrete stressor that is easily identified. During participation, it replaces ambiguous or nonspecific psychosocial stress. Exercise is also an avenue for the release of excess energy. The social support, the positive sources of stimulation, motivation, feedback, and nurturing that one may receive from family and friends as well as from fellow participants also seems to be useful to mind and body.

Eustress (good stress) occurs when one accepts and successfully meets a challenge. Exercise is both a stressor and a challenge but one that can be recognized and quantified by participants. This builds confidence, which leads to a sense of control over one's destiny. Sensible exercise graded in difficulty to periodically present a greater challenge provides a sense of accomplishment. Since success breeds success, newer challenges should be attainable to increase the likelihood of success. Exercise can cause distress when people have unreasonable expectations or objectives and aspirations that cannot be achieved. The rule for training is "train, don't strain" or "relax and enjoy it." When practiced in this manner, exercise is good stress. If exercise is not enjoyable, it may simply become another stressor.

People under chronic stress are constantly secreting adrenaline into the bloodstream. Continual activation of this response in the absence of physical activity results in adrenaline storage in the heart muscle and a probable increase in diastolic blood pressure. Circulating adrenaline contributes to the processes involved in cholesterol buildup in the arteries. The best antidote for stress is physical activity because it metabolizes adrenaline while recharging the psychological and emotional batteries.

Physical activity for the purpose of competition may become another stressor for some and a stress reliever for others. For some people, exercise is tolerable only when they are competing—running a road race, playing racquetball or tennis, and so on, and they might not participate unless there is competition. Whether competitiveness in physical activity and sports induces or reduces stress needs to be evaluated according to each individual.

According to the President's Commission on Mental Health, approximately 26 percent of Americans suffer from depression at any given time, and 80 percent of all people who commit suicide are depressed.[47] **Depression** is prolonged sadness that persists beyond a reasonable length of time. It is characterized by withdrawal, inactivity, and feelings of helplessness and loss of control. Exercise is now accepted as one component in a spectrum of possible treatments for depression. Several studies have shown that aerobic exercise eases clinical depression.[48] Some patients in these studies were "essentially well" after three weeks of training, while others were able to reduce their medication. Patients became less depressed with exercise, and those who exercised more frequently (five days a week) improved the most.

Meditation

Meditation is the generic name given to relaxation methods that emphasize quiet sitting along with breathing techniques. Transcendental meditation (TM), yoga, and Benson's relaxation response are some of the meditation techniques that have become popular. TM and yoga require the counsel of an instructor and are beyond the scope of this text. But Benson's method is quite easy to learn and to practice.

Herbert Benson and his colleagues evaluated various meditation techniques for their effectiveness in producing relaxation. Although the methods differ, Benson and his coworkers concluded that the methods all appeared to produce similar responses from the physiological systems of the body. Benson referred to these as the relaxation response. The attainment of the relaxation response has four common characteristics: (1) a quiet environment, (2) a comfortable physical position, (3) the mental repetition of a specific word or phrase (a mantra) designed to focus the mind's attention, and (4) a passive receptive mood.

The relaxation response can be learned without a significant investment in money, time, or training. Follow the simple guidelines below for a few weeks to determine whether this technique works for you. (Books, tapes, and other literature are available for those who wish to gain more insight into meditation techniques.)

1. Choose a quiet area and reduce the amount of light in the room.
2. Sit quietly in a comfortable chair, preferably one that will support your head.
3. Close your eyes but do not fall asleep—you cannot consciously experience the relaxation response if you are asleep.
4. Choose a word or phrase to focus on. Benson suggests the use of the word *one*, but any word will do. Some people are more comfortable with a positive word such as *peace, love,* or *joy*.
5. Concentrate on your breathing by repeating the word or phrase every time you exhale. Try to slow your breathing rate.
6. After 15 minutes of this exercise, open your eyes and sit quietly for a couple of minutes and then stand and stretch by reaching for the ceiling.
7. Meditate at least once a day—twice would be better.
8. Beginners should begin with 5-minute sessions and progress to 15 minutes per session.

Autogenic Relaxation Training

The term *autogenic* means self-generating. Autogenic relaxation training is based on six basic autosuggestions that are repeated while the subject is in a quiet comfortable environment and either sitting or lying down with the eyes closed. While in one of these two positions, slowly repeat the following phrases three times:

1. My arms and legs are heavy.
2. My arms and legs are warm.
3. My heart rhythm is calm and regular.
4. My lungs are filling and emptying slowly and rhythmically.

5. My abdomen is warm.

6. My forehead is cool.

Many similar types of phrases are available for other body parts, but these six are adequate to produce the relaxation response. Practice this technique several times a day.

Progressive Relaxation

Progressive relaxation employs the alternate contraction and relaxation of muscles. The technique capitalizes upon the muscles' natural inclination to relax after they contract. This concept can be selectively applied to relax the entire body. The complete program as devised by physician Edmund Jacobson consists of more than 200 muscle-contraction and relaxation exercises.

The technique requires that you lie on your back in comfortable surroundings. Your eyes are closed, arms at your sides with palms up, feet slightly apart. All muscle contractions are developed slowly and held for five seconds before the tension is released. Your purpose is to learn the differences between the contracted and relaxed states and, from this, appreciate the feeling associated with relaxed muscles. The premise is: if the muscles relax, the mind will relax. E. Jacobson suggested that an anxious mind cannot exist in a relaxed body. Since this technique is rather lengthy and involved, only a couple of examples of the method are presented. For the complete program, read E. Jacobson, Progressive Relaxation, Chicago: University of Chicago Press, 1956.

1. Point your left foot as far away from your body as possible. You should notice the tension in your calf muscle. Hold for five seconds, release the tension and repeat with the other foot.

2. Point your left foot in the opposite direction; that is, toes are pointing back toward your head. Note the tension in the front portion of the lower leg. Hold for five seconds, release the tension, and repeat with the other foot.

PERSONALITY TYPES

In 1969, physicians Myer Friedman and Ray Rosenman introduced the concept of behavior type as a risk factor for coronary heart disease. They identified a coronary–prone personality, which they labeled type A. Type A people are characteristically competitive, aggressive, time-conscious, tense, and oftentimes hostile. They also identified a more relaxed type B personality, who is easygoing and less time oriented. The researchers classified 3,000 healthy men by personality type and followed them for eight years. They found that type A people had twice as many heart attacks as type B people. Since then, other researchers using the same instruments and techniques to categorize behavior type have been unable to duplicate the results of Friedman and Rosenman. In fact, since the original study, the majority of the evidence indicates that type A behavior per se does not increase the risk of heart disease, nor does it confirm a protective effect between type B and coronary heart disease. However, there is some agreement that type A personality coupled with hostility does increase the risk for coronary heart disease.

Scientists who are presently trying to unravel the mysteries associated with the emotional effects of exercise have more questions than answers. But the people who have been exercising consistently voice their opinions unreservedly. They report feeling more relaxed, sleeping more soundly, having more energy, and feeling better than at any other time in their lives. To them, these are the important benefits; how and why they occur are of little consequence. The average participant is not concerned with whether the effect is elicited from the endorphins or the feeling of well-being associated with exercise or the feeling of taking charge of this aspect of their lives or some other reason that has yet to be identified. The important factor is that these effects do occur, and the feelings expressed by faithful exercisers are genuine and, in their perceptions, are tied in a causal way to their exercise program. Too many people report similar experiences for it to be in the realm of coincidence. In time, scientists will resolve the whys and hows, but for now we should place some deserved emphasis upon the subjective feelings connected with physical activity. We can predict that they will occur in an appropriately planned and executed exercise program. Perhaps those of us who are involved in motivating others to exercise have relied too much upon objective data focusing upon physiological responses and have slighted to some degree those subjective perceptions that convey to participants that a physically active life is the preferred way to live.

 POINTS TO PONDER

1. Respond to this statement: Exercise causes and worsens osteoarthritis.
2. Asthma sufferers should not exercise. Do you agree or disagree and why?
3. What is cancer, and why is it a deadly disease?
4. How might exercise boost the immune system?
5. Describe the general adaptation syndrome.
6. What are the warning signs of stress overload?
7. Identify and describe several strategies for coping with stress.
8. Describe the role of exercise as a stress-management technique.
9. Discuss the effect of type A and type B personalities as a risk factor for cardiovascular disease.

CHAPTER HIGHLIGHTS

- Osteoporosis results in a gradual loss of bone mass so that the bones weaken and become susceptible to breaking.
- Type I osteoporosis affects eight times more women than men, and vertebral crush fractures are the most common injury.
- Type II osteoporosis affects twice as many women as men, and hip fractures are the most common injury.
- Prevention of osteoporosis includes estrogen replacement for women, calcium supplementation for older women, and exercise for all.
- The spinal column is the only bony connection between the upper and lower halves of the body.
- Kyphosis, lordosis, and scoliosis are three abnormal curves of the spine.
- Strategies for preventing low-back problems include the maintenance of normal body weight, strength development exercises for the back and abdominals, flexibility exercises for the back, hips, and legs, correct posture, and correct lifting techniques.
- Osteoarthritis is a degenerative joint disease characterized by the deterioration of articular cartilage, particularly in the weight-bearing joints.
- Obesity is the major cause of osteoarthritis of the knees.
- Nine million Americans have asthma, and nearly 5,000 of them die annually of this disorder.
- Swimming and other water activities seem to be the best forms of exercise for asthmatics.
- Cancer involves a number of diseases characterized by abnormal and uncontrolled cellular growth.

- Malignant tumors are cancerous tumors.
- Early detection is the key to curing cancer.
- Exercise may prevent some forms of cancer because it reduces body fat and boosts the immune system.
- Stress is produced by any event, condition, or situation that results in change, threat, or loss.
- The ultimate effect of life change events is dependent on one's reaction to the events as well as to one's approach to coping with and constructively managing the events.
- The general adaptation syndrome consists of the body's response to stress in three stages: (1) alarm, (2) resistance, and (3) exhaustion.
- Chronic stress suppresses the immune system, increasing the likelihood of becoming ill.
- Techniques for managing stress include exercise, meditation, autogenic relaxation training, and progressive relaxation.
- It appears that the type A personality is at an increased risk for heart disease only if it is coupled with hostility.

● REFERENCES

1. "Osteoporosis: The Silent Thief," *Worldview* 3, no. 2 (Summer 1991): 1.
2. F. Munnings, "Osteoporosis: What Is the Role of Exercise?" *The Physician and Sportsmedicine* 20, no. 6 (June 1992): 127.
3. R. Papazian, "Osteoporosis Treatment Advances," *FDA Consumer* 25, no. 3 (April 1991): 29.
4. B.L. Riggs and L.J. Melton III, "Evidence for Two Distinct Syndromes of Involutional Osteoporosis," *American Journal of Medicine* 75 (1983): 899.
5. C.C. Johnston and C. Slemeda, "Osteoporosis: An Overview," *The Physician and Sportsmedicine* 15 (1987): 64.
6. R. Papazian, "Osteoporosis Treatment," (April 1991): 31.
7. E.L. Smith and C. Gilligan, "Effects of Inactivity and Exercise on Bone," *The Physician and Sportsmedicine* 15 (1987): 91.
8. N.E. Lane et al., "Long Distance Running, Bone Density, and Osteoarthritis," *Journal of the American Medical Association* 255 (1986): 1147.
9. E.L. Smith and C. Gilligan, "Effects of Inactivity," (1987): 96.
10. H.H. Jones et al., "Humeral Hypertrophy in Response to Exercise," *Journal of Bone and Joint Surgery* 59 (1977): 204.
11. P.C. Jacobson et al., "Bone Density in Women: College Athletes and Older Athletic Women," *Journal of Orthopedic Research* 2 (1985): 328.
12. E.L. Smith et al., "Physical Activity and Calcium Modalities for Bone Mineral Increase in Aged Women," *Medicine and Science in Sports and Exercise* 13 (1981): 60; A. Rundgren et al., "Effects of a Training Programme for Elderly People on Mineral Content of the Heel Bone," *Archives of Gerontology and Geriatrics* 3 (1984): 243.
13. "Low Back Pain," *Mayo Clinic Health Letter* 7 (February 1989): 4.
14. L. Root and T. Kiernan, *Oh, My Aching Back,* New York: David McKay, 1973.
15. "Low Back Pain," (February 1989): 4.
16. C. Cinque, "Back Pain Prescription: Out of Bed and into the Gym," *The Physician and Sportsmedicine* 17, no. 9 (September 1989): 185.
17. W. Liemohn et al., "Unresolved Controversies in Back Management—A Review," *Journal of Orthopedic and Sports Physical Therapy* 9 (1988): 239.
18. "Osteoarthritis: A Joint Endeavor," *Harvard Health Letter* 17, no. 6 (April 1992): 1.
19. M. Pascale and W.A. Grana, "Does Running Cause Osteoarthritis?" *The Physician and Sportsmedicine* 17 (1989): 156.
20. "Osteoarthritis," *Mayo Clinic Health Letter* (Supplement) 10, no. 2 (February 1992).
21. R.W. Moskowitz, "Primary Osteoarthritis: Epidemiology, Clinical Aspects, and General Management," *American Journal of Medicine* 83 (1987): 5.
22. N.E. Lane et al., "Aging, Long-Distance Running and the Development of Musculoskeletal Disability," *American Journal of Medicine* 82 (1987): 772.
23. N.E. Lane et al., "Long Distance Running," (1986): 1148.
24. D.T. Felson, "Obesity and Knee Osteoarthritis. The Framingham Study," *Annals of Internal Medicine* 109 (1988): 18.
25. R.S. Panush et al., "Is Running Associated with Degenerative Joint Disease?" *Journal of the American Medical Association* 255 (1986): 1152.
26. "Osteoarthritis," (February 1992): 6.
27. E.R. McFadden, "Fatal and Near-Fatal Asthma," *New England Journal of Medicine* 324, no. 6 (1991): 409.
28. R. Afrasiabi and S.L. Spector, "Exercise-Induced Asthma," *The Physician and Sportsmedicine* 19, no. 5 (May 1991): 49.
29. S.K. Ludwich et al., "Normalization of Cardiopulmonary Endurance in Severely Asthmatic Children After Bicycle Ergometry Therapy," *Journal of Pediatrics* 109 (1986): 446.
30. American Cancer Society, *Cancer Facts and Figures* 1992, Atlanta, Ga.: American Cancer Society, 1992.
31. J. McKenna and J. Shea, "How to Cut the Risk of Cancer," *Annual Editions—Health 89/90,* Guilford, Ct.: The Dushkin Publishing Group, 1989.
32. P.H. Raven and G.B. Johnson, *Understanding Biology,* St. Louis: Mosby Year Book, 1991.

33. R.S. Paffenbarger et al., "A Natural History of Athleticism and Cardiovascular Health," *Journal of the American Medical Association* 252 (1984): 491.

34. R.E. Frisch, "Lower Prevalence of Breast Cancer and Cancers of the Reproductive System Among Former College Athletes Compared to Non-Athletes," *British Journal of Cancer* 52 (1985): 885.

35. M. Gerhardsson et al., "Sedentary Jobs and Colon Cancer," *American Journal of Epidemiology* 123 (1986): 775.

36. S.N. Blair et al., "Physical Fitness and All-Cause Mortality," *Journal of the American Medical Association*, November 3, 1989, p. 2395.

37. A.P. Simopoulous, "Obesity and Carcinogenesis: Historical Perspective," *American Journal of Clinical Nutrition* 45 (1987): 271; L.N. Kolonel, "Fat and Colon Cancer. How Firm Is the Epidemiological Evidence?" *American Journal of Clinical Nutrition* 45 (1987): 336.

38. R.E. Frisch, "Lower Prevalence," (1985): 887.

39. A. Viti et al., "Effect of Exercise on Plasma Interferon Levels," *Journal of Applied Physiology* 59 (1985): 426.

40. J.G. Carmon et al., "Physiological Mechanisms Contributing to Increased Interleukin-1 Secretion," *Journal of Applied Physiology* 61 (1986): 1869; E.R. Eichner, "The Marathon: Is More Less?" *The Physician and Sportsmedicine* 14 (1986): 183.

41. C.C. Johnston and C. Slemeda, "Osteoporosis," 1987; H.H. Jones et al., "Humeral Hypertrophy," (1977): 17.

42. H.D. Simon, "Derailing Cancer," *The Walking Magazine* 4 (March/April 1989): 17.

43. D.J. Crews and D.M. Landers, "A Meta Analytic Review of Aerobic Fitness and Reactivity to Psychosocial Stressors," *Medicine and Science in Sports and Exercise* 19 (Supplement 1987): 5114.

44. D. Brown, "Exercise, Fitness, and Mental Health," in C. Bouchard et al., (Eds.), *Exercise, Fitness and Health,* Champaign, Ill: Human Kinetics, 1990.

45. S. Petruzello et al., "A Meta-Analysis on the Anxiety-Reducing Effects of Acute and Chronic Exercise," *Sports Medicine* 11 (1991): 143.

46. J.N. Howard et al. "Physical Activity As a Moderator of Life Events and Somatic Complaints: A Longitudinal Study," *Canadian Journal of Applied Sports Science* 9 (1984): 194.

47. T. Monahan, "Exercise and Depression: Swapping Sweat for Serenity?" *The Physician and Sportsmedicine* 14 (1988): 192.

48. E. Martinsen, "Physical Fitness, Anxiety and Depression," *British Journal of Hospital Medicine* 43 (1990): 195; J. Raglin, "Exercise and Mental Health: Beneficial and Detrimental Effects," *Sports Medicine* 9 (1990): 323.

The Basics of Nutrition

CHAPTER OUTLINE

INTRODUCTION

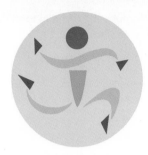

Carbohydrates, fats, protein, vitamins, minerals, and water are the basic nutrients that, when taken in proper amounts, allow the body to perform its many functions. They provide fuel for muscle contraction, maintain and repair body tissues, regulate chemical reactions at the cellular level, conduct nerve impulses, and contribute to growth and reproduction. Carbohydrates, fats, and protein supply the calories in the diet.

Metabolism is the sum total of chemical reactions whereby the energy liberated from food is made available to the body. Two processes are involved: anabolism, in which substances are built into new tissues or stored in some form for later use; and catabolism, which involves the breakdown of complex materials to simpler ones for the release of energy for muscular contraction.

Catabolism occurs when food is combined with oxygen. This process, referred to as oxidation, transforms food materials into heat or mechanical energy. The energy value of food is expressed as a calorie. The term calorie will represent the large calorie (kCal), the unit commonly used to assign the caloric value to food.

Three Self-Assessment activities appear in Appendix C that apply directly to the contents of this chapter:

9.1 Nutrition Inventory

9.2 Assessing Protein Requirements

9.3 Two-day Food Plan

Miniglossary

Amino Acids   The building blocks of proteins.

Carbohydrate   An organic compound composed of one or more sugars that are derived from plants.

Celsius Scale   A temperature scale based on the freezing point of water at 0° and the boiling point at 100°.

Crude Fiber   The fiber that remains in food after it has been treated with harsh chemicals during laboratory analysis.

Dietary Fiber   The fiber that remains after food is digested in the human body.

Disaccharides   A combination of two simple sugars.

Electrolyte   A substance capable of conducting an electrical current.

Fats   Organic compounds that are composed of glycerol and fatty acids.

Fiber   The indigestible polysaccharides that are found in the stems, leaves, and seeds of plants.

Insoluble Fiber   Cellulose, lignin, and hemicellulose add bulk to the contents of the intestine, accelerating the passage of food remnants through the digestive tract. They reduce the risk of colon cancer as well as other diseases of the digestive track.

Kilocalories (kCals)   The amount of energy found in food, it is the quantity of heat needed to raise the temperature of one kilogram of water one degree Celsius.

Minerals   Inorganic substances that exist freely in nature.

Monosaccharides   Simple sugars, such as table sugar, honey, and molasses.

Continued

—Continued

Phospholipids Similar to a triglyceride, except that one of the fatty acids is replaced by a phosphorous-containing acid.

Polysaccharides The joining of three or more simple sugars to form starch and glycogen.

Protein A food substance formed from amino acids.

Saturated Fats Found primarily in animal flesh and dairy products. Chemically, it carries the maximum number of hydrogen atoms.

Soluble Fiber Pectin, gums, and other substances

that add bulk to the contents of the stomach. They lower blood cholesterol levels.

Sterol One of the three major fats with a structure similar to cholesterol.

Triglycerides Consist of three fatty acids attached to a glycerol molecule.

Unsaturated Fats Fatty acids in which one or more points is free of hydrogen atoms.

Vitamins Organic compounds found in food that are essential to normal metabolism.

THE FOOD GUIDE PYRAMID

In April of 1992, the U.S. Department of Agriculture took a giant step forward in redirecting the nation's nutritional objectives by replacing the four basic food groups with the food guide pyramid (see Figure 9.1). The pyramid graphically illustrates (1) the types of food that the bulk of the diet, should comprise (2) the number of servings that should come from each category, and (3) the relative amount of fat and sugar that is naturally occurring as well as that which is added to each category. This later information is attained from the squares and triangles (representing fat and sugar) that are sprinkled about in each of the categories.

The food pyramid emphasizes the importance of carbohydrates. This food group is represented by the bottom two layers of the pyramid which form the foundation of a healthy style of eating.

While the pyramid is a significant improvement over previous food choice recommendations, it is not without its flaws.[1] First, the apex of the pyramid shows that fats, oils, and sweets should be used sparingly, but there is just a mild suggestion that dairy products and meat represent the primary sources of fat and satu-

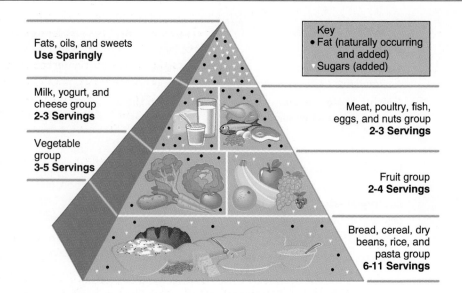

Fats, oils, and sweets **Use Sparingly**

Key
- Fat (naturally occurring and added)
- Sugars (added)

Milk, yogurt, and cheese group **2-3 Servings**

Meat, poultry, fish, eggs, and nuts group **2-3 Servings**

Vegetable group **3-5 Servings**

Fruit group **2-4 Servings**

Bread, cereal, dry beans, rice, and pasta group **6-11 Servings**

rated fat in the average American diet. Second, dry beans and meat are categorized together because both have some nutrients in common. The intent is that beans are a substitute for meat and not the other way around. People who are misinformed may substitute meat for beans. On the basis of fat content, beans do not belong in the meat category. Other than these two potential problems, the food pyramid illustrates quite well the direction that the American diet should take for better health.

Various health and nutrition agencies have been recommending changes in the diet that coincide with those that appear in the food pyramid. Table 9.1 is presented as a supplement to the pyramid because the latter expresses food substances by serving rather than as a percentage of the total. Table 9.1 presents the disparity between current and recommended consumption of carbohydrates, fats, and protein as well as the percentage that each represents of total consumption.

In addition to promoting the Food Guide Pyramid, the federal government has enacted new food-labeling laws that should make it easier for consumers to understand the nutritional content of all processed foods. The reading entitled "Finally—Food Labels That Make Sense" presents more information.

FINALLY—FOOD LABELS THAT MAKE SENSE

New food-labeling laws that will benefit consumers have finally been enacted by the federal government. All processed foods must display the new labels by May 1994. Although not perfect, the new labels will be an improvement over the labels currently in use and are regarded as a positive step in conveying nutritional information to the American consumer.

The upper half of the new label describes the nutritional information related specifically to the food in the package. (See the accompanying sample food label in Figure 9.2.) Included are serving size, total servings per container, total calories per serving, and number of calories from fat. The label also provides important information regarding the percent Daily Value (DV) of total fat, cholesterol, sodium, total carbohydrate, protein, vitamins A and C, calcium, and iron. By examining this portion of the food label, consumers can determine the percent of the daily intake that each food item contains. For example, a food containing 10 grams of fat contains 15% of the DV (based on a 2,000-calorie-per-day diet following the recommendation that fat should supply no more than 30% of the total calories). For a person consuming 2,500 calories per day, 10 grams of fat would constitute 12% of the DV. This information is produced for you; all you need to do is apply it.

Some authorities have suggested that foods containing more than 20% of the DV for a particular nutrient should be considered as a high supplier of that nutrient, while foods that have 5% or less of the DV for a particular nutrient should be considered as a low supplier of that nutrient.

The lower half of the new label will be the same for all food products. It describes the maximum daily amounts of selected nutrients based upon (1) a 2,000-calorie-per-day diet and (2) a 2,500-calorie-per-day diet. The former applies primarily to most women, children, and men older than 50; the latter applies to young men, teenage boys, and very active people. The very bottom of the label provides the number of calories in a gram of fat, carbohydrate, and protein.

The new labels represent a different way to present the nutritional contents of foods. The improved reporting system will allow a more enlightened comparison of foods by consumers.

CARBOHYDRATES

Carbohydrates (CHO) are organic compounds composed of carbon, hydrogen, and oxygen that are arranged as monosaccharides or multiples of monosaccha-

TABLE 9.1	Current and Recommended Consumption of Carbohydrates, Fats, and Protein	
FOOD SUBSTANCE	**CURRENT CONSUMPTION (% OF TOTAL KCALS)**	**RECOMMENDED CONSUMPTION (% OF TOTAL KCALS)**
Carbohydrate (CHO)	48%	58%
	a. ½ simple CHO	a. 10% simple CHO
	b. ½ complex CHO	b. 48% complex CHO
Fat	37%–38%	30%
	a. 17%–18% of saturated	a. *< 10% saturated
	b. 20% unsaturated	b. 10% monosaturated
		c. 10% polyunsaturated
Protein	15%	12%

* < less than

Data compiled from the American Heart Association, American Dietic Association, and the Nutrition and Diet Therapy Dictionary.

rides. Carbohydrates are found almost exclusively in plant sources. The only animal source containing an appreciable amount is milk.

Carbohydrates are classified as simple or complex. Simple carbohydrates consist of monosaccharides (glucose, fructose, and galactose) and disaccharides (sucrose, lactose, and maltose). **Monosaccharides** are single sugars (mono = one; saccharide = sugar); **disaccharides** consist of two sugars bonded together (di = two; saccharide = sugar). Glucose and fructose are the most commonly occurring single sugars in nature. Sucrose, lactose, and maltose consist of two single sugars bonded together. Table sugar (sucrose) is a combination of glucose and fructose. Lactose, a double sugar made from the bonding of galactose and glucose, is the major sugar found in milk.

The complex carbohydrates **polysaccharides** are made of many single sugars that are strung together to form starch and most of the fibers. Starch comes entirely from plant sources, the richest of which are seeds such as grains, peas, and beans. Legumes—butter beans, kidney beans, black-eyed peas, chickpeas (garbanzo beans), and soybeans—are about 40 percent starch by weight.[2] Root vegetables (yams), tubers (potatoes), and rice are examples of other sources of starch.

The most common polysaccharide fibers are cellulose, hemicellulose, pectin, and gums—the nonstarch polysaccharides in foods. **Crude fiber** is the fiber that remains in food after it has been treated with harsh chemicals during laboratory analysis. **Dietary fiber** is the fiber that remains after food is digested in the human body. Dietary fiber is the type that is of interest in this discussion.

Table sugar, corn syrup, molasses, and honey are some examples of simple sugars. Americans, active and inactive, consume too much of these substances. Most of this is in the form of hidden sugar; that is, it is included in processed foods. Canned soups and vegetables, canned meats, cereals, dairy products, soft drinks, and many other items are laden with sugar. Simple sugars are called empty calories because they are rich in calories but provide little or no nutrition.

The question that has been asked and investigated is whether the consumption of simple sugars is harmful. The evidence indicates that sugar becomes a problem only if it replaces more nutritious foods. In this case, deficiencies may eventually surface that are harmful to health. There is no credible research evidence to support the allegation that sugar intake causes heart disease, diabetes, obesity, or other problems. On the other hand, the calories from sugar may secondarily contribute to these disorders if and when they contribute to obesity.

Sugar intake does lead to dental caries (cavities). Sugar is metabolized to acid by bacteria that live on the teeth. The acid dissolves the tooth's protective enamel

FIGURE 9.2

Standardized Food Label

Source: "Food Labeling—Finally" *Nutrition Action Health Letter* 20, no. 1 (January/February 1993): 3.

Nutrition facts

Serving size 1/2 cup (114 g)
Servings per container 4

Amount per serving

Calories 90	Calories from fat 30

	Percent Daily Value *
Total fat 3 g	5%
Saturated fat 0 g	0%
Cholesterol 0 mg	0%
Sodium 300 mg	13%
Total carbohydrate 13 g	4%
Dietary fiber 3 g	12%
Sugars 3 g	
Protein 3 g	

Vitamin A	80%	Vitamin C	60%
Calcium	4%	Iron	4%

*Percent Daily Values are based on a 2,000 calorie diet. Your daily values may be higher or lower depending on your calorie needs:

	Calories	2,000	2,500
Total fat	Less than	65 g	80 g
Saturated fat	Less than	20 g	25 g
Cholesterol	Less than	300 mg	300 mg
Sodium	Less than	2,400 mg	2,400 mg
Total carbohydrate		300 g	375 g
Fiber		25 g	30 g

Calories per gram:

Fat 9	Carbohydrates 4	Protein 4

One 6-ounce potato contains 40 percent of the daily requirement of vitamin C. It is also high in fiber, niacin, and potassium. Many of the nutrients are located in or near the skin. It contains only 180 Kcals.

as well as its underlying structure. The worst offenders are sugary foods that stick to the teeth, such as raisins and caramels.

It is only in the past 50 years that simple sugars have become so readily available. When consumed, simple sugars make their way rapidly into the blood stream. This triggers an exaggerated insulin response and causes large swings in blood sugar level.

Starches such as rice, potatoes, cereal grains, and unprocessed vegetables are some of the complex carbohydrates. They supply energy, vitamins, minerals, fiber, and water. They are broken down through complex digestive processes to simple sugar for absorption by the body.

Carbohydrates had received bad press until 10 to 15 years ago, and many misconceptions about this most valuable source of nutrition still exist. Many uniformed dieters delete or severely reduce their consumption of such carbohydrates as bread, potatoes, rice, and other starches in the mistaken belief that these foods are primarily responsible for weight gain. Actually, these complex carbohydrates (starch and fiber) should be increased because they are filling, high in water content and nutrients, and low in calories. Simple or concentrated sugars such as table sugar, honey, and molasses are the carbohydrates to avoid because they are calorie-dense while lacking in fiber and nutrients.

The old perception that starches were fattening resulted not from the starches per se but because they were vehicles for the addition of fat calories. For example, a medium-size baked potato has about 100 to 110 calories, but if a tablespoon each of margarine and sour cream is added, the caloric value may increase by two to three times. The potato itself is a low-calorie item, as are other starches such as rice, macaroni, and pasta, but if the latter are loaded down with rich sauces and gravies, their calorie count rises substantially. In other words, the starches are not fattening, but what is added to them causes the problems.

Diets that are low in carbohydrates promote lean tissue and water loss. Each gram of glycogen (the stored form of carbohydrate) is stored with two to three grams of water. If the glycogen stores are depleted and not replenished, the lost water is also not replaced. Diet vendors capitalize on this knowledge to effect quick but ineffective water weight loss. Low-carbohydrate diets can lead to dehydration. When dieters return to pre-diet eating patterns, glycogen and all of the water needed to store it are returned so that the dieter quickly regains some of the lost weight.

Complex carbohydrates are looked on favorably by the nutritional and medical communities. They are low in fat and high in fiber, both of which can help protect against heart disease and certain types of cancer.

When oxidized, carbohydrates yield approximately 4 calories per gram. Because the calories are oxygen rich, they constitute our most efficient source of fuel. About 30 percent to 40 percent of the body's energy needs at rest are supplied by carbohydrates.[3] Mild to moderate exercise, such as walking 4 mph, jogging 1.7 to 3.4 miles in 20 to 40 minutes, and cycling at 10 mph, relies on carbohydrates to contribute up to 50 percent of the energy. More vigorous exercise relies principally on carbohydrates, while very intense exercise relies almost exclusively upon carbohydrates.

FIBER

Dietary fiber consists of a number of different substances that appear to affect the body in various ways. Fiber is classified as soluble or insoluble. **Soluble fiber** (pectin, gums, and other substances) comes from a wide variety of grains, fruits, and vegetables. Excellent sources include prunes, pears, oranges, apples, legumes, cauliflower, zucchini, sweet potatoes, and oat and corn bran. Soluble fibers add bulk to the contents of the stomach. This slows stomach emptying, prolongs the sense of feeling full, and reduces the desire to eat for a longer period of time. It also slows the absorption of sugars from the small intestine so that the blood sugar level rises moderately, resulting in a more precise insulin response. Regarding cardiovascular health, the soluble fibers lower blood cholesterol levels.

Most **fibers** are indigestible polysaccharides found in the stems, leaves, and seeds of plants. Human digestive enzymes are incapable of breaking the bonds that hold the units of fiber together, but bacteria in the digestive tract can dismantle a few of the fibers so that a small amount of absorbable energy is derived. Fiber is therefore not totally devoid of kilocalories (kCals), although their contribution to total body energy is negligible.

The amount of energy found in food is measured in **kilocalories,** the amount of heat needed to raise the temperature of a kilogram of water (about one quart) one degree **Celsius.** People simply refer to these as calories, but this is technically

Toasting bread removes much of the moisture but none of the calories.

incorrect. Since there are 1,000 calories in one kilocalorie, the energy in food is measured in thousands of calories. All food energy values in this text refer to kilocalories.

Insoluble fiber includes cellulose, lignin, and hemicellulose. Significant sources of insoluble fiber include bran (the outer layer of wheat and corn), the skins of fruits and root vegetables, and leafy greens. Foods such as these add bulk to the contents of the intestine, accelerating the passage of food remnants through the digestive tract and decreasing tissue exposure to toxins and carcinogenic substances. Insoluble fiber reduces the likelihood of developing colon cancer. Also, some insoluble fibers attract water, thus softening stools and preventing constipation, while others solidify watery stools, helping to alleviate diarrhea. The improved motility of the digestive contents contributes to the health and tone of the intestinal muscles and increases their resistance to the formation of pouches that signify the onset of diverticulitis. Diverticulitis is characterized by pouchlike formations in the intestinal wall that are subject to serious infection should they rupture.

Virtually all fruits, vegetables, and whole grain products contain some of each type of fiber. If you need to increase your consumption of fiber—and most Americans do—you must also increase your intake of fluid. Without a corresponding increase in fluid, the stool would become hard, resulting in painful and difficult elimination. Table 9.2 lists some common foods and their fiber content. Dietary fiber is always an estimate rather than an exact value because of the variability inherent in food samples and because no standardized test method has been developed for simulating the human digestive process. The estimates in Table 9.2 are in grams (gm).

Most authorities agree that Americans should increase their fiber intake from the current 10 to 13 grams per day to 20 to 35 grams per day. Still other authorities suggest that 40 to 50 grams per day would produce better results. This is the amount that most vegetarians safely consume. However, an increase in fiber intake should occur gradually to avoid the bloating, intestinal gas, and cramps caused by the fermentation of fiber and indigestible sugars in the colon. This is not a serious problem but rather an uncomfortable one that will eventually subside as the bacteria in the system adjust to the fiber increase.

A high-fiber intake poses a potential problem because of its ability to bind and inhibit the absorption of trace minerals such as zinc, iron, and magnesium. The effect is minimal, however, because high-fiber foods are rich enough in minerals to compensate for any possible losses that occur.

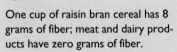

One cup of raisin bran cereal has 8 grams of fiber; meat and dairy products have zero grams of fiber.
—Nutrition Action Health Letter

FATS

Fats are energy dense organic compounds that yield approximately 9 calories per gram. They have a relatively low oxygen content compared to carbohydrates and consequently are not as efficient as sources of fuel. It takes more than twice the amount of oxygen to liberate energy from fat than from carbohydrates. However, we store at least 50 times more energy in the form of fat than in carbohydrates. Table 9.3 presents the caloric yield per gram (gm) of the energy-containing nutrients. There are 28.4 grams per ounce and 454 grams in a pound. There are 4086 kCals in a pound of fat if the water is removed (454 g × 9 kCal = 4086). But fat as it is stored in the body contains some water. Water is noncaloric and heavy. A pound of stored fat with its water content contains approximately 3500 kCals.

Fats (lipids) consist of three major types: triglycerides, sterols, and phospholipids. The triglycerides are the most abundant type of fat, representing at least 95 percent of the fat that is eaten as well as that which is stored within the body. The **sterols** have a structure similar to cholesterol. The **phospholipids** are similar to a triglyceride, except that one of the fatty acids is replaced by a phosphorous-

TABLE 9.2 Selected Sources of Fiber

	DIETARY FIBER (gm)
1. Cereals	
100% Bran (½ cup)	8.4
All Bran (⅓ cup)	8.5
Bran Buds (⅓ cup)	7.9
Bran Chex (⅔ cup)	4.6
Corn Bran (⅔ cup)	5.4
Cracklin' Oat Bran (⅓ cup)	4.3
Bran Flakes (¾ cup)	4.0
Oatmeal, cooked, 1 cup	2.2
2. Grains (1 ounce)	
Brown rice, cooked (½ cup)	2.4
Millet, cooked (½ cup)	1.8
Whole wheat bread (1 slice)	1.0
Spaghetti, cooked (½ cup)	0.8
White bread (1 slice)	0.6
White rice, cooked (½ cup)	0.1
3. Legumes (½ cup)	
Kidney beans	5.8
Pinto beans	5.3
Split peas	5.1
White beans	5.0
Lima beans	4.9
4. Vegetables (½ cup)	
Sweet potato (1 large)	4.2
Peas	4.1
Brussels sprouts	3.9
Corn	3.9
Potato, baked (1 medium)	3.8
Carrots (1 raw; ½ cup cooked)	2.3
Collards	2.2
Asparagus	2.1
Green beans	2.1
Broccoli	2.0
Spinach	2.0
Turnips	1.7
Mushrooms (raw)	0.9
Summer squash	0.7
Lettuce (raw)	0.3
5. Fruits	
Blackberries (½ cup)	4.5
Prunes, dried (3)	3.7
Apples with skin (1)	2.6
Banana (1 medium)	2.0
Strawberries (¾ cup)	2.0
Grapefruit (½ med.)	1.7
Peach (1 med.)	1.6
Cantaloupe (¼ small)	1.4
Raisins (2 tablespoons)	1.3
Orange (1 small)	1.2
Grapes (12)	0.5

Adapted from J. Anderson, *Plant Fiber in Foods,* Lexington, Ky.: HFC Diabetes Research Foundation, Inc., 1986; *Nutrition Action Healthletter* (April 1986); and E. Lanza and R. R. Butram, "A Critical Review of Food Fiber Analysis and Data," *Journal of the American Dietetic Association* 86 (1986): 732.

TABLE 9.3

The Energy-Containing Nutrients

NUTRIENTS	ENERGY YIELD (gms)
Carbohydrates (CHO)	4 kCals
Fats	9 kCals
Proteins	4 kCals

containing acid. The **triglycerides** are composed of three fatty acids attached to a molecule of glycerol. Fatty acids are classified as saturated or unsaturated, based upon their chemical structure. A fatty acid is a long chain of carbon atoms (C) bonded to hydrogen atoms (H), with an acid group at the end of the molecule. Fatty acids are saturated when all of the bonds between the carbon atoms are single bonds (see Figure 9.3a). Monounsaturated fatty acids have one double bond between carbon atoms (See Figure 9.3b). Polyunsaturated fatty acids have two or more double bonds between the carbon atoms (See Figure 9.3c).

The major sources of **saturated fats** are animal flesh, dairy products, and tropical oils (coconut, palm, and palm kernel oil). Saturated fats have a high melting point and solidify at room temperature. Bacon or sausage grease that stands at room temperature will solidify, signifying that it is saturated. Monounsaturated and polyunsaturated fats remain liquid at room temperature. Some food sources that are high in monounsaturated fats are avocados, canola oil, cashew nuts, olives, olive oil, peanuts, peanut oil, and peanut butter. Polyunsaturated fats are found in almonds, corn oil, cottonseed oil, filbert nuts, fish, pecans, safflower oil, sunflower oil, soybean oil, and walnuts.

Hydrogenated Fats

Unsaturated fats should be refrigerated to keep them from becoming rancid. They are vulnerable to spoilage when left to stand at room temperature because oxygen attacks those points in the chain that are unoccupied by hydrogen. To counteract spoilage, the food industry adds hydrogen to some of the free bonds through the process of hydrogenation. The fat then loses its polyunsaturated characteristics as well as its health benefits. Hydrogenation converts many double bonds to single bonds. The end product is the conversion of unsaturated fatty acids to trans fatty acids. Margarine is the major source of trans fatty acids in the American diet.

Vegetable oils are liquid and must be made more saturated if they are to be solidified into margarine. The harder the product (stick margarine)—versus softer margarines (tub and squeeze bottle)—the greater the effect of hydrogenation. The question to be answered is, Does the conversion of unsaturated fatty acids to trans fatty acids result in an unhealthy product? The evidence on this point is far from conclusive. A recent Dutch study found that trans fatty acids increased both cholesterol and LDL cholesterol while lowering HDL cholesterol.[4] This represents an unhealthy change. However, the subjects in this study were given 33 grams of trans fatty acids per day, compared to the U.S. average consumption of 4 to 7 grams per day. Is the lower U.S. consumption also harmful? The answer is not known at this time. Until more definitive studies are completed, the advice regarding all fat in general, and trans fatty acid consumption specifically, remains the same: (1) cut back total fat to less than 30 percent of the dietary calories, and (2) consume at least twice as much unsaturated fat as saturated fat.

Eating a fat-free diet is virtually impossible. Even vegetarian diets supply 5 percent to 10 percent of their calories from fat. Although some fat in the diet is necessary for good health, the problem in the United States is that we consume too

The 3½ percent fat in whole milk supplies 50 percent of the calories. Fat supplies 30 percent of the calories in 2 percent milk, 18 percent of the calories in 1 percent milk, and 2 percent of the calories in skim milk.

A diet high in monounsaturated fats (olive oil, canola oil, peanut oil) increases LDL cholesterol's resistance to oxidation moreso than a diet high in polyunsaturated fats (corn oil and most other vegetable oils).
—Nutrition Action Health Letter

FIGURE 9.3

Categories of Fatty Acids

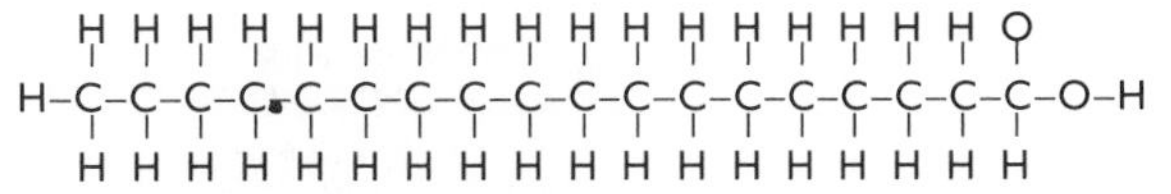

(a) Saturated fatty acid—no double bonds; all carbons are occupied.

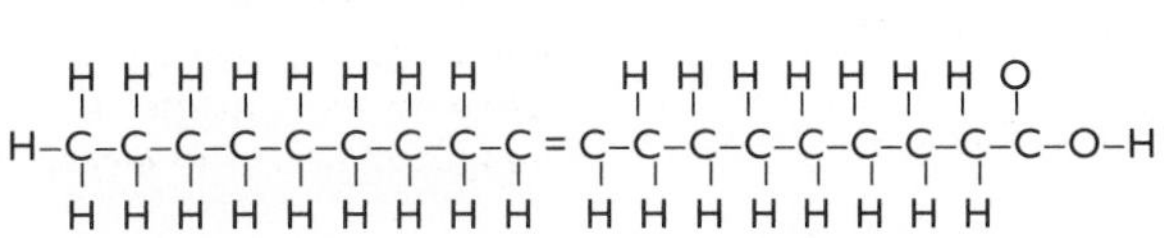

(b) Monounsaturated fatty acid—one double bond; two hydrogens missing at that site.

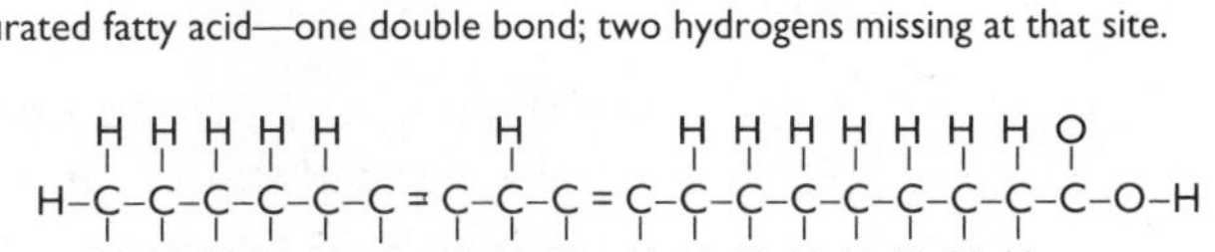

(c) Polyunsaturated fatty acid—two double bonds; four hydrogen missing at the site.

much fat. The human body can synthesize its fat requirements from carbohydrates, fats, and proteins, with the exception of two fatty acids. Linoleic acid and linolenic acid are categorized as essential fatty acids because they cannot be manufactured in sufficient amounts within the body to meet physiological needs. Both are polyunsaturated fatty acids that can be supplied only through the diet. These fatty acids are widely distributed in plant and fish oils. Linoleic acid is an omega-6 fatty acid found mostly in plants, while linolenic acid is an omega-3 fatty acid found in fish. The fatty acids in coldwater fish are the most polyunsaturated of the fats.[5]

Seafood

Seafood consumption in the United States averaged a paltry 15 pounds per person in 1991. During that same year, meat and poultry consumption averaged 112 and 58 pounds per person, respectively. Increasing seafood intake while decreasing meat consumption would benefit the health of the nation. Most seafood is very low in saturated fat and low in cholesterol and total calories. Eating seafood is nutritious and heart healthy. Only shrimp, Eastern oysters, and blue crabs have relatively high levels of cholesterol. Seafood is the only food that contains omega-3 fatty acids. These fish oils may reduce the risk of heart disease by making blood less sticky (less viscous) and therefore less likely to clot.

Which fish are richest in omega-3 fatty acids? In general, the fatter the fish, the higher the content of omega-3s. Table 9.4 lists some sources of omega-3 fatty acids.

Fat serves many vital functions. It is a significant energy source that provides up to 70 percent of the calories needed while the body is at rest. It is the major supplier of energy during mild exercise and low-intensity exercise of long duration. It is responsible for the storage, transport, and absorption of the fat-soluble vitamins. Fat is an essential component of nerve fibers and cell walls and protects vital organs from physical trauma by acting as a shock absorber. Fat also acts as an insulator against the loss of body heat. Excessive amounts of dietary or stored fat are not required to support these functions.

Shrimp and crayfish have about as much cholesterol as meat but they contain less fat than meat. Their fat is essentially unsaturated and includes heart-healthy omega-3 fatty acids.
—Univerwsity of California at Berkeley Wellness Letter

PROTEIN

Protein is an essential nutrient that yields approximately 4 calories per gram. Its energy is liberated for building and repairing body tissues; forming enzymes, hormones, antibodies, and hemoglobin; transporting fats and other nutrients to the blood; maintaining acid-base balance in tissue fluids; and supplying energy for muscular work when there is a shortage of carbohydrates and fat.

Protein is one of the most misused and abused of the nutrients. It has been advertised as a high-energy food. In the Roman Empire, gladiators were fed large amounts of animal muscle tissue in the belief that this practice would build

---

TABLE 9.4 **Sources of Omega-3 Fatty Acids***

The following have approximately 2 grams of omega-3 fatty acids per 4-ounce serving:

- Sablefish
- Herring
- White fish
- Atlantic or pink salmon
- Mackeral

The following have approximately 1 gram of omega-3 fatty acid per 4-ounce serving:

- Sea bass
- Smelt
- Trout
- Bluefish
- Bluefin tuna
- Altlantic mackerel
- Eastern oysters
- Sockeye salmon

*Since all fish have some omega-3 fatty acids, all are acceptable. The exceptions are fish sticks and fast-food sandwiches, which have none. Farm-raised grain-fed catfish have less than one tenth of a gram of omega-3s per four-ounce serving.

---

1. Most males should consume no more than 5 teaspoons of saturated fat in one day. One Burger King Double Whopper contains this much.
2. The consumption of fresh potatoes from 1960 to 1990 declined by 40%, but the consumption of frozen potatoes during the same period increased by 557%.
3. The average cost of ingredients in an Arby's sandwich costs 54 cents, while the average price is $2.02.
4. In 1965, 335 million pounds of synthetic pesticides were applied to farm crops; in 1989, 806 million pounds were applied.
5. A national survey of high school students indicated that only 10% of the females consumed five or more servings of fruits and vegetables the day before the survey, while 15% of the males consumed this amount.
6. Vitamin loss from cooking can be minimized by
   - cutting vegetables in large pieces or cooking them whole (small pieces increase the loss).
   - cooking vegetables quickly and in little water or steaming them.
   - eating vegetables immediately after cooking, not letting them sit.
7. Vitamin C is quickly degraded by exposure to air as well as by overcooking:
   - 63% of vitamin C is left if one cup of spinach is boiled in one cup of water, while only 36% is left if this amount is boiled in 2 cups of water.
   - 79% of vitamin C is left if broccoli is steamed, 77% if stir-fried, 74% if boiled in a covered pot with a small amount of water, 57% of microwaved, and 45% if covered with water in an uncovered pan.
   - 80% of the vitamin C is left in a baked potato, 53% if the potato is boiled, 23% if it is mashed, and 0% if mashed potatoes are kept on a steam table for 45 minutes.

human muscle tissues. Many of today's bodybuilders, weightlifters, and power lifters continue this practice. They consume quantities of protein-rich foods and supplements in the belief that active people cannot obtain too much protein.

Protein is a major supplier of energy only during starvation. In this state, the body consumes its own protein, the majority of which comes from the muscles to meet the body's energy needs. As a result, the body takes on a wasted appearance, exemplified by the "concentration-camp look." For an endurance athlete, protein can supply up to 15 percent of the energy required to fuel long-distance events (marathon distance and beyond).

Protein Sources

Proteins are complex chemical structures containing carbon, oxygen, hydrogen, and nitrogen. These elements are combined into chains of different structures called **amio acids.** There is general agreement that the proteins of all living tissue consist of 20 different amino acids. Two other rare amino acids have been identified but are found in very few proteins. Eight of the amino acids are essential because they cannot be manufactured in the body and can be obtained only through the diet.

To build body tissue, all of the essential amino acids must be present simultaneously. This is analogous to building a house. Construction progresses unimpeded as long as all of the building materials are at the site, but if there isn't any mortar for laying the bricks, construction stops until it is supplied. Similarly, the building of body tissue progresses to completion when all of the amino acids (the body's building blocks) are present, but if one or more is missing, construction stops at that point. Complete proteins—those containing all the essential amino acids—are found in meat, fish, poultry, and dairy products. The proteins found in vegetables and cereal grains generally do not contain all of the essential amino acids, but complementary foods from these two groups may be selected so that one supplies those amino acids missing in the other. See Table 9.5 for combinations of food that together provide complete proteins.

Legumes, such as kidney and lima beans, black-eyed peas, garden peas, lentils, and soybeans, are excellent sources of proteins. Although their protein is not quite

TABLE 9.5   Complete Proteins from Vegetable Combinations

CATEGORIES OF FOODS	EXAMPLES
Beans/wheat	Baked beans and brown bread
Beans/rice	Refried beans and rice
Dry peas/rye	Split pea soup and rye bread
Peanut butter/wheat	Peanut butter sandwich on whole wheat or whole grain bread
Cornmeal/beans	Cornbread and kidney beans
Legumes/rice	Black-eyed peas and rice
Beans/corn	Pinto beans and corn bread
Legumes/corn	Black-eyed peas and corn bread

Adapted from A. C. Grandjeans, *The Vegetarian Athlete* 15 (1987): 191.

the caliber of that of meat, they are rich in fiber, iron, and B-vitamins, and they are low in fat.

Protein Requirements

Daily protein requirements vary according to one's position in the life cycle. Infants require about 2.2 grams of protein per kilogram of body weight to support growth. Adolescents require 1.0 gram per kilogram, and adults need 0.8 gram per kilogram. Table 9.6 summarizes the protein requirements by age.

The typical American diet contains more than adequate amounts of protein. There seems to be no advantage in consuming more than 12 percent of the total calories in the form of protein. Excessive intakes have altered the body composition of children[6] and enlarged the kidneys and livers of animals.[7] They can cause dehydration because extra water is needed to rid the body of unused or wasted nitrogen. This can be a significant problem for active people because they lose additional fluid in perspiration during a workout. Another problem associated with excessive protein intake is that it is usually accomplished by increasing the consumption of animal products, which are also high in saturated fat. This increased consumption may displace fiber in the diet, possibly leading to constipation. In addition, such foods are expensive. Ingesting larger than normal amounts of protein does not enhance physical performance; but then, that is not the function of protein.

A 170-pound adult might consume 2,600 kCals/day. How much protein is consumed, and how much is actually needed?

The following illustrates the typical protein consumption by a 170-pound adult in the United States whose protein intake is about 15 percent of the total calories consumed.

1. Convert body weight in pounds to kilograms (kg):

$$\frac{170}{2.2 \text{ (lbs. per kg)}} = 72.3 \text{ kg}$$

2. 2,600 kCals consumed
   $\times .15$ percentage of protein in the diet
   390 kCals of protein

3. 1.0 gram of protein yields 4 kCals; therefore,

$$\frac{390}{4} = 97.5 \text{ grams protein}$$

4. Protein required is 0.8 gram per kg of body weight:

   72.3 kg
     .8

   57.8 grams of protein required

Skinless turkey contains about 33 percent less fat than skinless chicken. Skinless dark turkey and chicken meat contains twice as much fat as skinless white meat, 20 percent more calories, and 10 percent less protein.

TABLE 9.6

Recommended Daily Allowance (RDA) for Protein

AGE	RDA (GRAMS/ KILOGRAM*)
0–2 months	2.2
6 months–1 year	2.0
1–3 years	1.8
4–10 years	1.1
11–14 years	1.0
15–18 years	0.9
19 and beyond	0.8

*Pregnancy increasese the protein requirement by 30 grams per day, and lactation increases the protein requirement by 20 grams per day.

5. Difference between protein consumed and protein required:

97.5 consumed
<u>57.8</u> required
39.7 grams of extra protein

6. This person is consuming an excess of approximately 40 grams of protein per day.

Many people—competitors and noncompetitors alike—who are striving to develop strength and power have been taking amino acid supplements to build larger and more powerful muscles. Selected amino acids do not build larger muscles; only exercise can do that. However, these and other unfounded notions proliferate among uninformed participants who are constantly attempting to enhance performance with substances that might give them an edge beyond that achieved with training. William Evans, Chief of the Physiology Laboratory in the Human Nutrition Research Center on Aging at Tufts University stated, "If you have an intestine, you don't need amino acid supplements. The intestine breaks down protein perfectly well. Furthermore, no research indicates that amino acid supplements improve strength, power, or muscle mass."[8]

There is evidence that athletes who participate in vigorous aerobic activities or who are involved in strength or power events require twice as much protein as the average person.[9] Even if this proves to be correct, protein supplements are not necessary, since most athletes consume more than this amount from their food intake. Suppose a 220-pound male athlete consumes 4,800 kCals/day. His protein intake represents 17 percent of his total calories—about average for athletes. How many grams of protein does he consume, and how many does he actually need if his requirement is double the RDA?

1. Convert body weight in pounds to kilograms (kg)

$$\frac{220 \text{ lbs}}{2.2} = 100 \text{ kg}$$

2. 4,800 kCals consumed
<u>× .17</u> percentage of protein in the diet
816 kCals/protein

3. 1 gram of protein yields 4 kCals; therefore,

$$\frac{816}{4} = 204 \text{ grams protein}$$

4. Protein required is 1.6 grams per kg of body weight

100 kg
<u>× 1.6</u>
160 grams

5. Difference between protein consumed and protein required:

204 consumed
<u>160</u> needed
44 grams of extra protein

In light of the preceding example, protein supplementation or amino acid supplements are unnecessary and a waste of money.

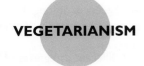

VEGETARIANISM

Vegetarianism, with its biblical origins, is probably the oldest form of diet known. There are many reasons for pursuing such a style of eating, from those that are health related to those that are philosophical and cultural. Regardless of the reason, vegetarianism requires some basic nutritional knowledge to meet the recommended daily allowances for normal nutrition. The amount of knowledge required depends on the restrictiveness of the diet. This is reflected by the type

Continued

—Continued

of vegetarian diet that is practiced. Vegetarianism runs the gamut from strict adherence to plant foods to other less restrictive forms that allow animal products. The types of vegetarian diets are as follows:

1. Fruitarians: food choices consist of raw or dried fruits, nuts, honey, and vegetable oil.
2. Vegan: all plant food diet without animal foods, milk products, or eggs.
3. Lacto-vegetarian: plant food diet plus milk, milk products.
4. Lacto-ovo-vegetarian: plant food diet plus milk, milk products, and eggs.
5. Semivegetarian: plant food diet plus some groups of animal products.
6. New vegetarian: plant food diet plus some groups of animal products, with emphasis on foods that are organic, natural, and unprocessed or unrefined.

Active people who are strict vegetarians (vegans) many times have difficulty obtaining enough calories to meet their daily caloric expenditure.[10] Their diet consists of foods that are nutritionally dense and high in fiber but low in calories. They may need to supplement with high-calorie foods such as nuts, seeds, legumes, and vegetable margarine. The problem with strict vegetarian diets is not limited only to low-calorie intake. Since vitamin B12 is found almost exclusively in animal products, the vegan will need to get this vitamin either from supplements or soybean milk fortified with B12. Also, the vegan can get complete proteins by matching appropriate foods as suggested in Table 9.5. In addition, the high-fiber content of vegetable diets interferes with the absorption of iron. Although legumes are a good source of iron, the iron contained in them is less absorbable than that found in meats. Vegans can triple the absorption of iron from legumes by eating vitamin C-rich foods at each meal.

Since plant foods have no practical source of vitamin D, regular exposure to the sun should prevent a deficiency. However, vegetarians need to be aware of the relationship between skin cancer and exposure to the sun's rays. It may be better for them to take a one-a-day vitamin/mineral supplement than to sunbathe. Vegetarians can obtain calcium from calcium-fortified soy milk, stone ground meal, legumes, almonds, sesame seeds, collards, mustard greens, and okra. The absorption of zinc is inhibited by fiber.[11] Sources of zinc include legumes, soy products, nuts, and seeds.

Vegetarianism as practiced by informed people constitutes a very healthy style of eating. On the average, knowledgeable vegetarians are leaner, have lower cholesterol levels, and have lower blood pressures than meat eaters. They also have lower rates of certain kinds of cancer, lower mortality from cardiovascular diseases, and greater longevity than their meat-eating counterparts.

POINTS TO PONDER

1. Define anabolism, catabolism, and metabolism.
2. What is the food guide pyramid, and how is it meant to change the eating habits of Americans?
3. Define simple and complex carbohydrates and give some examples of each.
4. What are the major functions of soluble and insoluble dietary fiber?
5. How much fiber should people consume on a daily basis?
6. Name the major categories of fats and discuss the differences among them.
7. Define essential fatty acids. Why are they classified as essential? Identify the two essential fatty acids.
8. What are the health implications associated with the different categories of fats?
9. Discuss the role of fish oil as it relates to cardiovascular health.

Continued

Continued
10. Describe the daily protein requirements of children, adolescents, and adults.
11. What is a complete protein?
12. Identify and describe the different types of vegetarianism.
13. Discuss the advantages and disadvantages of following a vegetarian diet.

VITAMINS

Vitamins are noncaloric organic compounds found in small quantities in most foods. All vitamins are either fat soluble or water soluble. The fat-soluble vitamins (A, D, E, and K) are stored in the liver and fatty tissues until they are needed. The water-soluble vitamins (C and the B complex group) are not stored for any appreciable length of time and must be replenished daily.

Vitamins function as coenzymes that promote the many chemical reactions that occur in the body around the clock. Since vitamin deficiencies result in a variety of diseases, an adequate daily intake is necessary for optimal health. The recommended daily allowances (RDA) have been established for most of the vitamins. Although these amounts are needed to prevent the occurrence of diseases that are the result of vitamin deficiencies, they do not represent optimal values. However, the RDA are based on the best available evidence. The recommended levels actually cover the nutritional needs of 98 percent to 99 percent of the American population.[12] An alarming trend—the practice of taking megadoses of vitamins in the mistaken belief that extremely large doses will prevent or cure anything—has surfaced in recent years. Manufacturers and advertisers have convinced the public that the American diet is so deficient in vitamins that supplementation is a necessity. Those who supplement heavily may experience vitamin toxicity, particularly from overindulgence in the fat-soluble group. When vitamins are taken in very large amounts, they cease to function as vitamins and begin to act like drugs. Also, large doses interfere or disrupt the action of other nutrients. See Tables 9.7 and 9.8 for problems associated with vitamin megadoses.

Are synthetic vitamins inferior to natural vitamins? Promoters of vitamin products that come from natural sources adamantly proclaim that this is correct, but see the following for another viewpoint.

One cup of broccoli or cauliflower contains more vitamin C than an orange. Broccoli and cauliflower are also high in fiber and, as with other cruciferous vegetables, may protect against certain forms of cancer.

TABLE 9.7 Vitamin, RDA, Sources, and Toxic Symptoms (Fat-Soluble)

VITAMIN (U.S. RDA)	SOURCES	TOXIC SYMPTOMS
Vitamin A (1000 RD)	Fortified milk and margarine, cream, cheese, butter, eggs, liver, spinach and other dark leafy greens, broccoli, apricots, peaches, cantaloupe, squash, carrots, sweet potatoes, and pumpkin.	Red blood cell breakage, nosebleeds, abdominal cramps, nausea, diarrhea, weight loss, blurred vision, irritability, loss of appetite, bone pain, dry skin, rashes, hair loss, cessation of menstruation, growth retardation.
Vitamin D (400 IU)	Self-synthesis with sunlight, fortified milk, fortified margarine, eggs, liver, fish.	Raised blood calcium, constipation, weight loss, irritability, weakness, nausea, kidney stones, mental and physical retardation.
Vitamin E (30 IU)	Vegetable oils, green leafy vegetables, wheat germ, whole-grain products, butter, liver, egg yolk, milk fat, nuts, seeds.	Interference with anticlotting medication, general discomfort.
Vitamin K (no U.S. RDA)	Bacterial synthesis in digestive tract, liver, green leafy and cruciferous vegetables, milk.	Interference with anticlotting medication; may cause jaundice.

TABLE 9.8 Vitamin, RDA, Sources, and Toxic Symptoms (Water-Soluble)

VITAMIN (U.S. RDA)	SOURCES	TOXIC SYMPTOMS
Thiamin B1 (1.5 mg)	Meat, pork, liver, fish, poultry, whole-grain and enriched breads, cereals, pasta, nuts, legumes, wheat germ, oats.	Rapid pulse, weakness, headaches, insomnia, irritability
Riboflavin B2 (1.7 mg)	Milk, dark green vegetables, yogurt, cottage cheese, liver, meat, whole-grain or enriched breads and cereals.	None reported, but an excess of any of the B vitamins could cause a deficiency of the others.
Niacin B3 (20 mg)	Meat, eggs, poultry, fish, milk, whole-grain and enriched breads and cereals, nuts, legumes, peanuts, nutritional yeast, all protein foods.	Flushing, nausea, headaches, cramps, ulcer irritation, heartburn, abnormal liver function, low blood pressure.
Vitamin B6 (2.0 mg)	Meat, poultry, fish, shellfish, legumes, whole-grain products, green leafy vegetables, bananas.	Depression, fatigue, irritability, headaches, numbness, damage to nerves, difficulty walking.
Folcain (Folic acid) (400 micrograms)	Green leafy vegetables, organ meats, legumes, seeds.	Diarrhea, insomnia, irritability; may mask a vitamin B12 deficiency.
Vitamin B12 (cobalamin) (3g)	Animal products: meats, fish, poultry, shellfish, milk, cheese, eggs, nutritional yeast.	None reported.
Pantothenic acid (10 mg)	Widespread in foods.	Occasional diarrhea.
Biotin (300g)	Widespread in foods.	None reported.
Vitamin C (Ascorbic acid) (60 mg)	Citrus fruits, cruciferous vegetables, tomatoes, potatotes, dark green vegetables, peppers, lettuce, cantaloupe, strawberries, mangos, papayas.	Nausea, abdominal cramps, diarhhea, breakdown of red blood cells in persons with certain genetic disorders; deficiency symptoms may appear at first on withdrawal of high doses.

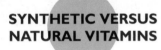

SYNTHETIC VERSUS NATURAL VITAMINS

It should be repeated that the body's cells can't tell the difference between the synthesized vitamin and the "natural" vitamin, even though the marketers of "natural" vitamins would like you to believe otherwise. The word synthetic sometimes implies fake, as in a synthetic (fake) fur coat. To the chemist, however, to synthesize means to put together—and the product is not fake, it is identical to the real thing.

Vitamins sold as natural often have synthetics added anyway. For example, vitamin C pills made from rose hips would have to be as big as golf balls to contain significant amounts of the vitamin. The manufacturer therefore adds synthetic vitamin to the small amount of "natural" vitamin and sells the product for many times the original price.

As we said earlier, a cell picking up vitamins from the bloodstream can't tell the difference between the vitamins from pills and those from foods. However, the digestive tract often does respond to the vehicle in which nutrients arrive. For some reason, synthetic vitamin C seems to be better retained than "natural" vitamin C when both are supplied in pill form. But because the body evolved to utilize foods, not pills, we might guess that vitamin C would be retained even better if it came from foods. The lesson in this must be that it really is not natural to take any kind of pills.

Reprinted by permission from *Nutrition: Concepts and Controversies,* 2d ed. Copyright © 1982 by West Publishing Company. All rights reserved.

Studies too numerous to mention in this text have shown that a deficiency in one or more water-soluble vitamins has a negative effect on performance. Work output deteriorates, fatigue occurs more rapidly, and there is a tendency toward muscular soreness as a result. Work output returns to normal when vitamin intake is restored, but above-normal amounts do not appear to promote further increases in work output, muscular strength, or resistance to fatigue.

The results of an excellent double-blind, crossover placebo study with 30 competitive male runners (average age 32 years) were recently reported.[13] For three months, 15 of the subjects were given daily vitamin and mineral supplements, while the other 15 received placebo pills. This was followed by a three-month "washout" period; that is, neither group received the true supplement. This was followed by a three-month crossover trial in which the original placebo group was switched to the vitamin and mineral supplement and the original supplement group was switched to the placebo. This occurred without the knowledge of the subjects or the researchers who administered the supplements. The results indicated that vitamin and mineral supplementation did not significantly change performance. Unchanged were aerobic capacity, peak running speed on the treadmill, and peak blood lactate concentrations, and there was no significant change in the time required to run 15 km (9.3 miles).

Active people get more vitamins in their diet than sedentary people because they consume more calories. If you are concerned about not getting enough vitamins in your diet but are unwilling to make appropriate dietary changes, a one-a-day brand should do. More than this amount is unnecessary and costly.

ANTIOXIDANTS—THE NEW GOOD GUYS

The recommended daily allowance (RDA) for vitamins is based upon the amounts needed to prevent vitamin-deficiency diseases. Today, the interest in vitamins by the scientific community goes beyond that. A substantial research effort is currently going on as investigators attempt to determine the role of selected antioxidants (Vitamins C and E and beta carotene) in the prevention of cardiovascular diseases and cancer. The early evidence is promising, and the vitamins being investigated are safe even when taken in larger doses than those that are recommended.

The preventive potential of the antioxidants centers around their ability in inhibit the action of free radicals (produced as by-products of molecular oxidation). Free radicals can be very destructive to electron-dense areas of the cell, such as DNA (the master plan for all cellular function) and cellular membranes. The violent collisions of free radicals with healthy cellular material produces "subatomic cracks" or scratches in the cells and their interior structures. If the damage is not repaired, the cell's normal function is disrupted, and it becomes vulnerable to cancer, atherosclerosis, cataracts, and aging. (The antioxidants protect the cells from free radicals by blocking the process of molecular oxidation that leads to their formation.)

Cancer Free radicals are capable of causing mutations in bacteria and other single-cell organisms. In much the same way, they damage the genetic material of human cells that can ultimately become cancerous.

Atherosclerosis Free radicals can combine with or oxidize LDL cholesterol beneath the lining of the coronary arteries. The oxidized LDLs damage the arteries, making them vulnerable to the development of atherosclerosis.

Cataracts Sunlight-induced free-radical formation in the eye damages the tissue of the lens until it becomes opaque.

Aging The processes of cellular repair are less efficient as we age. The bombardment of DNA by free radicals over the years seems to be involved in the aging of the cell.

Free radicals are formed by a variety of external and internal factors. Some of the external factors include heat, radiation from the sun as well as other radiation sources, cigarette smoke, alcohol, environmental pollutants and burns. The

Continued

internal factors center around the generation of free radicals by the cells themselves without external provocation.

Combating the free radicals are the antioxidants—the "chemical good guys." Should this translate to the consumption of antioxidant supplements to derail the free radicals? The evidence to date does not support supplementation, but there is considerable evidence that supports the notion that we should consume more fruits and vegetables—the natural sources of antioxidants. This is the preferred method of intake because scientists are not sure whether it is the antioxidants alone or antioxidants in combination with other substances present in the foods in which they are located that protects the cells. The best advice at this point is to follow the food guide pyramid to get the antioxidants that you need.

MINERALS

Minerals are inorganic substances that exist freely in nature. They are found in the earth's soil and water, and they pervade some of the earth's vegetation. Minerals maintain or regulate such physiological processes as muscle contraction, normal heart rhythm, body water supplies, acid-base balance of the blood, and nerve impulse conduction. Calcium, phosphorous, potassium, sulphur, sodium, chloride, and magnesium are the major minerals. They are classified as major because they occur in the body in quantities greater than five grams. The trace minerals, or micronutrients, number a dozen or more. The distinction between the major and trace minerals is one of quantity rather than importance. Deficiencies of either can have serious consequences.

Sodium, potassium, and chloride are the primary minerals lost through perspiration. Sodium, the positive ion in sodium chloride (table salt), is one of the body's major **electrolytes** (ions that conduct electricity). Americans consume three to seven grams of sodium daily, but only one to three grams are recommended.[14] Approximately 70 percent of the salt consumed in the United States is located in processed foods such as canned and instant soups, smoked meats and fish, cheeses, and deep-fried snacks. Salt is a cheap preservative and flavor enhancer. Read the labels on all canned and packaged foods to get an idea of the amount of salt that the product contains. The other thirty percent of our salt intake results from using the salt shaker and from naturally occurring salt in the foods that we eat.

Sodium is found in the fluid outside of the cells, while potassium is found within cellular fluid. The temporary exchange of sodium and potassium across the cell's membrane permits the transmission of neural impulses and the contraction of muscles. Low potassium levels interfere with muscle cell nutrition and lead to muscle weakness and fatigue. Potassium is essential for the maintenance of the heartbeat. Starvation and very low calorie diets for prolonged periods can produce sudden death from heart failure as potassium storage drops to critically low levels. Vomiting, diarrhea, and diuretics (substances to rid the body of excess water) reduce potassium levels. Chronic physical activity that produces heavy sweating probably will not diminish potassium stores unless the diet is woefully lacking in this mineral. It is hard to lose potassium because potassium is contained in most foods. It is particularly abundant in citrus fruits and juices, bananas, dates, nuts, fresh vegetables, meat, and fish.

As with vitamins, mineral intake can be abused. Excess amounts of both major and trace minerals produce a variety of symptoms (see Tables 9.9 and 9.10).

WATER

People can survive for a month or more without food, but a few days without water will result in death. Since all body processes and chemical reactions take

Older people who don't get enough vitamins and minerals in their daily diet should be able to bolster the immune systems and stay healthier by taking modest supplements.
—Harvard Health Letter

TABLE 9.9 **RDA, Sources, and Toxic Symptoms (Major Minerals)**

MINERALS (U.S. RDA)	SELECTED SOURCES	TOXIC SYMPTOMS
Calcium, Phosphorus (1000 mg)	Calcium: milk and milk products, small fish (with bones), tofu, greens, legumes, Phosphorus: all animal tissues.	Excess calcium is excreted except in hormonal imbalance states. Excess phosphorous can create relative deficiency of calcium.
Magnesium (400 mg)	Nuts, legumes, whole grains, dark green vegetables, seafoods, chocolate, cocoa.	Not known.
Sodium (no U.S. RDA)	Salt, soy sauce, moderate quantities in whole (unprocessed), foods, large amounts in processed foods.	Hypertension.
Chloride (no U.S. RDA)	Salt, soy sauce, moderate quantities in whole (unprocessed), foods, large amounts in processed foods.	Normally harmless (the gas chlorine is a poison but evaporates from water), disturbed acid-base balance, vomiting.
Potassium (no U.S. RDA)	All whole foods: meats, milk, fruits, vegetables, grains, legumes.	Causes muscular weakness, triggers vomiting; if given into a vein, can stop the heart.
Sulfur (no U.S. RDA)	All protein-containing foods.	Would occur only if sulfur amino acids were eaten in excess; this (in animals) depresses growth.

place in a liquid medium, it is imperative to be fully hydrated and to make a special effort to replace water when it is lost. Under normal conditions, adults drink 1.2 to 1.4 liters of fluid each day. More is needed when the weather is hot and humid or when one is physically active regardless of weather conditions.

Approximately 40 percent to 60 percent of the body's weight consists of water. A sizable amount is stored in the muscles, and some is stored in fat. By virtue of his larger muscle mass, the average male stores more water than the average female. Sixty-two percent of the total amount is found in the intracellular com-

TABLE 9.10 **RDA, Sources, and Toxic Symptoms (Trace Minerals)**

MINERALS (U.S. RDA)	SELECTED SOURCES	TOXIC SYMPTOMS
Iodine (150 g)	Iodized salt, seafood.	Very high intakes depress thyroid activity.
Iron (18 mg)	Red meats, fish, poultry, shellfish, eggs, legumes, dried fruits.	Iron overload: infections, liver injury.
Zinc (15 mg)	Protein-containing foods: meats, fish, poultry, grains, vegetables.	Fever, nausea, vomiting, diarrhea.
Copper (2 mg)	Meats, drinking water.	Unknown except as part of a rare hereditary disease (Wilson's disease).
Flouride (no U.S. RDA)	Drinking water (if naturally flouride containing or fluoridated), tea, seafood.	Fluorosis: discoloration of teeth.
Selenium (no U.S. RDA)	Seafood, meat, grains.	Digestive system disorders.
Chromium (no U.S. RDA)	Meats, unrefined foods, fats, vegetable oils.	Unknown as a nutrition disorder. Occupational exposures damage skin and kidneys.
Molybdenum, Manganese (no U.S. RDA)	Molybdenum: legumes, cereals, organ meats. Manganese: widely distributed in foods.	Molybdenum: enzyme inhibition. Manganese: poisoning, nervous system disorders.
Cobalt (no U.S. RDA)	Meats, milk, and milk products.	Unknown as a nutritional disorder.

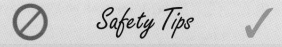
HEALTHY EATING

The following dietary guidelines will enable you to evaluate your current eating habits. These guidelines differ from dieting per se in that they provide a sensible approach to healthy, low-calorie eating that can be maintained for life rather than for only a few weeks or months.

1. Eat more fresh fruits, vegetables, and cereal grains. They are nutritionally dense, low in calories, and high in fiber. Olives, avocados, and coconuts are exceptions in that the first two are high in fat, while the latter is high in saturated fat.
2. Substitute high-fiber foods for high-fat foods. Do this gradually to avoid gastric upset.
3. Consume whole-grain breads—be sure to include pita bread, because it contains no fat.
4. Don't load bread down with butter, margarine, jellies, jams, creamed cheese, and peanut butter, because these substances can double or triple the number of calories in a slice of bread. When you use these toppings, spread them lightly.
5. Increase consumption of rice, potatoes, macaroni, and pastas, but don't drown them in rich sauces, margarine, butter, or sour cream.
6. Eat at least two fish meals per week.
7. Increase consumption of white-meat chicken and turkey. Do not eat the skin.
8. Decrease consumption of red meat (beef and pork). Select the cheaper cuts, such as round steak, because they are lower in fat.
9. Use sparingly smoked, salty, and chemically cured meats such as bacon, sausage, and ham.
10. Select low-fat (97 percent fat-free at least) luncheon meats and low-fat or no-fat hot dogs.
11. Organ meats are high in nutrition but also high in cholesterol, so eat them only occasionally.
12. Emphasize low-fat dairy products—skim or 1% milk and low-fat cheeses.
13. Consume no more than four eggs per week. Be sure to count eggs that are used as ingredients in other products.
14. Choose shortenings, salad dressings, and mayonnaise that are made from unsaturated fats or choose nonfat substitutes.
15. Nuts and seeds are nutritious but high in fat. Two whole walnuts or 10 large peanuts contain 5 grams of fat. This is equivalent to the fat calories in a teaspoon of butter or margarine—45 calories.
16. Reduce consumption of high-calorie snacks that are rich in sugar and/or fat, such as candy, cakes, pies, ice cream, and commercially fried foods such as potato chips.
17. Limit intake of cola drinks, coffee, and tea. These have substantial amounts of caffeine (see Table 9.11 for sources and amounts of caffeine).
18. Drink alcohol moderately or not at all. Alcohol is high in calories (7 kCals per gram—second only to fat), with little or no nutrition.
19. Reduce consumption of processed foods, which may be high in fat, sugar, and salt.
20. Patronize fast-food restaurants less frequently because their menus are generally high in salt and fat. Select their low-fat, low-calorie items.
21. Eat fried foods sparingly because frying adds to the caloric content of food. Broiling, boiling, steaming, stewing, baking, roasting, or grilling does not add calories and may actually reduce the fat content.

partment (water within the cells), while the remaining 38 percent is extracellular (water in the blood, lymph system, spinal cord fluid, saliva, etc.).

Water level in the body is maintained primarily by drinking fluids, but solid foods also contribute to water replenishment. Many foods—fruits, vegetables, and meats—contain large amounts of water. Even seemingly dry foods such as bread contain some water. Solid foods add water in another way—they contribute metabolic water, one of the by-products of their breakdown to energy sources.

Most water loss occurs through urination, while small quantities are lost in the feces and in exhaled air from the lungs. Insensible perspiration (that which is not visible) accounts for a considerable amount of water loss. Since exercise and hot humid weather increase sweating, more water must be consumed during these times. Exercise in hot weather and water replacement guidelines were discussed in Chapter 3.

TABLE 9.11 Selected Sources of Caffeine

BEVERAGES	SERVING SIZE (oz)	CAFFEINE (mg)
Coffee, drip	5	110–150
Coffee, perk	5	60–125
Coffee, instant	5	40–105
Tea, 5-minute steep	5	2–5
Tea, 3-minute steep	5	40–100
Coca-Cola	12	45
Hot cocoa	5	2–10
Coffee, decaffeinated	5	2–10

FOODS	SERVING SIZE	CAFFEINE (mg)
Milk chocolate	1 oz	1–15
Bittersweet chocolate	1 oz	5–35
Chocolate cake	1 slice	20–30

OVER-THE-COUNTER DRUGS	DOSE	CAFFEINE (mg)
Anacin, Empirin, or Midol	2	64
Excedrin	2	130
NoDoz	2	200
Aqua-Ban (diuretic)	2	200
Dexatrim (weight control aid)	1	200

 OINTS TO PONDER

1. Name the fat- and water-soluble vitamins.
2. Discuss the validity of this statement: Natural vitamins are more effective in promoting and maintaining good health than the synthetic vitamins.
3. Discuss the potential harmful effects of taking megadoses of vitamins.
4. Identify some foods and beverages that contain caffeine.
5. What effect does caffeine have upon the body?
6. Identify the major nutritional drawbacks associated with the consumption of fast foods.

CHAPTER HIGHLIGHTS

- The food guide pyramid is the latest attempt to direct the American diet along more healthy lines.
- Carbohydrates are organic compounds composed of one or more sugars derived from plant sources.
- Complex carbohydrates contain fiber and are low in calories and high in nutrition.
- Average fiber consumption in the U.S. is 10–13 grams/day; recommended level is 20–35 grams/day.
- Soluble fiber is an aid in the prevention of cardiovascular diseases; insoluble fiber helps prevent colon cancer, constipation, and diverticulitis.
- Fats are energy-dense compounds that yield 9 kCals/gm.
- Saturated fats come from animal flesh, have low melting points, have single-bond carbon atoms, and are used to manufacture cholesterol.

- Unsaturated fats come from vegetable sources, have low melting points, have one or more carbon atoms with double bonds, and have lower total and LDL cholesterol.
- Hydrogenation turns unsaturated fats into trans fatty acids, which may be harmful to the cardiovascular system.
- Seafood contains omega-3 fatty acids that may protect against heart disease by inhibiting the clotting of blood.
- Protein is needed to build and repair body tissues.
- Complete proteins—those that contain all of the essential amino acids—are found in animal flesh and dairy products.
- Vegetarianism as practiced by knowledgeable people constitutes a very healthy style of eating.
- Vitamins are classified as water soluble (C and B complex) or fat soluble (A, D, E, K).
- Antioxidant vitamins—beta carotene and vitamins C and E—may play a role in the prevention of heart disease, cancer, and cataracts. They may also delay cellular aging.
- Minerals are inorganic substances that exist freely in nature.

● REFERENCES

1. "Pyramid Scheme Foiled," *Nutrition Action Healthletter* 19, no. 6 (July/August 1992): 3.
2. M.A. Boyle and E.N. Whitney, *Personal Nutrition*, St. Paul: West, 1989.
3. M.H. Williams, *Nutrition for Fitness and Sport*, Dubuque, Iowa: Wm. C. Brown, 1983.
4. B. Liebman, "Trans in Trouble," *Nutrition Action Healthletter* 17, no. 8 (October 1990): 7.
5. L. Lamb (Ed.), "Current Thinking About Fish Oil," *The Health Letter*, September 9, 1988, p. 1.
6. "Infections and Undernutrition," *Nutrition Reviews* 40 (1982): 119.
7. J. Klug, "Overeating Possible Cause of Renal Disease," *Internal Medicine News*, December 1982, p. 1.
8. L.E. Koszuta, "Experts Speak Out on Fitness and Nutrition," *The Physician and Sportsmedicine* 16 (1988): 42.
9. G.M. Wardlaw and P.M. Insel, *Perspectives in Nutrition*, St. Louis: Times Mirror/Mosby, 1990.
10. A.C. Grandjean, "The Vegetarian Athlete," *The Physician and Sportsmedicine*, 15 (1987): 191.
11. J.H. Freeland-Graves et al., "Zinc Status of Vegetarians," *Journal of the American Dietetic Association* 77 (1980): 655.
12. E.N. Whitney, E.N.M. Hamilton, and S.R. Rolfes, *Understanding Nutrition*, St. Paul: West, 1990.
13. L.M. Wright et al., "Vitamin and Mineral Supplementation: Effect on the Running Performance of Trained Athletes," *American Journal of Clinical Nutrition* 47 (1988): 192.
14. *Nutrition and Your Health: Dietary Guidelines for Americans*, Hyattsville, Md.: U.S. Dept. of Agriculture and U.S. Dept. of Health and Human Services, 1990.

The Reduction Equation: Exercise + Sensible Eating = Fat Control

CHAPTER OUTLINE

INTRODUCTION

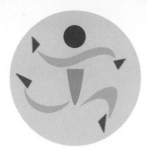

This chapter covers the effects of diet and exercise on weight reduction and weight maintenance. It begins with the definition of body composition, lean body mass, and essential and storage fat. Overweight and obesity (which are *not* synonymous) are discussed and their differences delineated. The connection between wellness and the maintenance of optimal body composition is established.

Exercise is an important component for reducing body weight (specifically fat weight) while sparing or enhancing muscle tissue. Exercise uses calories, stimulates metabolism, and brings appetite in line with energy expenditure. On the other hand, dieting without exercise produces diminishing returns because metabolism slows down as caloric needs decrease. After a few weeks of dieting, the body goes into a survival mode and adapts to the reduced caloric intake. The diet becomes less effective, and continued weight loss is more difficult to accomplish. Eventually, the diet will end, some or all of the old eating patterns will be reestablished, and the lost weight will be regained. If dieting becomes cyclical, each attempt at losing weight may take longer, but the lost weight may be regained quicker, and the likelihood that additional weight will be gained increases. Very-low calorie diets should be avoided. Without supplementation, it is impossible to receive the required nutrients, and the effect of low caloric intake on metabolism is devastating.

In addition, this chapter discusses anorexia nervosa and bulimia—two different eating disorders or appetite disorders with some common characteristics.

Finally, the chapter presents several methods for assessing body composition. These methods are accompanied by a method for determining optimal body weight based upon the body composition measurement.

Miniglossary

Adipose Tissue   Fat cells.

Amenorrhea   Failure to menstruate.

Android Obesity   Male pattern of fat deposition in the abdominal region.

Anorexia Nervosa   A psychological and emotional disorder characterized by excessive underweight.

Basal Metabolic Rate (BMR)   The energy required to sustain life while in the rested and fasted state.

Bioelectrical Impedence   A noninvasive method for estimating body fat by measuring the speed that an electrical current travels through the body.

Body Composition   The percentage of lean versus fat tissue in the body.

Body Mass Index   A method of estimating weight status by dividing body weight in kilograms by body height in meters squared.

Bulimarexia Nervosa   An eating disorder characterized by episodes of secretive binge eating followed by purging.

Gynoid Obesity   Female pattern of fat deposition in the thighs and gluteal areas.

Hydrostatic Weighing   A method for determining specific gravity and percent body fat by underwater weighing.

Obesity   The excessive accumulation of body fat.

Continued

—Continued

Overweight   Excess weight for one's height without regard for body composition.

Resting Metabolic Rate (RMR)   The conditions for measuring BMR are difficult to achieve and when they are approximated the term resting metabolic rate is used. It is an approximation of the energy required to sustain life while in the resting state.

Skinfold Measurement   A method for determining percent body fat by measuring a pinch of skin at selected sites with a skinfold caliper.

Thermogenic Effect of Food (TEF)   The energy required to digest and absorb food.

Very-low Calorie Diet   Diets that contain 800 or fewer kCals per day.

Weight Cycling   Repeated cycles of weight loss followed by weight gain.

Five Self-Assessment activities appear in Appendix C that apply directly to the contents of this chapter:

10.1   Estimating the Caloric Cost of Exercise

10.2   Estimating Cardiovascular Risk With BMI

10.3   Estimating Desirable Body Weight from BMI

10.4   Calculating Resting Metabolic Rate (RMR) and Total Energy Expenditure

10.5   Calculating Your RMR

BODY COMPOSITION DEFINED

When considered in its simplest form, **body composition** refers to the amount of fat in the body versus the amount of lean tissue in the body. Lean tissue includes all tissue exclusive of fat: muscles, bones, organs, fluid, and so on. Fat includes both essential and storage fat. Essential fat, found in the bone marrow, organs, muscles, intestines, and central nervous system, is indispensable to normal physiological functioning. The amount of essential fat in the male body is equal to approximately 3 percent to 5 percent of the total body weight. The amount of essential fat in the female body is equal to about 11 percent to 14 percent of the total body weight. The disparity in the amount of essential fat between the sexes is probably because of sex-specific essential fat stored in a female's breasts, pelvic area, and thighs. Essential fat constitutes a lower limit beyond which fat loss is undesirable and unhealthy because of the possibility of impaired normal physiological and biological functioning from such loss.

Storage fat is found in adipose tissue. For most Americans, this represents a substantial energy reserve. **Adipose tissue** is found subcutaneously (under the skin) and around the organs, where it acts as a buffer against physical trauma. It is desirable to reduce excess storage fat for health and aesthetic reasons. Reasonable goals for total body fat (essential plus storage fat) differ for both sexes. Excellent values for males and females are 12 percent and 18 percent, respectively.

Females who become excessively lean (below 12 percent to 14 percent fat), such as long-distance runners and ballerinas, often experience menstrual dysfunction. Irregular menses (menstrual cycle), oligomenorrhea (infrequent menses), and **amenorrhea** (no menses) are frequent problems for exercising women who reduce their total body weight and/or fat excessively. Loss of body weight and fat are among several factors associated with menstrual dysfunction. Emotional stress, inadequate nutrition, hypothyroidism, and pituitary tumors are some other factors related to the onset of menstrual problems.[1]

A paradox exists in that females who exercise heavily strengthen their bodies, but those who develop athletic amenorrhea lose calcium from their bones, especially those of the vertebrae.[2] Bone responds to exercise by acquiring more calcium and growing stronger, but highly intense exercise carried out on a regular basis that leads to excessive fat loss tends to weaken the bones. "By lowering hormone levels, regular heavy exercise leads to loss of calcium from bones and thus weakens them. Which bones are affected, and in what way, depends on the type and intensity of exercise."[3] A woman's menstrual cycle will return to normal when the amount of exercise is reduced and weight is gained.[4] Bone mineral content loss is probably reversible and returns to normal values as well, but this has not been clearly established.

Excessive leanness has been implicated in the death of 14 young and middle-aged marathon runners. A common element shared by these runners was a very restricted diet coupled with vigorous exercise.

LEAN RUNNERS AT RISK?

Many serious runners have tried to improve their racing times by increasing their level of training while reducing their food consumption. These runners know that every extra pound that they carry costs them in terms of the energy needed to transport their body weight from start to finish lines in a race. Losing weight theoretically enhances performing times. Problems occur when this is pursued excessively. The practice of severe dieting with very heavy training has proven to be fatal for several runners.

Autopsies performed on twelve marathon runners, average 44 years of age showed no evidence of fatty deposits in their coronary arteries, yet they died of heart attacks. Pathologist and marathon runner, Thomas Bassler, M.D., concluded that these runners died from heart rhythm disturbances brought on by deliberate weight loss—from heavy training accompanied by severe dieting—to enhance running performance. Bassler described these victims as having a wasted, sallow appearance due to a general lack of nutrition. He concluded that they died from "nutritional arrhythmias."

The message is clear regarding the effect of endurance performance on health status. A person in heavy training must supply the calories needed to support the energy demand of vigorous physical activity plus the demands of daily living. There is nothing wrong with being lean—in fact it is an asset, but it should not be carried to the extreme. A diet must provide enough energy to keep the body from consuming its own protein to make up the energy deficit. The body stores of protein used for energy comes from the protein containing organs such as the liver, heart, and muscles. As the organs and systems shrink in size their function is impaired. If enough protein is lost from the heart it becomes irritable and abnormal arrhythmias occur, possibly resulting in death.

To repeat, severely cutting calories while increasing the level of training is hazardous to one's health and a misguided way to improve physical performance.

"Lean Runners and Fatal Heart Irregularities," *The Health Letter*, 24, No. 5, September 14, 1984, p. 1.

▲ DEVELOPMENT OF ADIPOSITY

Overweight and obesity have complex physiological and psychological causes, but the principles involved in weight loss are very simple. Energy cannot be destroyed; it is either used for work or converted into another form for storage. Individuals are in equilibrium when the calories consumed equal the calories used. Weight maintenance is lost when the equation is unbalanced in either direction. If the calories consumed exceed those that are used, the excess is converted into fat and stored. If the calories used exceed those that are consumed, weight will be lost because a portion of the stored fat must be mobilized to supply the extra need for fuel.

Scientifically, the principle is beautifully uncomplicated. We have made the process complex by inventing hundreds of ways to achieve weight loss painlessly and rapidly. Unfortunately, most of these methods are fruitless; some are actually dangerous and usually benefit only those who invent and promote them. The preferred course of action is to prevent obesity from occurring rather than treating it after the fact. From this standpoint, it might be useful to know some basics about the development of adipose cells. As with other organs, adipose tissue (fat cells) normally grows by increasing in number (hyperplasia) or size (hypertrophy). Fat-cell number and size vary from one body part to another.

Fat cells enlarge significantly during the initial six months of postnatal (after birth) life and by the end of the first year are similar in size to those of adolescents.[5] It appears that fat-cell size remains fairly stable one year of age to puberty, but fat-cell number increases progressively during this time. During puberty, males and females experience substantial increases in both fat-cell size and fat-cell number. However, there are gender differences in regional fat distribution. Males distribute fat primarily in the upper half of the body, and females deposit it in the lower half of the body. Further, the percentage of fat reaches peak values during early adolescence for males and then declines during the remainder of adolescent growth, while females show a continuous increase in the percentage of fat from the onset of puberty through age 18.

Excess fat storage is the result of hypertrophy and/or hyperplasia of adipose cells. Obese children beyond two years of age have a greater number of fat cells than children of normal weight. Not long ago, it was hypothesized that the number of adipose cells was fixed soon after birth. This controversial theory no longer appears to be credible. Early research suggested that overfeeding in infancy promoted the formation of fat cells and, further, predisposed affected children to later obesity. Current evidence indicates that obesity later in life is unaffected by overfeeding in early life, and conversely, underfeeding in early life does not prevent or preclude the development of obesity or adipose cell number later in life.[6] The consequences of early feeding patterns on later obesity are not clear.

Neonatal adiposity is not a good predictor of adult obesity. Most obese infants normalize their weight by the age of 9. However, the correlation between childhood obesity and adult obesity is positive and quite high.[7] Approximately 80 percent of the obese children either remain or become obese during adulthood. Obviously, certain forces accompanying growth become operative between the periods of infancy and childhood that contribute to adult obesity. Overweight adolescents have a higher probability of becoming overweight adults than normal weight adolescents.[8] The heaviest adolescents are 1.6 to 2.5 times more likely than the lightest adolescents to become overweight adults.

Overweight in adolescence seems to have a broad range of adverse health effects later in life.[9] A 55-year followup of adolescents indicated that those who were overweight had an increased mortality risk from all causes even if they normalized their weight as adults. The only exception was that those who managed to normalize their weight in adulthood were at less risk for type II diabetes.

The term *overweight* is inadequate for describing body composition or for identifying risk to health. If the extra weight for an overweight individual is in the form of muscle and bone, as is the case with most active people, it does not pose a risk. **Overweight** may be defined as excessive weight for one's height without regard to body composition. Body weight becomes a risk when a substantial portion of it is in the form of fat. **Obesity** is the term that refers to the excessive accumulation and storage of fat. Obesity is gender linked. Men are considered to be obese if fat comprises more than 25 percent of their total weight, and women are obese if fat comprises more than 32 percent of their total weight.[10]

Childhood and adolescent obesity are usually the result of the combined effects of hypertrophy and hyperplasia of fat cells. Eighty percent to 90 percent of adult onset obesity is hypertrophic, but extreme obesity may be hyperplastic as well.[11]

Adipose cells have a long life span. A reduction in body weight does not reduce the number of fat cells; it just reduces their cells' size. This affects one's ability to attain and maintain normal weight, because evidence indicates that the more fat cells there are, the greater the body's reluctance to reduce its fat stores. It may be that adipose cells require at least minimal amounts of stored fat for them to maintain their biological function. The minimum fat saturation level of adipose cells make it very difficult for those who have a higher than average number to reduce their stored fat below a certain level. It is also possible that a large number of adipose cells stimulate the hunger drive.[12] If both of these assumptions are correct, an increase in the number of fat cells would influence appetite and require more fat storage, thus resulting in greater difficulty in losing and maintaining weight.

BODY COMPOSITION AND THE WELLNESS CONNECTION

The majority of Americans of all ages and both sexes can avoid obesity. It is a matter of choice, effort or lack of it, awareness of the hazards of obesity and a commitment to do something about it. High-level wellness cannot be attained by the obese, and the quality of their lives is diminished as a result.

The National Institutes of Health (NIH) convened a panel of experts to develop a consensus statement regarding the health implications of obesity. While this was a formidable task, and while segments of the study were criticized, the fact remains that for the majority of people, the higher their weight escalates, the greater the risk of developing health problems. The panel cited the strong association between obesity and high blood pressure, type II diabetes, and high blood cholesterol levels.[13] Obese women are more likely than normal weight women to die from cancer of the uterus, breast, ovaries, and gallbladder. Obese men are more likely to die from cancer of the colon, prostate, and rectum.

As a result of its effect on longevity and its high positive association with severe chronic disease, obesity should be regarded as a serious medical and psychological problem. In 1985, the NIH formally elevated obesity to disease status.[14] Obesity is a disease with health implications of its own, but additionally, it coexists with risk factors that are associated with other chronic diseases and combines with them to increase the probability and incidence of these diseases.

The regional distribution of fat also appears to affect the risk. Fat distributed in the abdomen, chest, nape of the neck, and lower back increases the risk for heart disease, stroke, type II diabetes, and some forms of cancer. This is the android pattern, or the masculine pattern, of fat deposition. This pattern, while predominantly male, is not confined to males. Some women deposit fat in the android pattern, and the pattern's prevalence increases as women move through menopause.[15] **Android obesity** is characterized by hypertrophy of existing fat cells.

Fat distributed primarily in the buttocks, hips, and thighs is **gynoid obesity.** This pattern represents less of a risk than the android pattern. Gynoid obesity is typical of the female distribution of fat, but some men carry their excess weight in this manner as well. Gynoid obesity is characterized by hyperplasia of fat cells.

Abdominal fat is a hazard to health for several reasons. First enzyme activity is very active in abdominal adipose cells, so that fat moves in and out of these cells quite easily. Acute or chronic stress produced by emotions or exercise enhances the activity level of the abdominal enzymes, further facilitating the movement of fat into and out of adipose cells. This can be "good" or "bad." The "bad" is that emotional stress releases adrenaline (epinephrine), which in turn encourages the release of fat from the abdominal region. Abdominal fat enters the blood stream

According to the National Institutes of Health, one-fourth to one-third of American adults are overweight. At any given time nearly twice this number are dieting. Losing weight, even when it may not be necessary, seems to be a national obsession.

—Worldview

and is routed directly to the liver, where it becomes the raw material for the manufacture of cholesterol. (Figure 10.1 illustrates the cardiovascular effect of android obesity.) Second, abdominal fat cells are associated with blood sugar intolerance and excessive insulin in the blood. In time, this can lead to type II diabetes. Third, excessive insulin promotes the reabsorption of sodium by the kidneys. Ineffective removal maintains a high sodium content in the body that can ultimately lead to hypertension.

The "good" associated with abdominal fat is that exercise-induced stress also mobilizes fat from storage, but unlike emotional stress, fat-rich blood is shunted to the exercising muscles, where it is burned for fuel. Exercise thus prevents the conversion of fat to harmful cholesterol. In addition, the turnover rate for abdominal fat is high. The implications of this for weight loss are enormous. Android fat can be lost more easily than gynoid fat. In fact, this is one of the primary reasons that many men can lose weight with exercise without dietary restriction. Conversely, most women must supplement exercise with caloric restriction to produce weight loss. Gynoid fat is highly resistant to removal. It takes more effort to get rid of fat that is deposited in this manner. While it can be done, those who deposit fat in the lower half of the body may not be able to reshape their figures to suit their desires.

The deposition pattern of fat as a risk can be determined by calculating the waist/hip ratio (WHR). Ideally, the hips should be larger than the waist. (Self-Assessment 7.3 gives directions for calculating your waist/hip ratio).

The obese also suffer from economic and social discrimination, poor body image, and a depressed self-concept. A survey of 1,500 executives revealed that body weight was inversely related to earning power. Only 10 percent of the executives in the upper income bracket were more than ten pounds overweight, while 40 percent of those in the lower bracket were more than ten pounds overweight. Excessive weight seems to be hazardous to purse and wallet. Fat people are victims of discrimination because our culture is "slim" oriented. We have become enamored with the thin silhouette. Advertisements cater to the young and the slim. Clothing is made for and modeled by thin people. Fat people pay higher insurance premiums, obese children are ridiculed by their slim peers, and armed forces personnel are drummed out of service if they gain weight beyond an acceptable level.

FIGURE 10.1

Cardiovascular Hazards of Android Obesity

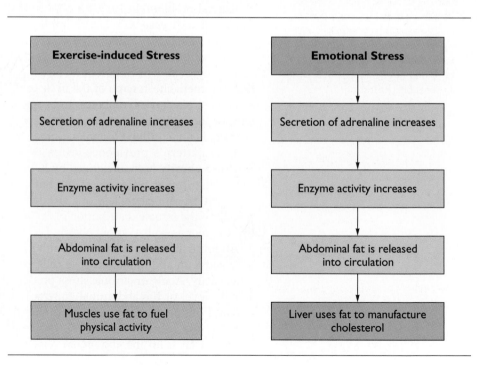

Fortunately, obesity is reversible, as are many of the risks with which it is associated. As with any disease or condition, the preferred course of action would be to prevent obesity rather than trying to deal with it after the fact. This requires knowledgeable management of dietary and exercise habits both by individuals and by their parents. Parents should teach and practice sound nutritional and exercise habits so that their children can have a model of desirable lifestyle behaviors to emulate.

FAT DISTRIBUTION— MORE BAD NEWS

A study of 41,837 women ages 55–69 that began in 1986 indicated that fat in the abdomen was a significant risk for premature death. Five years after the start of the study, 1,504 of the subjects had died—52% from cancer and 32% from cardiovascular disease.

While mortality rates were higher for the very heavy and very thin, a better predictor of death was the waist-to-hip ratio. The higher the ratio, the greater the risk. A woman with a 32-inch waist and 40-inch hips has a waist/hip ratio of 0.8 (32/40). A ratio of 1.0 (40-inch waist/40-inch hips) increased the risk of death by 60%. The women with the highest ratios experienced a 2.5 times greater increase of dying than women with the lowest ratios. Even thin people with high waist-to hip ratios had an increased risk of dying.

There is a growing sense in the medical community that a measurement of the waist-to-hip ratio should be included in all routine medical exams.

Source: "Fat Distribution and Morality" *Harvard Heart Letter* 3 no. 10 (June 1993): 8.

Facts, Fallacies, and Timely Tidbits

1. Nutrition plays a key role in 4 of the 10 leading causes of death in the U.S.
2. If Americans reduced their fat intake from its present 37% of total calories to 30%, it would result in an increase of only 4 months of life expectancy for the average person. Is this enough incentive for people to make the necessary dietary changes? The answer is somewhat complex, but the reasons advanced for making such an effort include the following:
   - Eating a low-fat diet reduces the incidence of cardiovascular disease and cancers of the breast, colon, and prostate and may control or prevent type II diabetes.
   - Dropping below 30% has reversed atherosclerosis in cardiac patients.
   - It is difficult to increase the life expectancy of a nation that is already living into its seventies and eighties.
   - A low-fat diet could delay the onset of a nonfatal heart attack, thus allowing individuals to enjoy more quality years.
3. What is the ideal diet for humans that would lead to the lowest risk of heart disease, cancer, and other chronic disorders? There is still considerable disagreement among the experts regarding this question. Differences and

agreements by authorities about some important nutritional issues are summarized below:
   - Saturated fat. All agree that saturated fat should constitute less than 10% of total calories. A few suggest 0%, while some others have suggested 5% to 6%.
   - Total fat. Most agree that total fat should make up less than 30% of total calories, with some of the experts recommending no more than 10% of total calories.
   - Cholesterol. Less than 300 mg per day, but several of the experts suggested 100 mg per day, with at least two suggesting 0 mg of cholesterol.
   - Fiber-rich foods. The ideal may be 40 to 50 grams of fiber per day. The average American consumes only 11 to 12 grams per day. We should consume a minimum of 5 servings of fruits and vegetables every day, but on any given day only 9% of Americans eat two or more servings of fruit and three or more servings of vegetables.
   - Sodium. 1,800 mg is a reasonable goal to shoot for.
   - Sugar. Since sugar has calories but no nutrients, the experts agree that its consumption should be limited. Also, sugar can raise triglycerides in overweight people whose bodies don't use insulin efficiently. And, of course, sugar causes tooth decay.

THE CAUSES OF OBESITY

Obesity is a multifactorial disease. Its cause can be genetic, dietary, lack of exercise, or behavioral.

Heredity

Studies of Adoptees Researchers classified 540 adoptees as thin, medium weight, overweight, and obese.[16] They compared these subjects to their biological and adoptive parents to determine which parents they resembled. The subjects were reared and learned the lifestyle of the adoptive parents while carrying the genes of their biological parents. The researchers used **body mass index** (BMI— body weight in kilograms divided by body height in meters squared) to measure body composition. (The calculation of BMI is discussed later in the chapter.) According to this technique, the adoptees resembled their biological parents more than their adoptive parents. This is just one of several studies that has established the influence of genetic factors in human obesity.

Studies of Twins Identical twins (monozygotic twins) are excellent subjects for determining and quantifying the contribution of heredity to obesity. Identical twins emanate from the same egg and share the same genetic makeup. Researchers can examine the differences and similarities between identical twins reared together (shared environment) and identical twins reared apart (different environments) and gain an idea of the effects of genetics and environment. Any physical differences that occur in one of a pair of such twins can be attributed to environmental and/or lifestyle factors.

In one study the BMIs of identical and fraternal twins (dizygotic twins—emanating from separate eggs) were calculated when the twins entered the military and again 25 years later.[17] The similarity in weight gain among the identical twins was twice that observed in the fraternal twins. Each member of the identical twins gained about the same amount of weight and at about the same time during the 25 years.

The influence of genetics appears to extend across the body weight continuum from very thin to very obese.[18] An excellent study of identical and fraternal twins, some of whom were reared together and some of whom were reared apart, provided further evidence of the hereditary effects on body composition.[19] The researchers found that the differences in BMIs between identical twins reared together and those who were reared apart were very small, illustrating the powerful influence of heredity on body size. Height and weight were not influenced by separation, age of separation, or degree of separation.

In another study, twelve pairs of male identical twins were overfed 1,000 calories (kCals) a day, six days a week, for 100 days.[20] This was a well-controlled study in which the kCals consumed and the physical activity prescribed were closely supervised. The men consumed an extra 84,000 kCals during the 100-day period of the study. They were each expected to gain 24 pounds. However, the actual weight gain averaged 18 pounds. The range of weight gain was surprising—as little as 9 1/2 pounds gained to as much as 30 pounds gained. Why such a disparity when caloric intake and caloric expenditure were similar for all pairs of twins? The researchers indicated that some of the twin pairs were more efficient in converting calories consumed to stored fat while others were very inefficient. The least efficient of the subjects were able to deposit only 40 percent of the extra kCals as body tissue. The intrapair similarity in weight gain and fat deposition was primarily accounted for by heredity factors. Each member of the set gained a similar amount of weight, and the weight was distributed similarly for each.

If you have overweight parents, before throwing your hands up in despair, it is important for you to realize that heredity is not destiny. Being the offspring of overweight parents does not necessarily mean that you will be overweight. You may have to work a little harder to attain and maintain normal weight, but you can do it. Regular exercise and sound nutritional habits cannot negate heredity, but they can modify its consequences considerably.

The Setpoint Theory The setpoint theory indicates that all humans have a natural weight that the body will defend and protect quite vigorously. According to this theoretical concept—it is not an actual physiological mechanism—each person has an internal setpoint for body weight and degree of relative fatness. This model assumes that the setpoint is regulated by the hypothalamus (one of the parts of the brain) through the signals that it receives from the fat that is stored in adipose cells, glucose level in the blood, and body weight. The input is used to regulate calorie consumption—either decreasing or increasing it—in order to maintain the setpoint. Dieting does not change the setpoint. If it did, all dieters would stabilize at post-diet weights. The fact that 95 percent of dieters return to their prediet weight levels in a few years suggests that the original setpoint did not change.

The setpoint is lowered, however, by consistent exercise. Exercise reduces body fat and encourages the hypothalamus to defend the new level and new setpoint. This is a good example of a genetic inclination being modified through an appropriate lifestyle behavior.

THE EFFECTS OF EXERCISE ON BODY COMPOSITION

The often neglected factor in a weight loss attempt is exercise. Exercise and diet are not mutually exclusive. They are complementary in that each has a unique contribution to make to weight loss. The role of exercise was addressed in 1985 at an international meeting on obesity. The unanimous consensus of the experts was that "if you are about to start a weight reduction program or if you are trying to maintain your present weight, success or failure can depend on whether or not you exercise."[21] Exercise contributes to weight loss and is essential for weight maintenance because of its ability to burn kCals, increase metabolism, build muscle tissue, and balance appetite with energy expenditure.

Exercise Burns Calories

A persistent misconception regarding exercise is that it does not burn enough kCals to make the effort worthwhile. Actually, consistent participation in aerobic exercise (walking, jogging, cycling, rowing, aerobic dance, etc.) will burn substantial amounts of kCals. Anaerobic activities such as weight training do not burn many kCals during the workout, but they build the muscle tissue that will require more kCals later on. Muscle-building activities are an investment in future weight control. In the long run, the increase in muscle mass increases metabolism so that the body's kCal requirements increase even at rest. This is why activities for both cardiorespiratory development and muscular development are suggested for weight loss or weight maintenance or for any well-rounded physical fitness program.

The kCal expenditure of weight-bearing activities (walking, jogging, cross-country skiing, and most games) is dependent upon the body weight of participants. If two people, one weighing 120 pounds and the other 200 pounds, walk one mile together, the heavier person will burn more kCals because it requires more energy to transport a heavier weight from point A to point B. Table 10.1 provides an estimate of the caloric cost of selected activities on a per-minute basis according to body weight. There are 3,500 kCals in one pound of fat as it is stored in the human body. (Self-Assessment 10.1 presents a problem that challenges your knowledge and ability to apply the contents of Table 10.1.)

The American College of Sports Medicine (ACSM) suggests that the minimal threshold of exercise for weight loss is 300 kCals per exercise session performed at least three times a week or 200 kCals per session performed at least four times a

TABLE 10.1 Estimated Caloric Cost of Selected Activities

ACTIVITY	CAL/MIN/LB*	ACTIVITY	CAL/MIN/LB*
Aerobic dance (vigorous)	.062	Jogging (5mph)	.060
Basketball (vigorous, full-court)	.097	Laundry (taking out and hanging)	.027
Bathing, dressing, undressing	.021	Mopping floors	.024
Bed making (and stripping)	.031	Peeling Potatoes	.019
Bicycling (13 mph)	.071	Piano Playing	.018
Canoeing (flat water, 4 mph)	.045	Rowing (vigorous)	.097
Chopping wood	.049	Running (8 mph)	.104
Cleaning windows	.024	Sawing wood (crosscut saw)	.058
Cross-country skiing (8 mph)	.104	Shining shoes	.017
Gardening		Shoveling snow	.052
Digging	.062	Snowshoeing (2.5 mph)	.060
Hedging	.034	Soccer (vigorous)	.097
Raking	.024	Swimming (55 yd/min)	.088
Weeding	.038	Table tennis (skilled)	.045
Golf (twosome carrying clubs)	.045	Tennis (beginner)	.032
Handball (skilled, singles)	.078	Walking (4.5 mph)	.048
Horseback riding (trot)	.029	Writing while seated	.013
Ironing	.029		

*Multiply cal/min/lb times your body weight in pounds and then multiply that product by the number of minutes spent in the activity.

From *Physical Fitness for Practically Everybody: The Consumers Union Report on Exercise*, Mount Vernon, N.Y.: Consumers Union of the U.S., 1983.

week.[22] You should understand that these suggested workouts reflect minimum levels of exercise. The ACSM recommends that weight loss could be accomplished more effectively by burning more kCals per exercise session and by increasing the number of sessions per week. They also suggest that low-intensity exercises be selected to avoid possible injury.

The kCals burned during recovery from exercise contribute marginally to weight loss. The body does not shut off completely after exercise; it recovers gradually. Extra kCals are burned during this period until metabolism returns to normal resting level. A rule of thumb is that 15 kCals are burned in recovery for every 100 kCals burned during exercise.[23] If 400 kCals are used during exercise, an extra 60 kCals will be used during the recovery period. Exercising at this level five days a week will result in approximately 4 1/2 pounds lost in one year from the kCals burned in recovery from exercise. This is illustrated by the following:

$$60 \text{ kCals} \times 5 \text{ days} = 300 \text{ kCals/wk} \times 52 \text{ wks}$$
$$= 15{,}600 \text{ kCals/yr} \div 3{,}500 \text{ kCals}$$
$$= 4.45 \text{ lbs}$$

Admittedly, this amount is not much, but it is a bonus that supplements the kCals lost directly through exercise.

Physical activity is the most effective way to rid the body of kCals, but it is not the only way that the body uses kCals. The process of digesting and absorbing food requires energy and represents another source of using kCals. The energy for these processes, known as the **thermogenic effect of food (TEF),** is supplied by some of the food that is eaten.[24] Research interest in TEF has resurfaced as investigators attempt to piece out the influence of various factors involved in energy storage and utilization. Metabolism may be elevated for as long as several hours following a meal. What would happen to metabolism if aerobic exercise were combined with the TEF effect, since both individually boost metabolism? Some authorities suggest that mild exercise, such as walking, be performed shortly after ingesting a meal because such activities potentiate the TEF.[25] This concept is attractive. From a weight-loss perspective, it is certainly much better than taking a nap after a meal. However, since there is substantial individual variation in TEF, its effectiveness in weight management has yet to be determined.

Dietary fat is most efficient in promoting storage fat in the body because of its low TEF. One hundred extra kCals of dietary fat require only 3 kCals to convert it to storage fat. In other words, 97 of the original 100 kCals are converted to body fat. If those same 100 kCals of fat are eaten with something sweet, such as a cola beverage, even more of them will be stored. However, 100 extra kCals of carbohydrate consumed require 23 kCals to convert it to storage fat; therefore only 77 of the original 100 kCals are converted to storage fat. This is another powerful incentive to select a diet low in fat and high in carbohydrates. Not only is this a healthy diet, but it is preferred for weight loss and weight management.

Exercise and Appetite: Eat More, Weigh Less

To the uninitiated, the title of this section must seem at least paradoxical if not impossible. How can one eat more and weigh less? It sounds like a bit of alchemy or a get-rich-quick sales pitch. But wouldn't it be nice to eat what you want without gaining weight? This is especially intriguing since it is known that Americans are eating less and getting fatter. Since weight gain and loss are a combination of kCals consumed and kCals expended, it is obvious that the reduction in caloric consumption has been accompanied by a greater reduction in kCals expended. This explains our continued weight gain.

The results of animal and human studies during the past 35 years have been equivocal and confusing regarding the effect of exercise on appetite. The data have shown that exercise may decrease, increase, or have no effect upon food intake. Just a few short years ago, the scientific community adopted the position that one hour of mild to moderate exercise would exert an anorexigenic effect (reduction in appetite). The theory was that food intake would decrease during the early days of exercise as one was making the transition from inactivity to moderate exercise and persist until the level of exercise increased to above moderate levels. At this point, the appetite would increase to be in balance with energy expenditure. Other researchers tested these assumptions but were unable to produce similar results. Exercise did not seem to suppress the appetite, except temporarily immediately after exercise.

Most studies indicated that people either continued to eat the same amount or increased their food intake when they began exercising and were allowed to eat freely. In one study, the food intake and energy expenditure of military cadets was carefully monitored for 14 days.[26] The cadets' food intake was depressed during exercise days and increased during the off days. The researchers concluded that moderate exercise undertaken regularly tends to be accompanied by a slight increase in food intake.

P. D. Wood investigated the effect of a year of jogging on previously sedentary middle-aged males.[27] The subjects were encouraged not to reduce their food intake or to attempt to lose weight during the course of the study. At the end of one year, the men who ran the most miles lost the most fat. The more miles they ran, the more they increased their food intake. Those who jogged the most miles (up to 25 miles per week) lost the most fat and the most weight and had the greatest increase in food intake. Many studies have shown that active people consume more kCals and are leaner than inactive people.

Two studies at St. Luke's Hospital in New York showed that the effect of exercise on the appetite is regulated to some extent by the degree of obesity at the start of the program.[28] Fifty-seven days of moderate treadmill exercise resulted in a 15-pound weight loss by obese female subjects. The women's caloric intake during exercise compared to the preexercise period was essentially unchanged. This study was repeated with women who were close to ideal weight according to insurance company charts. The results were very different. Moderate treadmill exercise produced an immediate surge in appetite, and the women maintained their "ideal body weight."

Muscle atrophies and metabolism slows with diet-only strategies. All muscles are adversely affected, including that of the heart, and the more severe the diet, the greater the muscle loss. Data that illustrated this effect were presented at the 1987 Scientific Session of the American Heart Association convention. Twenty-one obese women ages 18 to 40 were put on diets of 800 to 1,000 kCals per day (low-calorie diet) or 1,300 to 1,600 kCals per day (moderate-kCal diet).[29] Some of the subjects remained sedentary, some did aerobic exercise, and some combined aerobic exercise with circuit weight training. All of the women lost weight during the 12 weeks of the study. Those on the low-calorie diet lost 26 pounds, while those on the moderate-calorie diet lost 15 pounds. Echocardiographic assessments showed that all of the low-kCal subjects experienced a reduction in left ventricular mass (the heart chamber that pumps blood to all tissues of the body), but the loss was greater in the nonexercising group. Exercising subjects on the moderate-kCal diet had an increase in left ventricular size. It seems that the harmful effects of low-kCal diets cannot be offset entirely even with exercise, but heart muscle increased when exercise was combined with only moderate kCal restriction.

Weight loss attempts in the United States have emphasized dietary restriction with continued sedentary living. This combination has led to consistent failure. Weight loss with this method is temporary, and the majority of these weight watchers lose and gain weight many times during their lives. The eating patterns established during the diet period are short-lived.

At any given time, approximately 24 percent of American men and 40 percent of United States women are attempting to lose weight for reasons of health or physical appearance. These people average 2.3 diet attempts per year. Unfortunately, 90 percent to 95 percent of all dieters regain all or most of the weight that they lost within five years.[30] Eat-less approaches to weight loss and permanent weight control have not worked and probably never will. It is notable that people repeatedly utilize weight-loss strategies that have failed them in the past. New attempts may feature new "diets," but calorie restriction remains the method of choice. It is time to forget dieting as an effective weight-loss technique. The appropriate nutritional approach emphasizes sensible modifications in eating behavior that can be followed for a lifetime, not for just a few weeks or a few months. This combined with sensible, progressive, and consistent exercise for a lifetime should produce the permanent weight loss and control that people want.

Exercise Stimulates Metabolism

Approximately 65 percent to 70 percent of the energy liberated from food is expended to maintain the essential functions of the body.[31] The energy to accomplish these functions is the **basal metabolic rate (BMR)**—the amount of energy that the body expends to sustain life while at complete rest. The BMR is measured while the person is fasted (at least 12 hours since the last meal), rested (in the morning after 8 hours of sleep), and in a thermally neutral environment (at a comfortable room temperature). Since these conditions are difficult to satisfy, they are often approximated, so that the BMR is estimated by the **resting metabolic rate (RMR).** The RMR requires that measurements be taken three to four hours after the last meal, following a 30-minute rest period in a thermally comfortable environment on a day in which the subject has not participated in vigorous physical activity.

Because of less muscle tissue, the RMRs of females is five to 10 percent lower than males and 15 percent lower than that of very muscular males. Males who are overweight primarily because of heavy musculature have higher RMRs and higher TEF and respond more readily to exercise/diet approaches to weight loss than overweight men whose excess weight is primarily fat.[32] The energy needed to sustain the RMR constitutes a significant amount of the total number of daily calories expended by the average adult. Then, from a weight-management perspective, it is advantageous to preserve and/or enhance the RMR and to do nothing to reduce it. Exercise fits the bill very nicely.

In the past, the decline in RMR was presumed to be a natural aspect of aging. But age per se has relatively little effect. It seems that the acquired changes accompanying aging are primarily responsible for the decline in RMR. H.A. deVries stated that "it has been shown that the loss in human muscle tissue with age can entirely account for the downward trend in basal metabolism."[33] Muscle tissue uses more energy than fat during rest or physical activity. Authorities estimate that we lose 3 percent to 5 percent of our active protoplasm (mostly muscle tissue) each decade after 25 years of age. This loss is directly attributed to physical inactivity as we age and results in the all too common negative changes that are seen in body composition.

Physical activity is the key to weight management because it uses calories and accelerates metabolism. It also prevents or attenuates the weight-loss plateau that the majority of dieters experience. This plateau represents a period of time when weight loss decelerates substantially or stops temporarily.[34]

Researchers measured the food intake and energy expenditure of a group of three-month-old infants. The measurements were repeated when the infants were one year old.[35] Infants who were overweight by their first birthday were expending 21 percent less energy than normal-weight infants, even though the two groups did not differ in food intake. It is difficult to control and distinguish between genetics (all overweight infants in this study had overweight mothers) and environmental influences in studies such as these. However, the researchers strongly suggest that encouraging physical activity may be more effective than food restriction in preventing obesity in vulnerable infants. Low energy expenditure is also a major contributor to obesity in adults.

Young and middle-aged subjects who were within plus or minus 5 percent of their ideal weight as determined by height, weight, and frame size charts illustrated the body composition changes that occur with age. Although both groups were within the ideal range for weight, the middle-aged subjects had twice as much body fat as the young subjects. These data show quite well that lost muscle weight that is replaced by a gain in fat weight produces negative changes in body composition even in the absence of weight gain. Since fat is less dense than muscle, it occupies more room in the body; hence, the change in the configuration of the body. Table 10.2 illustrates some of the changes in the body composition that occur as Americans age. The examples are hypothetical, but they are based upon fact.

Subject 1 typifies the inactive person who maintains his body weight while aging but experiences a change in body composition. His bathroom scales provide no clues regarding the change, but the mirror and the fit of his clothes do. This man must hold a tight rein on appetite because his resting caloric requirements have diminished. Subject 2 is inactive and chooses to lose weight with age to keep from becoming fatter—rare in our society. He loses one quarter to one half a pound per year after age 30. This individual has lost muscle tissue and has

TABLE 10.2 Effects of Physical Inactivity on Body Composition

Subject	Body Weight at Age 20 (lb)	Body Weight at Age 60 (lb)	Activity Level	Lean Tissue*	Fat	Body Composition
1	150	150	Inactive	Lost 12%–20%	Gain	Changed
2	150	135	Inactive	Lost 12%–20%	No gain	Changed
3	150	165	Inactive	Lost 12%–20%	Gain	Changed
4	150	150	Active	No Loss	No gain	Unchanged

*The lean tissue values in the table apply to males, but the same trend is evident to a lesser degree in females because women have less lean tissue to lose.

Source: Adapted from M. Williams *Nutrition for Fitness and Sport*, Dubuque, Iowa: Wm. C. Brown, Publishers, 1992.

reduced his body weight. His body composition has changed as a result—he is smaller all over. Because of the decline in metabolism from the loss of muscle along with a lower body weight, which diminishes the caloric cost of any weight-bearing movement, this individual must eat progressively less as the years pass to prevent a gain in fat tissue. Hunger would be a constant companion with this strategy. Subject 3 is probably most representative of the typical American who gains both fat and total weight with age. Subject 4 is physically active throughout life. He has little muscle loss and no gain in fat weight. Many examples of this modern-day phenomenon continue to jog, cycle, swim, and so on. Programs that build and maintain muscle tissue preserve the RMR and perpetuate a youthful body composition.

POINTS TO PONDER

1. Define the terms *body composition, overweight,* and *obesity.*
2. Differentiate between essential and storage fat and describe the influence of gender on each.
3. Discuss the development of adipose tissue.
4. Can a nonsmoking obese individual with normal cholesterol and blood pressure be considered in a state of high-level wellness? Defend your answer.
5. Why should exercise be an integral part of a weight-loss program? How would you convince a dieter who is reluctant to exercise?
6. What evidence can you cite to support the notion that exercise increases metabolism over the long term?

THE EFFECTS OF DIET ON BODY COMPOSITION

Metabolism is adversely affected by calorie restriction. In its quest for homeostasis (the tendency to maintain a constancy of internal conditions), the body adapts to the reduced-calorie intake by lowering the metabolic rate. This effort to economize in response to less food intake is a survival mechanism that protects people during lean times. Because the body learns to get by with less, the difference between calories eaten and calories needed narrows. This defense mechanism makes it possible for prisoners of war to survive internment in concentration camps. This same defense mechanism is operative in individuals who voluntarily reduce their food intake with the same result: a drop in RMR. As the RMR decreases, so too does the effectiveness of dieting. Regular vigorous exercise has the opposite effect: it accelerates the metabolic processes and increases body temperature during and after physical activity. The RMR may remain elevated for some time after exercise. Under exercise conditions, the body is spending rather than hoarding.

Diet programs continue to proliferate. Some of today's most popular diets are evaluated in Table 10.3. Diet systems not included in Table 10.3 include Nutri Systems, Diet Center, and Physicians Weight Loss Center. Programs such as these are generally less desirable for the average person because they are expensive, require either mandatory diet food and/or supplements (usually purchased from them), and incorporate intensive counseling. These systems do not allow for an easy transition to healthy normal eating later on. When the dieter leaves these programs, the likelihood of regaining the lost weight is very high.

The Never-Say-Diet Diet was created by Richard Simmons of television fame. It is a low-kCal diet (about 900 kCals/day) with limited food choices. It is also lacking in important vitamins and minerals. Only those who are highly motivated can adhere to this diet for any length of time.

Some of the best-selling diets have made absurd assumptions. For example, Fit for Life by the Diamonds proposes that meat will not be digested if it is eaten with potatoes! They also state that fruits should only be eaten before noon! The Body Principal by Victoria Principal alleges that foods containing more than one letter "e", such as beets, cheese, lettuce, celery, and beef, are unhealthy and should be avoided. Dr. Berger's Immune Power Diet makes the claim that 30 percent of all Americans have food allergies and that these are responsible for obesity and other diseases. Supposedly, if your food allergies can be identified, you can avoid those

TABLE 10.3 Guide to Selected Popular Diets

Type	Description	Weight Loss	Health Drawbacks	Pros/Cons
Balanced (available in book stores) • Weight Watchers Quick Success Program (Weight Watchers International) • Take Off Pounds Sensibly (TOPS) • Overeaters Anonymous • Jane Fonda's New Workout & Weight Loss Program • I Don't Eat (But I Can't Lose Weight) • Complete University Medical Diet • Jane Brody's Nutrition Book • Fit or Fat Target Diet • Popcorn Plus Diet • Getting Thin • Setpoint Diet • Nautilus Diet	Recommends 1,000 or more calories/day. At least 50% carbohydrate, less than 30% fat, 15% to 20% protein. Variety of foods from four basic food groups. (Regular exercise and lifestyle changes.)	1 to 2 lb./week. Promotes permanent loss of fat, especially if combined with regular exercise.	None (no side effects in healthy people). Diet includes an adequate amount of food in all the major food groups. No specialized medical supervision necessary in healthy people.	Provides variety and good nutrition. Combined with exercise, diet can be used as a basis of lifelong weight control. No supplementation necessary. Weight loss is fat, not muscle.
High Carbohydrate • Bloomingdale's Eat Health Diet • Pritkin Permanent Weight Loss Manual	Calorie level varies. Encourages increasing carbohydrate intake to more than 60% of diet. Can severely restrict protein and fat intake. Some advocate exercise and positive lifestyle changes.	Gradual or rapid, depending on calorie intake.	May be too low in protein and require vitamin and mineral supplements.	If protein level and calorie intake are adequate high-carbo hydrate diets are safe and effective. However, they may be so restrictive that they can be hard to stick to.
Formula/Rx (available through a physician or hospital-run program) • HMR (Health Management Resources) • Medifast • Optifast	Suggests only 800 or fewer calories/day. Requires dieters to forgo food for about 12 weeks and eat only a protein supplement. After initial fast, food is gradually reintroduced. May encourage exercise and lifestyle changes.	Vary rapid. 3 to 4 lb./week. Protein supplements claimed to reduce loss of muscle tissue. Unknown: whether dieters keeps weight off.	Can produce severe metabolic disturbances, heartbeat irregularities, hair loss, dehydration, kidney problems, and sense of feeling cold. Vitamins and mineral supplements required.	Expensive, Cost can run as high as $500 per month. Only for obese people (20% or more overweight), to offset a weight-related health problem, or for people who have failed on other diets. Requires close medical supervision.
Formula OTC (over the counter) • Nutrament • Slender • Slim Fast	May advocate fewer than 1,000 calories/day. Replaces one or more meals with a low-calorie shake or food bar that contains some combination of protein, carbohydrates, fats, vitamins, minerals.	Can be rapid, 3 or more lb./week if daily calorie level falls below 1,000. May promote water and muscle loss. Weight often regained.	May be low in protein, carbohydrates, vitamins, or minerals. Can be dangerous if used for sole source of nutrition.	Teaches reliance on patented products, not on sound, life-long eating habits.

Continued

TABLE 10.3 Guide to Selected Popular Diets—*Continued*

Type	Description	Weight Loss	Health Drawbacks	Pros/Cons
Low Carbohydrate/High Protein • Dr. Atkins' Diet Revolution • Complete Scarsdale Medical Diet • Doctor's Quick Weight Loss Diet (Stillman, "water diet") • 35-Plus Diet for Women • Calories Don't Count • Drinking Man's Diet	Calorie level varies. Severely restricts carbohydrates, such as bread, cereals, grains, starchy vegetables.	Rapid, 3 or more lb./week. Promotes loss of water and muscle tissue. Weight usually regained.	Usually unbalanced. May be very high in saturated fat and cholesterol. Can cause fatigue, headaches, nausea, dehydration, and dizziness.	Does not promote good eating habits. Nutritional claims are unsound.
Very-Low Calorie • Diet Principal • Rotation Diet • Cambridge • Genesis • Last Chance Diet	Suggests fewer than 1,000 calories/day for part of diet or for its entirety. Based on low-fat, high-carbohydrate foods.	Rapid, 3 or more lb./week. Initial loss of water and muscle, not fat. Weight usually regained.	May be unbalanced and require vitamin and mineral supplements.	Usually does not teach long-term good eating habits.
Food Combination • Beverly Hills Diet • Fit for Life • Rice Diet Report	Usually fewer than 1,000 calories/day. Often makes false claims that specific foods or combinations burn fat; suggests eating one type of food to exclusion of others.	Can be rapid, depending on calorie intake, Weight generally regained.	Unbalanced. May be dangerously low in protein: often deficient in vitamins and minerals. Can result in dizziness, diarrhea, gas, hair loss, brittle nails, and loss of vital muscle tissue.	Based on unsound nutritional guidelines. Weight is lost because of reduction in calories, not magic food formula; can be dangerous. May be extremely restrictive and monotonous.

Compiled from information from *The Walking Magazine,* June 1989, and G. M. Wardlaw and P. M. Insel, *Perspectives in Nutrition,* St. Louis: Times Mirror/Mosby, 1990.

that are causative and normalize your weight. There is no scientific evidence to support the claims made by the developers of these fad diets.

Dieting reduces basal heat production. In one study, the basal heat of dieting obese subjects dropped to 91 percent of prediet levels in two weeks on a 500-kCal-per-day diet.[36] After the initial two weeks, the subjects switched to 20 to 30 minutes of exercise at 60 percent of their aerobic capacity. Basal heat production increased to normal values in three to four days and continued to increase for the next two weeks to a value equal to 107 percent of the prediet level. Meanwhile, the basal heat production of sedentary controls on a 500-kCal-per-day diet for the four weeks dropped to 81 percent of their prediet levels. This drop in heat production or energy expenditure partially explains why the actual weight lost by dieting is often less than the predicted weight loss.

More restrictive diets produce greater losses of lean tissue. Fasting or starvation results in substantial losses of lean tissue. The brain and central nervous system require glucose (sugar) as their only source of fuel. Glucose is produced from the breakdown of dietary carbohydrates, but fasting or starvation means zero nutrient intake. Under these circumstances, the body's protein from muscles, liver, and other organs is converted to glucose for the brain and central nervous system. Ninety percent of the body's glucose is formed in this manner, and the other 10 percent comes from glycerol (fat).

The conversion of protein to glucose is a wasteful process because only half of the amino acids (the structure of protein) are used, while the other half must be removed. Ninety-five percent of all fat cannot be converted to glucose. The body adapts to fat as a major supplier of fuel by converting fatty acids to ketone bodies (organic acids that disturb the acid-base balance of the blood). Ketone bodies are the product of the incomplete breakdown of fat when carbohydrates are not available. The brain and central nervous system partially adapt and receive 50 percent

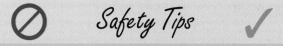

RECOGNIZING FAD DIETS

Fad diets usually

1. Promote quick weight loss requiring little effort by the dieter.
2. Feature limited food selections.
3. Suggest that foods must be eaten in a particular order.
4. Use testimonials from famous people.
5. Assert that their diet plan is the best available and is not accepted by the scientific community because it doesn't want to lose its clientele to an outsider.
6. Involve a secret ingredient unknown to science that is responsible for the success of the program.
7. Feature expensive supplements that usually must be purchased from them.
8. Show little concern for educating people regarding proper nutrition and healthy eating patterns.

of their fuel from ketones. The other 50 percent continues to come from the breakdown of the body's protein. Consequently, the RMR decreases significantly during the time of deprivation as the body attempts to conserve its lean tissue and fat stores. As the protein-containing organs progressively shrink, they perform less and less metabolic work and reduce the body's energy needs. The slowed-down metabolic engine results in less fat loss while body weight continues to fall rapidly. Concurrently, ketone bodies accumulate in the blood because they are produced in quantities that outstrip the body's ability to use or excrete them. The increase in blood acid level is potentially dangerous. Death often occurs from heart rhythm irregularities rather than starvation. Starvation should be avoided except for the extremely obese, and then only under hospitalized medical supervision.

Very-low kCal diets (800 or fewer kCals/day), including those that have been promoted as having a "protein-sparing effect," have often been associated with medical complications if they are followed long enough to produce substantial weight loss. The consequences of these diets include cardiac arrhythmias and sudden death.[37] These diets produce distinctive EKG (electrocardiogram) patterns that depict abnormal rhythm disturbances that are probably caused by protein depletion of the myocardium and/or cell membrane instability from rapid weight loss.[38] In addition to these risks, such crash dieting typically results in a return to prediet weight when the diet ends.

Repeated weight loss and gain is referred as **weight cycling** (cycle dieting) or yo-yo dieting. Some controversial issues regarding such dieting are in need of resolution. For example, (1) do cycle dieters find it more difficult to lose weight with each new attempt? (2) do they regain the weight faster after each attempt? (3) is more fat gained with each attempt? (4) are weight cyclers more inclined to store fat in the android pattern? (5) does cycle dieting slow metabolism? (6) does cycle dieting increase the risk for chronic disease and early death?

Rena Wing surveyed the literature on cycle dieting through 1991. Her investigation indicated that there appeared to be no negative effects of cycle dieting on total body fat and the distribution of fat in the body. Also, metabolism appeared to be unaffected, and subsequent attempts at losing weight did not appear to be more difficult.[39] However, there is evidence that weight cycling increases the risk of all-cause mortality, and cardiovascular death in particular.

The strongest evidence of the relationship between weight cycling and cardiovascular disease comes from a 32-year followup of 3,000 men and women ages 30 to 62 who are participants in the ongoing Framingham Heart Study.[40] When compared to subjects whose weight remained stable over the 32 years, the weight cyclers experienced an increase in the risk of heart disease, heart disease death, and all-cause mortality. Weight fluctuations appeared to be more of a risk to

The Reduction Equation: Exercise + Sensible Eating = Fat Control   **253**

health in the youngest age group—those who were 30 to 44 years of age. The people in this age group are more prone to use dieting to control their weight.

The Framingham researchers indicated that it was probably better, with respect to developing cardiovascular disease, to remain a little overweight than to lose and regain the same 15 pounds over and over again. Men who lost and regained 20 to 30 pounds during a given two-year period were at twice the risk of dying from cardiovascular disease than those whose weight remained reasonably constant. Women were at 1 1/2 times the risk of dying from cardiovascular disease if they lost and regained 15 to 20 pounds during a two-year period. Two long-term studies with thousands of subjects (the Multiple Risk Factor Intervention Trial and the Harvard Alumni Study) produced similar results.

Why is weight cycling associated with premature death? The mechanisms responsible for this relationship are not fully understood, but there is agreement that weight gain increases serum cholesterol, blood pressure, and serum glucose levels—all of which contribute to coronary risk.

The message is clear for those who need to lose weight: do it right the first time and commit to keeping the weight off. Cycle dieters, especially those with the greatest fluctuations, have the greatest risk.[41]

Zuti and Golding investigated the relationship between exercise, diet, and weight loss.[42] They analyzed the effects of three different strategies upon the quantity and quality of weight loss. Each strategy was designed to elicit a loss of one pound per week. The subjects were overweight women 25 to 45 years of age. A summary of the results of the study appears in Table 10.4.

The diet-only group reduced food intake by 500 kCals per day and did not exercise. The exercise-only group did not diet but increased their physical activity by 500 kCals per day. The diet-and-exercise group reduced their caloric intake by 250 kCals per day while increasing their caloric expenditure by the same amount. The aim of all three strategies was to lose one pound per week (500 kCals × 7 days = 3,500 kCals), and this objective was essentially accomplished by all three groups. But the significant outcome of this study was that 21 percent of the total loss experienced by the diet-only group was in the form of lean tissue. This occurred despite a nutritionally sound diet of modest calorie restriction. The other two groups lost fat (the true goal of weight-loss programs) and gained rather than lost lean tissue.

Following the Zuti and Golding approach, investigators recently examined the effect of dieting and weight training on body composition. The subjects were 40 obese females whose average age was 33 years.[43] The subjects were randomly assigned to one of four groups: (1) a control group who did not diet or exercise, (2) a diet-only group, (3) an exercise-only group, and (4) a diet-plus-exercise group. The exercise program consisted of supervised weight training, and the diet was designed so that each individual would lose two pounds per week. The diet-only group also received a protein supplement. Measurements taken at the end of the study showed that two groups—the exercise-only and the diet-plus-exercise—significantly increased their lean body weight and their strength. The researchers concluded that exercise and diet acted independently during weight loss. Weight training affected those variables associated with muscle components, while dieting affected those variables associated with fat components. This study reinforces

TABLE 10.4 Average Weight Lost by Groups

WEIGHT LOSS STRATEGY	FAT TISSUE LOSS (LB)	LEAN TISSUE LOSS (LB)	TOTAL WEIGHT LOSS (LB)
Diet only	−9.3	−2.4	−11.7
Exercise only	−12.6	+2.0	−10.6
Diet and exercise	−13.0	+1.0	−12.0

the need for including both sensible exercise and dietary modifications in a weight-loss program.

Some obese people seem to be diet resistant; that is, their weight remains stable even when they are following a low-calorie diet. This irony has been variously blamed upon an underactive thyroid, a slow metabolism, or a hereditary tendency toward obesity. A number of studies have shown that the actual reason for the majority of these cases is that these subjects tend to underreport their caloric intake and overestimate their physical activity. This dilemma was examined in a well-controlled study.[44] The researchers found that their diet-resistant subjects underestimated their food intake by 47 percent and overestimated their physical activity by 51 percent. The subjects perceived that their obesity was caused by genetic and metabolic factors rather then errors in their estimates of caloric intake and caloric expenditure.

The American College of Sports Medicine (ACSM) produced a position paper entitled "Proper and Improper Weight Loss Programs." In it, this organization provided sensible guidelines for weight loss. Although the paper was written in 1983, its tenets and guidelines, with some minor modifications as identified by statements in parentheses below, are still appropriate today. Some of the important concepts addressed by ACSM are found in the box entitled "Weight Loss-Tying Things Together."

WEIGHT LOSS-TYING THINGS TOGETHER

1. A diet should provide at least 1200 kCals/day to increase the likelihood of obtaining the necessary nutrients for the maintenance of good health. Diets that are calorically more restrictive are undesirable and potentially dangerous.

2. Food choices should be nutritionally balanced, palatable, and acceptable to the dieter.

3. Weight loss goals should be moderate—no more than 2 pounds per week. (Today there is support for limiting weight loss to 1 1/2 pounds per week.)

4. Behavior modification techniques should be employed in conjunction with dietary modification and exercise to form a well-rounded approach to weight reduction.

5. An endurance type exercise program is a must. The minimum amount of exercise recommended for weight loss includes participation 20 to 30 minutes per day, 3 times per week, at 60% of the maximum heart rate. (If you expend 200 kCals per exercise session, you should exercise 4 times per week; if you expend 300 kCals per exercise session you can exercise 3 times per week).

6. The dietary modifications and exercise program should be sustainable for a lifetime.

American College of Sports Medicine. "Proper and Improper Weight Loss Programs," *Medicine and Science in Sports and Exercise*, 15 (1983): IX.

EXERCISE AND THE UNDERWEIGHT

The focus thus far has been on weight loss rather than weight gain, but the purposeful gain of weight represents a real problem for the underweight. What constitutes underweight? This question has not been satisfactorily answered. Actuarial statistics indicate that those who are significantly below the average in body weight have a higher expected mortality rate. Marked underweight may be indicative of underlying disease and is as much of a risk as obesity for early death.

Being underweight may pose as much of a cosmetic problem for an affected individual as obesity is for an obese individual. An effective weight-gain program should include regular resistance exercise in conjunction with three well-balanced meals plus a couple of nutritious between-meal snacks. There are some commercial drinks that are useful for increasing caloric consumption. Protein supplementation is unnecessary and can be harmful if taken in excessive amounts. Despite Herculean efforts, many underweight people find it more difficult to gain a pound than it is for the obese to lose one. Very lean people should not attempt to gain weight by increasing the fat content of their diet. This is an unhealthy eating pattern for anyone regardless of body weight.

The amount and type of weight gain should be closely monitored. It is desirable to gain muscle tissue without increasing fat stores. Overeating without exercise will not accomplish this objective, nor will it enhance physical appearance. Body fat should not be increased unless affected individuals are so thin that they may be in danger of dipping into essential fat, which is necessary for the life processes. Essential fat constitutes 3 percent to 5 percent of the total weight of males and 11 percent to 14 percent of the total weight of females.[45] The higher quantity of fat in the female body is necessary for the maintenance of a regular menstrual cycle for the purposes of fertility and childbearing. For health-related purposes, it is suggested that adult men maintain 12 percent to 18 percent of their weight in the form of fat, while adult women should maintain 16 percent to 25 percent of their weight as fat. Athletes of all ages and both sexes are generally below these values, and they are very healthy. The preceding values are general guidelines only. Many male marathon runners are between 4 percent and 7 percent body fat with no harmful effects to health. Female athletes should maintain enough body fat so as not to disrupt their menstrual cycle.

EATING DISORDERS

Some people are obsessed with becoming and remaining thin. **Anorexia nervosa** and **bulimarexia nervosa** (bulimia) are two eating disorders reflective of the preoccupation with thinness. Although they share some common characteristics, anorexia and bulimia are different eating disorders. The major commonality between the two is an intense fear of becoming overweight. The anorexic stays thin primarily through starvation, while the bulimic gorges and then purges by vomiting or by using laxatives and diuretics.[47] Bulimics seldom starve to the point of emaciation; in fact, they are often moderately overweight.[48] Bulimia is characterized by episodes of secretive binge eating, menstrual irregularities, swollen glands, frequent weight fluctuation, and the inability to stop eating voluntarily. It is not caused by anorexia nervosa, and many bulimics do not become anorexic, although many anorexics practice bulimic behavior.

Young females account for more than 90% of the cases of anorexia and bulimia.[49] It is estimated that one in every 100 teenage girls is anorexic and that one in five college-bound and college-going females is bulimic. Victims affected by either of these disorders typically suffer from low-self esteem and depression, which is frequently the result of the conflict between their desire for perfection on the one hand and their feelings of inadequacy on the other. Another characteristic of eating disorders is that their victims are overly compliant people who rely on others for approval and validation.

Both anorexia and bulimia are serious eating disorders. Bulimia is seldom fatal, but for the 10 percent to 15 percent of the anorexics whose disease is episodic, the possibility of death is a grim reality. Anorexia is an insidious disease. Its practitioners are evasive, hiding their disease in deep denial even while under treatment.

Treatment usually involves a team approach that begins with the anorexic's admittance to a hospital. Nutritional and psychological counseling, behavior modification, and family counseling are employed concurring to provide insight for affected people and their families regarding the specific eating disorder.

Family counseling prepares the family for living with an eating-disordered person without expending all of their energies worrying about the person. Family members have their own lives to lead, and their lives should not revolve around the eating-disordered person. Bulimia is also treated by a team approach, but hospitalization is usually not necessary. Table 10.5 compares the warning signs and characteristics of anorexia and bulimia.

 ## ASSESSMENT OF BODY COMPOSITION

The assessment of body composition has presented some problems. The only direct method available involves the separation of lean from fat tissue in cadavers. Only a few cadavers have been dissected in this manner because of the difficulty in obtaining them, the amount of time and effort required by the process, and the limited usefulness of the ensuing data. Such problems have stimulated scientists to develop indirect methods of analysis. The techniques provide an estimate of body composition. Because they are estimates, some degree of error is associated with each. The following subsections discuss several of the indirect measures.

Body Mass Index (BMI)

Body mass index (BMI) is a very easy, useful, and quick method of estimating the body weight classification for the general public. It is not equally applicable to all groups of people. For example, very muscular athletes with a low level of body fat might fall into the overweight range. But this is deceiving. This athlete is overweight because of a high amount of muscle, not fat. The BMI calculation does not make allowances for such people, only body composition measures can do that. The calculation requires the accurate measurement of height and weight plus a few simple conversions. Body weight should be determined in the morning after voiding, before breakfast, with light clothing, and without shoes. Height should be taken in inches to the nearest one-quarter inch.

The BMI correlates fairly well (r = .70), with percent body fat derived from hydrostatic (underwater) weighing.[50] The following example serves to illustrate the method. What is the BMI of a male who is 72 inches tall and weights 170 pounds?

TABLE 10.5 Comparisons Between Anorexia and Bulimia

WARNING SIGNS AND CHARACTERISTICS	
Anorexia	*Bulimia*
• Preoccupation with body size and weight.	• Periodic consumptiom of large amounts of high-caloric food.
• Dramatic weight loss.	• Sneaking or hoarding food for later binges.
• Drastic reduction in food intake or refusal to eat at all.	• Repeated unsuccessful attempts to control weight by dieting.
• Extensive exercising.	• Overuse of laxatives or diuretics.
• Abnormal use of laxatives or diuretics.	• Periodic abuse of alcohol or other drugs.
• Food binges and/or purges.	• Excessive concern about physical appearance.
• Hoarding or concealing food.	• Excessive food bills.
• Peculiar behavior concerning food, such as preparation of elaborate meals for others which the anorexic does not eat.	• Frequent complaints of gastrointestinal problems.
• Complaints of being cold.	• Increased number of dental problems.
• Dizziness or fainting.	

1. The BMI formula is

$$\text{BMI} = \frac{\text{wt (kg)}}{\text{ht (m}^2)}$$

2. Weight in pounds is converted to kilograms (kg) by dividing it by 2.2:

$$\frac{170 \text{ lbs.}}{2.2} = 77.3 \text{ kg}$$

3. Height in inches is converted to meters (m) by multiplying it by 0.0254:

$$72 \text{ inches} \times 0.0254 = 1.83 \text{ m}$$

4. Insert the above conversions into the formula

$$\text{BMI} = \frac{\text{wt (kg)}}{\text{ht (m}^2)}$$
$$= \frac{77.3}{1.83^2}$$
$$= \frac{77.3}{3.34}$$
$$= 23.1 \text{ kg/m}^2$$

Body mass index standards have been suggested by the American College of Sports Medicine.[51] BMIs of 21 to 23 kg/m^2 are considered desirable for women; 22 to 24 kg/m^2 are desirable for men. The risk of cardiovascular disease increases substantially when BMIs equal or surpass 27.3 kg/m^2 for women and 27.8 kg/m^2 for men. See Self-Assessment 10.2 and 10.3 for problems involving BMI.

In addition to cardiovascular risk, body mass index also provides an estimate of one's weight classification ranging from underweight to morbid obesity (see Table 10.6). Turn to Self-Assessment activities 10.2 and 10.3 in Appendix C for practice using and interpreting BMI measurements.

If your BMI measurement falls in an undesirable category, you may wish to alter it. But how much weight should you lose or gain to accomplish your goal? Determining desirable body weight using BMI is relatively simple. Follow the example below that applies to a woman who is 5′ 6″ tall and weighs 185 lbs. Her BMI is equal to 29.8kg/m^2. Table 10.6 indicates that she is in the overweight category. The American College of Sports Medicine guidelines indicate that she is at an increased risk for heart disease. Her goals are to reduce body weight and risk by decreasing her BMI to 23 kg/m^2. How much weight should she lose to attain her goal? The problem is solved as follows:

1. Convert body weight in lbs. to kilograms

$$\frac{185}{2.2} = 84.1 \text{ kg}$$

TABLE 10.6 **BMI and Weight Classification for Males and Females**

BMI (MALES)	BMI (FEMALES)	CLASSIFICATION
*<20.7	*<19.1	Underweight
20.7–26.4	19.2–25.8	Acceptable Weight
26.5–27.8	25.9–27.3	Marginal overweight
27.9–31.1	27.4–32.2	Overweight
31.2–45.4	32.3–44.8	Severe overweight
**>45.4	**>44.8	Morbid Obesity

*< less than
**> greater than

Adapted from E. N. Whitney and S. R. Rolfes, *Understanding Nutrition*, St. Paul: West Publishing Co., 1993.

2. Convert height in inches to meters (m)

$$\begin{array}{r} 66 \\ \times \quad .0254 \\ \hline 1.68 \text{ m} \end{array}$$

3. Square the answer to number 2

$1.68^2 = 2.82$

4. Desired body weight (DBW) in kilograms = desired BMI × height (m2) so that:

$$\begin{aligned} \text{DBW} &= \text{desired BMI} \times \text{height (m}^2) \\ &= 23 \times 2.82 \\ &= 64.9 \text{ kg} \end{aligned}$$

5. Convert DBW in kg to lbs.

$$\begin{array}{r} 64.9 \\ \times \quad 2.2 \\ \hline 142.8 \text{ lbs.} \end{array}$$

6. Subtract DBW in lbs. from current body weight in lbs. to find out how much weight she should lose to reach her desired BMI.

$$\begin{array}{r} 185 \\ - \quad 143 \\ \hline 42 \text{ lbs to lose to reach a BMI of 23 kg/m}^2 \end{array}$$

7. Now turn to Self-Assessment activity 10-3 in Appendix C to calculate your desired BMI.

Skinfold Measurements

Skinfold measurements are based upon the assumption that 50 percent of the body's fat lies beneath the surface of the skin, that it can be separated from muscle tissue, and that it can be accurately and reliably measured. The thumb and index finger are used to pinch the loose skin over the site to be measured. This pinch, consisting of a double layer of skin plus subcutaneous fat, makes up the skinfold, which is measured with a special caliper. The most accurate calipers maintain a constant jaw pressure of 10 grams per square millimeter of surface area. The Lange and Harpenden calipers meet these criteria and have been two of the most popular devices for measuring skinfolds. In recent years, several inexpensive calipers have merged that are relatively accurate when used by well-trained technicians. They range in price from $10 to $30, while the Lange and Harpenden are in the 220-dollar to 400-dollar range.

The technique for taking skinfold measurements is not complicated, but to become proficient, one must practice measuring the different sites for all ages and both sexes. One can standardize the method by observing the following suggestions:

1. Mark each site according to the directions given in Figures 10.2 through 10.6.

2. Take two measurements at each site, unless there is a difference of more than one millimeter between the two; if there is, take a third measurement and average the two closest readings.

3. The calipers should be applied about one quarter to one half of an inch below the fingers. This allows the calipers rather than the fingers to compress the skinfold.

4. The calipers should maintain contact with the skinfold for two to five seconds so that the reading can stabilize.

Use Tables 10.7 (page 262) and 10.8 (page 263) to convert millimeters of skinfold thickness to percent body fat. Table 10.7 uses the sum of chest, abdominal, and thigh skinfolds by age to estimate percent body fat for males. Table 10.8 uses the

FIGURE 10.2

Triceps Skinfold Take a vertical fold on the midline of the upper arm over the triceps, halfway between the tip of the shoulder and the elbow: The arm should be extended and relaxed when the measurement is taken. All skinfold measurements should be taken on the right side.

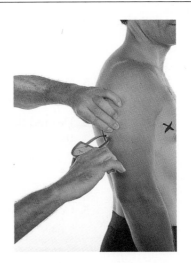

FIGURE 10.3

Suprailium Skinfold Take a diagonal fold above the crest of the ilium directly below the armpit.

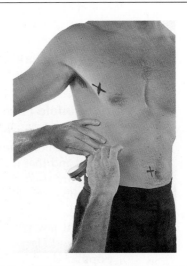

FIGURE 10.4

Thigh Skinfold Take a vertical fold on the front of the thigh midway between the hip and the knee joint. The midpoint should be marked while the subject is seated.

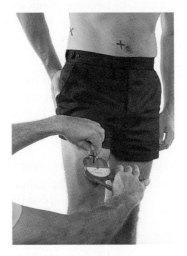

FIGURE 10.5

Chest Skinfold Take a diagonal fold one half of the distance between the anterior axillary line and the nipple.

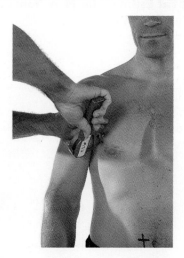

sum of triceps, suprailium, and thigh skinfolds by age to estimate percent body fat for females. The skinfold technique as a method for estimating body fat has an error of ± 3.5 percent when hydrostatic weighing is the standard for comparison.

Bioelectrical Impedence

Bioelectrical impedence is a relatively simple way to estimate percent body fat. The equipment required is portable and computerized, but it is expensive. This method is safe and noninvasive and yields a general assessment of body composition.

Bioelectrical impedence estimates body fat by measuring the speed that an electrical current travels through the body. The method is based on the principle that an electric current flows more rapidly through fat-free tissue because of its greater water and electrolyte content. Electrolytes are minerals such as sodium and potassium that conduct electrical impulses through the body's fluids. Impedence is measured as the resistance to electrical currents. Resistance is greatest in fat tissue, which is essentially anhydrous (contains 14 percent to 22 percent water).

Bioelectrical impedence measurements should be made under strict standardized conditions because there are factors that, if not controlled, can increase the error of measurement. Dehydration, whether from sweating or inadequate fluid

FIGURE 10.6

Abdominal Skinfold Take a vertical fold about one inch above the navel.

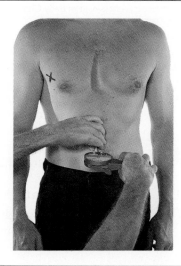

TABLE 10.7 Percent Fat Estimate for Men: Sum of Chest, Abdomen, and Thigh Skinfolds

SUM OF SKINFOLDS (MM)	AGE TO LAST YEAR								
	Under 22	*23–27*	*28–32*	*33–37*	*38–42*	*43–47*	*48–52*	*53–57*	*Over 57*
8–10	1.3	1.8	2.3	2.9	3.4	3.9	4.5	5.0	5.5
11–13	2.2	2.8	3.3	3.9	4.4	4.9	5.5	6.0	6.5
14–16	3.2	3.8	4.3	4.8	5.4	5.9	6.4	7.0	7.5
17–19	4.2	4.7	5.3	5.8	6.3	6.9	7.4	8.0	8.5
20–22	5.1	5.7	6.2	6.8	7.3	7.9	8.4	8.9	9.5
23–25	6.1	6.6	7.2	7.7	8.3	8.8	9.4	9.9	10.5
26–28	7.0	7.6	8.1	8.7	9.2	9.8	10.3	10.9	11.4
29–31	8.0	8.5	9.1	9.6	10.2	10.7	11.3	11.8	12.4
32–34	8.9	9.4	10.0	10.5	11.1	11.6	12.2	12.8	13.3
35–37	9.8	10.4	10.9	11.5	12.0	12.6	13.1	13.7	14.3
38–40	10.7	11.3	11.8	12.4	12.9	13.5	14.1	14.6	15.2
41–43	11.6	12.2	12.7	13.3	13.8	14.4	15.0	15.5	16.1
44–46	12.5	13.1	13.6	14.2	14.7	15.3	15.9	16.4	17.0
47–49	13.4	13.9	14.5	15.1	15.6	16.2	16.8	17.3	17.9
50–52	14.3	14.8	15.4	15.9	16.5	17.1	17.6	18.2	18.8
53–55	15.1	15.7	16.2	16.8	17.4	17.9	18.5	19.1	19.7
56–58	16.0	16.5	17.1	17.7	18.2	18.8	19.4	20.0	20.5
59–61	16.9	17.4	17.9	18.5	19.1	19.7	20.2	20.8	21.4
62–64	17.6	18.2	18.8	19.4	19.9	20.5	21.1	21.7	22.2
65–67	18.5	19.0	19.6	20.2	20.8	21.3	21.9	22.5	23.1
68–70	19.3	19.9	20.4	21.0	21.6	22.2	22.7	23.3	23.9
71–73	20.1	20.7	21.2	21.8	22.4	23.0	23.6	24.1	24.7
74–76	20.9	21.5	22.0	22.6	23.2	23.8	24.4	25.0	25.5
77–79	21.7	22.2	22.8	23.4	24.0	24.6	25.2	25.8	26.3
80–82	22.4	23.0	23.6	24.2	24.8	25.4	25.9	26.5	27.1
83–85	23.2	23.8	24.4	25.0	25.5	26.1	26.7	27.3	27.9
86–88	24.0	24.5	25.1	25.7	26.3	26.9	27.5	28.1	28.7
89–91	24.7	25.3	25.9	26.5	27.1	27.6	28.2	28.8	29.4
92–94	25.4	26.0	26.6	27.2	27.8	28.4	29.0	29.6	30.2
95–97	26.1	26.7	27.3	27.9	28.5	29.1	29.7	30.3	30.9
98–100	26.9	27.4	28.0	28.6	29.2	29.8	30.4	31.0	31.6
101–103	27.5	28.1	28.7	29.3	29.9	30.5	31.1	31.7	32.3
104–106	28.2	28.8	29.4	30.0	30.6	31.2	31.8	32.4	33.0
107–109	28.9	29.5	30.1	30.7	31.3	31.9	32.5	33.1	33.7
110–112	29.6	30.2	30.8	31.4	32.0	32.6	33.2	33.8	34.4
113–115	30.2	30.8	31.4	32.0	32.6	33.2	33.8	34.5	35.1
116–118	30.9	31.5	32.1	32.7	33.3	33.9	34.5	35.1	35.7
119–121	31.5	32.1	32.7	33.3	33.9	34.5	35.1	35.7	36.4
122–124	32.1	32.7	33.3	33.9	34.5	35.1	35.8	36.4	37.0
125–127	32.7	33.3	33.9	34.5	35.1	35.8	36.4	37.0	37.6

From A. S. Jackson and M. L. Pollock, "Practical Assessment of Body Composition," *The Physician and Sportsmedicine* 13, no. 5 (May 1988): 85.

intake, decreases resistance to electrical flow, leading to an underestimation of percent of body fat. Overhydration produces opposite results. Skin temperature, which is affected by ambient conditions, also affects the accuracy of this technique. Estimates of body fat percentage are lower in warm environments and higher in cold environments.

Studies have shown that bioelectrical impedence measures made under controlled conditions are about as accurate as skinfold techniques. See Figure 10.7 for an illustration of this technique.

Hydrostatic Weighing

Hydrostatic weighing, as the name implies, involves the weighing of subjects while they are completely submerged. It is one of the more accurate measures, provided that the subject is capable of a maximal exhalation of air from the lungs

TABLE 10.8 **Percent Fat Estimate for Women: Sum of Triceps, Suprailium, and Thigh Skinfolds**

SUM OF SKINFOLDS (MM)	AGE TO LAST YEAR								
	Under 22	23–27	28–32	33–37	38–42	43–47	48–52	53–57	Over 57
23–25	9.7	9.9	10.2	10.4	10.7	10.9	11.2	11.4	11.7
26–28	11.0	11.2	11.5	11.7	12.0	12.3	12.5	12.7	13.0
29–31	12.3	12.5	12.8	13.0	13.3	13.5	13.8	14.0	14.3
32–34	13.6	13.8	14.0	14.3	14.5	14.8	15.0	15.3	15.5
35–37	14.8	15.0	15.3	15.5	15.8	16.0	16.3	16.5	16.8
38–40	16.0	16.3	16.5	16.7	17.0	17.2	17.5	17.7	18.0
41–43	17.2	17.4	17.7	17.9	18.2	18.4	18.7	18.9	19.2
44–46	18.3	18.6	18.8	19.1	19.3	19.6	19.8	20.1	20.3
47–49	19.5	19.7	20.0	20.2	20.5	20.7	21.0	21.2	21.5
50–52	20.6	20.8	21.1	21.3	21.6	21.8	22.1	22.3	22.6
53–55	21.7	21.9	22.1	22.4	22.6	22.9	23.1	23.4	23.6
56–58	22.7	23.0	23.2	23.4	23.7	23.9	24.2	24.4	24.7
59–61	23.7	24.0	24.2	24.5	24.7	25.0	25.2	25.5	25.7
62–64	24.7	25.0	25.2	25.5	25.7	26.0	26.7	26.4	26.7
65–67	25.7	25.9	26.2	26.4	26.7	26.9	27.2	27.4	27.7
68–70	26.6	26.9	27.1	27.4	27.6	27.9	28.1	28.4	28.6
71–73	27.5	27.8	28.0	28.3	28.5	28.8	29.0	29.3	29.5
74–76	28.4	28.7	28.9	29.2	29.4	29.7	29.9	30.2	30.4
77–79	29.3	29.5	29.8	30.0	30.3	30.5	30.8	31.0	31.3
80–82	30.1	30.4	30.6	30.9	31.1	31.4	31.6	31.9	32.1
83–85	30.9	31.2	31.4	31.7	31.9	32.2	32.4	32.7	32.9
86–88	31.7	32.0	32.2	32.5	32.7	32.9	33.2	33.4	33.7
89–91	32.5	32.7	33.0	33.2	33.5	33.7	33.9	34.2	34.4
92–94	33.2	33.4	33.7	33.9	34.2	34.4	34.7	34.9	35.2
95–97	33.9	34.1	34.4	34.6	34.9	35.1	35.4	35.6	35.9
98–100	34.6	34.8	35.1	35.3	35.5	35.8	36.0	36.3	36.5
101–103	35.3	35.4	35.7	35.9	36.2	36.4	36.7	36.9	37.2
104–106	35.8	36.1	36.3	36.6	36.8	37.1	37.3	37.5	37.8
107–109	36.4	36.7	36.9	37.1	37.4	37.6	37.9	38.1	38.4
110–112	37.0	37.2	37.5	37.7	38.0	38.2	38.5	38.7	38.9
113–115	37.5	37.8	38.0	38.2	38.5	38.7	39.0	39.2	39.5
116–118	38.0	38.3	38.5	38.8	39.0	39.3	39.5	39.7	40.0
119–121	38.5	38.7	39.0	39.2	39.5	39.7	40.0	40.2	40.5
122–124	39.0	39.2	39.4	39.7	39.9	40.2	40.4	40.7	40.9
125–127	39.4	39.6	39.9	40.1	40.4	40.6	40.9	41.1	41.4
128–130	39.8	40.0	40.3	40.5	40.8	41.0	41.3	41.5	41.8

From A. S. Jackson and M. L. Pollock, "Practical Assessment of Body Composition," *The Physician and Sportsmedicine* 13, no. 5 (May 1985): 86.

and can remain submerged and still for 6 to 10 seconds. Accuracy is enhanced still further if the technician has the equipment to measure residual air (the amount of air remaining in the lungs following a maximal expiration). Without such equipment, residual air can be estimated from a table of constants that has been developed for age and sex.

The equipment for hydrostatic weighing includes an autopsy scale calibrated in grams with a capacity of approximately 8 kilograms. This is suspended over the shallow end of a swimming pool or tank at least three feet deep. A lightweight seat is attached to the scale. The subject is suspended chin-deep in the water, exhales completely and bends forward from the waist until entirely submerged. This position is maintained for 6 to 10 seconds—enough time for the scale's pointer to stabilize. Five to ten trials are needed, and the three heaviest readings are averaged. The individual's net underwater weight is calculated by subtracting the weight of the seat and its supporting structure (plus a weight belt if needed) from the gross underwater weight. The typical underwater weighing apparatus appears in Figure 10.8.

FIGURE 10.7

Bioelectrical Impedence

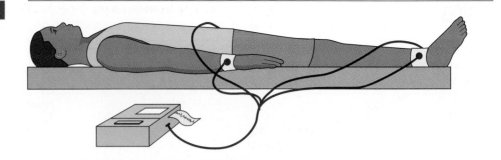

Standards for Body Fat Percentage

There is relative agreement among authorities regarding the standards and classification for percent body fat for both sexes (see Table 10.9). These standards apply to the general public.

Desirable Body Weight

Desirable body weight can be easily determined when percent body fat has been ascertained. For example, a 20-year-old male who weighs 195 pounds has a measured body fat of 26 percent. Reducing his fat weight to 15% would place him in an acceptable category for his age and sex. How much weight should he lose to accomplish this objective? The calculations are as follows:

1. Find fat weight (FW) in pounds. Convert 26 percent into its decimal form (.26) and multiply it by the subject's body weight:

   FW = 195 × .26
   = 50.7 lbs.

2. Find fat-free weight (FFW) by subtracting the FW from the total weight:

   FFW = 195 – 50.7
   =144.3 lbs.

FIGURE 10.8

Underwater Weighing Apparatus Subject in the ready position for underwater weighing. Subject in the process of being weighed.

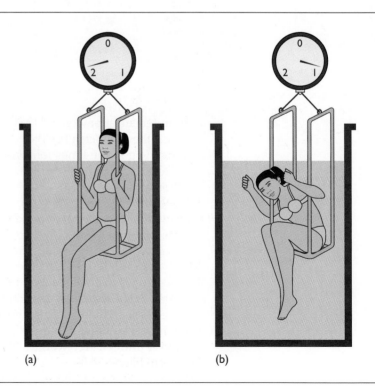

(a)   (b)

TABLE 10.9 Standards for Body Fat Percentage

MALE	FEMALE	CLASSIFICATION
*<8%	<13%	Lean
8–15%	13–20%	Optimal
16–20%	21–25%	Slightly overfat
21–24%	26–32%	Fat
**≥25%	≥32%	Obese

* < less than

** ≥ equal to or greater than

Adapted from D. C. Nieman, *Fitness and Sports Medicine,* Palo Alto: Bull Publishing Co, 1990.

3. Find desirable body weight (DBW) by dividing FFW by 1.0 minus the desired percent fat:

$$DBW = \frac{FFW}{1.0 - \% \text{ fat desired}}$$

$$DBW = \frac{144.3}{1.0 - .15}$$

$$DBW = \frac{144.3}{.85}$$

$$= 169.7 \text{ lbs.}$$

4. This subject needs to lose 25.3 lbs. (195 − 169.7) to get his percent body fat down to 15 percent.

This method is appropriate if the subject (1) is exercising to keep from losing muscle tissue, (2) loses no more than 1.5 lbs. per week, (3) is reevaluated two or three times during the weight-loss phase, (4) understands that all attempts to estimate body fat in a living human are indirect and that each contains some measurement error, and (5) understands that the measurement is an estimate that should be used with some degree of latitude.

EXERCISES FOR IMPROVING BODY COMPOSITION

Body composition can be improved by increasing muscle tissue and decreasing fat tissue. Exercise represents the only viable way to accomplish both of these objectives. Aerobic activities that use 200 to 300 calories per workout three to four times a week are the minimum for effecting a change in body composition. Such aerobic activities include walking, jogging, cycling, swimming, rowing, and aerobic dance. They can be performed individually or in combination. Court games such as handball, racquetball, squash, and badminton also can change body composition if played vigorously. This requires a fair degree of skill on the part of participants and entails singles competition against compatible opposition.

The potential to change body composition through exercise has led people to attempt to change only selected sites. Spot reduction implies that one can reduce the fat content of a particular body part by doing specific exercises related to that part. Sit-ups and leg-lifts have been commonly used to reduce abdominal fat and waist girth while leaving the remainder of the body unchanged. The attractiveness of this concept has led an unsuspecting public to believe that with a little effort people can sculpt their bodies to suit their fancies.

Spot reduction is a myth promoted by charlatans or unknowledgeable people who have a gimmick, gadget, or system to sell that is supposedly designed to achieve reductions in localized areas of the body. The truth is that buyers will probably reduce nothing but the contents of their wallets. Localized exercise produces muscle tone and strength, but it does not reduce the amount of fat at a given site. It may tighten up localized areas, resulting in a difference in girth. For example, sit-ups done over a long period of time will strengthen and tighten the abdominal area. The stronger abdominal musculature helps to hold back the viscera and in this respect may reduce waist girth, but fat content remains unchanged. To reduce fat stored in the abdominal region—or in the back of the arm or in the buttocks—a person must expend more calories than calories consumed. This way, fat is lost from everywhere in the body, including the site in question. If spot reduction were a reality, people with fat faces could chew gum every day and eventually become people with thin faces. It just doesn't work.

 OINTS TO PONDER

1. What physical problems are associated with very-low calorie diets?
2. Define weight cycling and discuss the reasons for its ineffectiveness as a weight-management technique.
3. Why is weight cycling a cardiovascular risk factor?
4. Discuss the genetic influence in weight control.
5. Discuss the roles of diet and exercise in weight control.
6. How should those who are underweight gain weight in a healthy manner?
7. Define anorexia nervosa and bulimarexia nervosa.
8. How do these two eating disorders differ? What do they share in common?
9. Define BMI. At what level is it a risk factor for cardiovascular disease?
10. What is the principle that bioelectrical impedence is based upon for the assessment of body composition?
11. Discuss the steps that should be followed for assessing body composition using skinfold calipers.
12. What is hydrostatic weighing? Give a brief description of the technique.
13. A female weighs 155 pounds and has 32 percent body fat. She would like to get down to 22 percent body fat. How much weight should she lose to achieve this goal?

CHAPTER HIGHLIGHTS

*   Body composition refers to the amount of fat versus lean tissue in the body.
*   Essential fat is found in bone marrow, organs, muscles, intestines, and the central nervous system.
*   Obesity in infancy is not a good predictor of adult obesity; however, childhood and adolescent obesity are highly correlated with adult obesity.
*   Obesity is a disease that also coexists with the risk factors for other diseases.
*   Android obesity is the male pattern of fat distributed in the upper half of the body; gynoid obesity is the female pattern of fat distributed in the lower half of the body.
*   Obesity is caused by a number of factors that include genetics, poor nutritional habits, lack of exercise, and inappropriate behaviors.
*   The setpoint theory is a theoretical concept that indicates that all humans have a natural weight that the body will defend.
*   Exercise contributes to weight loss and management by burning kCals, increasing muscle metabolism, building muscle tissue, and balancing appetite with energy expenditure.
*   The thermogenic effect of food (TEF) refers to the number of kCals that the body uses to digest and process the food that has been eaten.

- On the average, the resting metabolic rate of females is 5 percent to 10 percent lower than that of males.
- Cycle dieting increases the risk for cardiovascular disease in particular and all-cause mortality in general.
- Anorexia and bulimia are two eating disorders characterized by an intense fear of becoming overweight.
- Body mass index (BMI) is a useful and practical measure of body composition.
- Skinfold measurements are a relatively easy and accurate technique for measuring body fatness.
- Bioelectrical impedence estimates body fat by measuring the speed that an electrical current travels through the body.
- Hydrostatic weighing is one of the more accurate ways to measure body fat.

● REFERENCES

1. M. M. Shangold, "Athletic Amenorrhea," *Clinical Obstetrics and Gynecology* 28 (1985): 664.
2. Athletic Amenorrhea and Bone Density," *Harvard Medical School Health Letter* 10 (December 1984): 5.
3. Ibid.
4. F. Munnings, "Exercise and Estrogen in Women's Health: Getting a Clearer Picture," *The Physician and Sportsmedicine* 16 (1988): 152.
5. C. M. Poissonnet et al., "Growth and Development of Adipose Tissue," *Journal of Pediatrics* 113 (1988): 1.
6. F. X. Hausberger and J. E. Volz, "Feeding in Infancy, Adipose Tissue Cellularity and Obesity," *Physiology and Behavior* 33 (1984): 81.
7. A. Must et al., "Long-term Morbidity and Mortality of Overweight Adolescents," *New England Journal of Medicine* 327 (1992): 1350.
8. G. A. Bray, "Adolescent Overweight May Be Tempting Fate," *New England Journal of Medicine* 327 (1992): 1379.
9. A. Must et al., "Long-term Morbidity," (1992): 1351.
10. E. T. Howley and B. D. Franks, *Health Fitness Instructors Handbook*, Champaign, Ill.: Human Kinetics, 1992.
11. R. L. Leibel and J. Hirsch, "Metabolic Characteristics of Obesity," *Annals of Internal Medicine* 103 (1985): 1000.
12. G. M. Wardlaw and P. M. Insel, *Perspectives in Nutrition*, St. Louis: Times Mirror/Mosby, 1990.
13. "First, Understand What Causes Weight Gain," *Tufts University Diet and Nutrition Letter* 3 (January 1986): 3.
14. W. R. Foster and B. T. Burton (Eds.), "Health Implications of Obesity: National Institutes of Health Development Conference," *Annals of Internal Medicine* 103 (Supp. 6, Part 2): 977.
15. C. J. Ley, B. Lees, and J. C. Stevenson, "Sex-and-Menopause-Associated Changes in Body-fat Distribution," *American Journal of Clinical Nutrition* 55 (1992): 950.
16. A. J. Stunkard et al., "An Adoption Study of Human Obesity," *New England Journal of Medicine* 314 (1986): 193.
17. A. J. Stunkard et al., "A Twin Study of Human Obesity," *Journal of the American Medical Association* 256 (1986): 51.
18. T. I. A. Sorensen et al., "Genetics of Obesity in Adult Adoptees and Their Biological Siblings," *British Medical Journal* 298 (1989): 87.
19. A. J. Stunkard et al., "The Body-Mass Index of Twins Who Have Been Reared Apart," *New England Journal of Medicine* 322 (1990): 1483.
20. C. Bouchard et al., "The Response to Long-Term Overfeeding in Identical Twins," *New England Journal of Medicine* 322 (1990): 1477.
21. J. S. Stern, "Movement Makes the Difference," *Food and Fitness* 49 (1984): 3.
22. American College of Sports Medicine, "The Recommended Quantity and Quality of Exercise for Developing and Maintaining Cardiorespiratory and Muscular Fitness in Healthy Adults," *Medicine in Science and Sports* 22 (1990): 265.
23. D. C. Nieman, *Fitness and Sports Medicine: An Introduction*, Palo Alto, Calif.: Bull, 1990.
24. C. Pierre, "Maximizing Metabolism: Can Calorie Burning Be Increased?" *Environmental Nutrition* 12 (February 1989): 1.
25. A. R. Tagliaferro et al., "Effects of Exercise Training on the Thermic Effect of Food and Body Fatness of Adult Women," *Psychology and Behavior* 38 (1986): 703.
26. O. G. Edholm et al., "The Food Intake and Individual Expenditure of Individual Men," *British Journal of Nutrition* 9 (1955): 286.
27. P. D. Wood et al., "Increased Exercise Level and Plasma Lipoprotein Concentrations: A One-Year, Randomized, Controlled Study in Sedentary Middle-Aged Men," *Metabolism* 32 (1983): 31.
28. P. Wood, *California Diet and Exercise Program*, Mountain View, Calif: Anderson World Books, 1983.
29. L. Lamb (Ed.) "Exercise Protects Heart During Dieting," *The Health Letter*, February 12, 1988, p. 3.
30. "Yo-Yo Dieting: The Losing Game," Harvard Heart Letter 3 (January 1993): 1.
31. O. E. Owen et al., "A Reappraisal of Caloric Requirements in Healthy Women," *American Journal of Clinical Nutrition* 44 (1986): 1.
32. C. Pierre, "Maximizing Metabolism," (February 1989): 2.
33. H. A. de Vries, "Physical Fitness Guidelines for Older Adults," *President's Council on Physical Fitness and Sports Newsletter*, Washington, D.C.: March 1980.
34. M. Chinnici, "Picking the Perfect Diet," *The Walking Magazine* 4 (May/June 1989): 40; A.J. Siegel, "New Insights About Obesity and Exercise," *Your Patient and Fitness* 2 (January/February 1989): 12.
35. S. B. Roberts et al., "Energy Expenditure and Intake in Infants Born to Lean and Overweight Mothers," *New England Journal of Medicine* 318 (1988): 461.

36. C. Shultz et al., "Effects of Severe Caloric Restriction and Moderate Exercise on Basal Metabolic Rate and Hormonal Status in Adult Humans," *Federal Proceedings* 39 (1980): 783.

37. A. J. Moss, "Caution: Very-Low Calorie Diets Can Be Deadly." *Annals of Internal Medicine* 102 (1985): 121.

38. F. Munnings, "Exercise and Estrogen," (1988): 158.

39. R. R. Wing, "Weight Cycling in Humans: A Review of the Literature," *Annals of Behavioral Medicine* 14 (1992): 113.

40. L. Lissner et al., "Variability of Body Weight and Health Outcomes in the Framingham Population," *New England Journal of Medicine* 324 (1991): 1839.

41. R. R. Wing, "Weight Cycling in Humans," (1992): 116.

42. B. Zuti and L. Golding, "Comparing Diet and Exercise as Weight Reduction Tools," *The Physician and Sportsmedicine* 4 (1976): 49.

43. D. L. Ballor et al., "Resistance Weight Training During Caloric Restriction Enhances Lean Body Weight Maintenance," *American Journal of Clinical Nutrition* 47 (1988): 19.

44. S. W. Lichtman et al., "Discrepancy Between Self-Reported and Actual Caloric Intake and Exercise in Obese Subjects," *New England Journal of Medicine* 327 (1992): 1893.

45. G. E. Doxey et al., "Body Composition Roundtable: Part 1. Scientific Considerations," *National Strength and Conditioning Association Journal* 9 (1987): 14.

46. J. M. Isner et al., "Anorexia Nervosa and Sudden Death," *Annals of Internal Medicine* 102 (1985): 49.

47. A. E. Andersen, *American Anorexia/Bulemia Association Newsletter* 9 (1986): 9.

48. S. C. Lipnickey, "Beyond Dieting: A Preventive Perspective on Eating Disorders," in *Health 89/90,* Guilford, Conn: Dushkin Publishing Group, 1989.

49. J. Hendricks, "Anorexia Nervosa and Bulimia: Two Serious Eating Disorders," *Alternatives in Health and Wellness* (August 1991): 2.

50. D. A. Revicki and R. G. Israel, "Relationship Between Body Mass Indices and Measures of Body Adiposity," *American Journal of Public Health* 76 (1986): 992.

51. American College of Sports Medicine, *Guidelines for Exercise Testing and Prescription,* Philadelphia: Lea and Febiger, 1991.

The Consequences of Negative Choices

INTRODUCTION

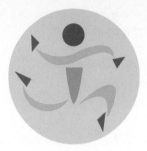

One of the characteristics of maturation is an increasing ability to make choices. Infants, although capable of letting people around them know when they are happy or unhappy, are unable to make a decision to change their current situation. They are dependent upon the adults and older children around them for assuring that their needs are met. Each year of life, children have more and more input into what happens in their lives. One-year-olds cry when they are hungry and hope they will be fed. When seven-year-olds are hungry, they do not have to wait for someone to bring them food—they can readily go to the refrigerator or cupboard and select something on their own. However, seven-year-olds may not always be capable of making wise or positive decisions. An unwise decision would be to experiment with a bottle of detergent or aspirin, the consequences of which can be disastrous.

When older children experience a need, they also have choices. Making an unwise choice can be just as disastrous for a 15-year-old—or a 20-year-old or a 50-year-old—as for a 7-year-old. Before making a positive decision, however, people must know the difference between a positive and a negative choice and have some understanding of the consequences involved in negative decision making.

This chapter focuses on two primary areas where people frequently make decisions that are not in their best interest: drug use and sexual activity. Often these choices lead to negative lifelong consequences. Indeed, some choices can lead to early death. For this reason, this chapter briefly discusses drug use and sexually transmitted diseases.

Two Self-Assessment activities appear in Appendix C that apply directly to the contents of this chapter: (1) 11.1 Why Do You Smoke? and (2) 11.2 Indications of a Problem with Alcohol.

Miniglossary

Abuse (of Drugs)   Use of any drug, whether legal or illegal, that results in behavior or action that is detrimental to the user's health or the health of others.

Addiction   A compulsion for a drug that results in abuse.

Alcoholism   Abusive use of alcohol characterized by emotional and physical dependence and a loss of control over its use.

Amotivational Syndrome   A collection of symptoms/behavior patterns that is associated with chronic use of marijuana where the user displays apathy towards life and a passive, introverted personality.

Blood Alcohol Concentration (BAC)   The concentration of alcohol in a specific amount of blood; a BAC of 0.10% is illegal intoxication in most states, although

some states use a BAC of 0.08%.

Crack   A solid form of cocaine, usually mixed with baking soda, that provides a strong temporary sense of euphoria.

Dependence   A physical or psychological desire for a drug resulting from some interaction between user and drug that causes the user to feel a compulsion or a need for the drug in order to function.

Drug   Other than food, any substance that enters the body and changes its usual function.

Drug Use   The wise, discriminate use of drugs.

Ectopic Pregnancy   An abnormal pregnancy where the embryo is implanted outside the uterus.

Continued

Miniglossary

—*Continued*

Epididymus   Long, coiled ducts in the male that carry sperm.

Fetal Alcohol Syndrome (FAS)   Birth defects associated with the consumption of alcohol by the mother during pregnancy.

Hallucinogen   Any drug that affects the user's sense of reality, alters visual and auditory perceptions and causes hallucinations.

Jaundice   Yellow coloring of the skin, mucus membrane, and whites of the eyes.

Misuse (of Drugs)   The using of any prescription or nonprescription drug for any reason other than that for which it was intended.

Neutrotransmitters   Chemical messengers within a nerve cell.

Passive Smoke   Also called sidestream or second hand smoke, the smoke emitted from the end of a burning cigarette.

Psychoactive Drugs   Drugs that alter perceptions, mood, thought, behavior, or consciousness.

Retrovirus   Viruses with the ability to interrupt the ordinary flow of genetic material.

Tolerance   The body's ability to adjust to the effect of a drug so that more and more of the drug is required to produce the same effect.

Urethra   Small, tubular structure that drains urine from the bladder in males and females.

Vulva   The external female genitalia.

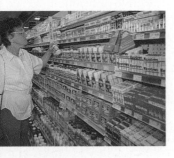

Wise appropriate use of drugs can improve quality of life.

© 1993 Martin/Custom Medical Stock

 ## DRUGS: THEIR USE, MISUSE, AND ABUSE

The term **drug** is frequently defined as "any substance other than food that alters any function of the body."[1] Many drugs serve a vital purpose, and without them, quality of life would be reduced. **Drug use** is the wise and discriminate use of drugs to improve quality of life. Antibiotics, anesthesia, analgesics, antihistamines, anti-inflammatories, and anti-cholesterol drugs are just a few of the many drugs that are beneficial to humanity. It is when drugs are **misused** (using a legal drug for a purpose other than originally intended, such as ingesting another person's medication) or **abused** (using any illegal drug or using a legal drug that results in physical, emotional, social, or intellectual detriment) that problems occur. It is not uncommon for people to use someone else's medicine for a time, but there is never any guarantee as to how anyone will react to any medication (even aspirin) or how medications will interact. Use of one drug while taking another can cause interactions that can be life threatening. Not only is drug abuse illegal, but the results of drug abuse can wreak havoc in the lives of the abuser and the abuser's friends and family.

 ## TOLERANCE, DEPENDENCE, AND ADDICTION

Tolerance describes the body's ability to adjust to the effect of a drug so that more and more of the drug is required to produce the same effect.[2] The first time an individual drinks alcohol, it usually requires very little to produce a change in how the person feels or reacts. Over time and with consistent use, more alcohol is needed to achieve the same effect.

Dependence on a drug is a psychological or physical desire for the drug resulting from some interaction between the user and the drug that causes the user to feel a compulsion or a need for the drug in order to function. Many people are dependent on caffeine—especially first thing in the morning. They feel that they cannot function well until they get that first cup of coffee or can of cola.

The distinction of exactly where dependence ends and **addiction** begins is somewhat nebulous. Addiction is a compulsion for a drug so that abuse results.

Excessive coffee drinking could be qualified as addiction. If anyone doubts it, let a heavy coffee drinker try to function without caffeine for a few days while experiencing the withdrawal of doing without. The problem with addiction is that some addictions are more detrimental than others. For instance, cocaine addiction is illegal and very expensive and requires increasingly larger amounts. When the drug is the most important factor in a person's life, its use has certainly become an addiction.

 ## LEGAL DRUGS

Over-the-counter (nonprescription) drugs can be bought by anyone at most any time. They include cold medications, cough syrups, analgesics, and a variety of other drugs. While commonly used and not difficult to acquire, it is easily possible to misuse these drugs by taking too much or using them in combination with other medications (or with alcohol) that might be unhealthy. Dependence can result. The person who must have a dose of sleeping pills in order to sleep at night is dependent; the drug is not intended for persistent use.

Prescription drugs are medications that must be obtained under medical supervision. Prescription drugs include, among others, more powerful pain relievers, antidepressants, and anti-anxiety drugs. They are drugs that can have more dangerous consequences if misused and are more likely to be abused.

 ## PSYCHOACTIVE DRUGS

Some drugs are more commonly misused or abused than others. **Psychoactive drugs** are drugs that alter perceptions, mood, thought, behavior, or consciousness; for this reason, they are the ones most likely to be abused.[3] Psychoactive drugs affect mood, emotion, and behavior because they are structurally similar to neurotransmitters, and as such, they alter the effect of neurotransmitters on brain cells (**neurotransmitters** stimulate or inhibit brain-cell function). Many psychoactive drugs have legal use, while others are strictly illegal. Table 11.1 lists several classifications of psychoactive drugs along with their physiological effects and examples of each classification.

TABLE 11.1 Psychoactive Drugs

DRUG	PHYSIOLOGICAL EFFECT	EXAMPLES
Stimulants	Speed up nervous system; increase alterness, excitability.	Cocaine, caffeine, amphetamines, nicotine
Depressants (sedatives, hypnotics)	Slow down the central nervous system; induce feelings of relaxation.	Alcohol, sleeping pills, mathaqualone, minor tranquilizers (Xanax, Valium)
Narcotics	Act as painkillers; induce feelings of euphoria.	Opium, codeine, heroin, morphine
Hallucinogens, Psychedelics	Alter perceptions of reality; induce unusual visual sensations.	LSD, mescaline, PCP, mushrooms, psylocybin
Inhalants	Create druglike effects.	Glue, gasoline, cleaning fluid, nitrous oxide
Marijuana and derivatives	Often produce a relaxant, depressive state; may induce hallucinations, altered perceptions.	Marijuana, hashish, THC

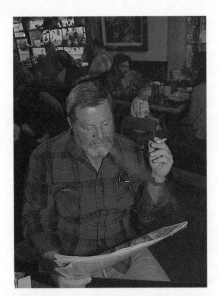

Cigarette smoke affects the user and other people both physically and is an example of a poor behavior choice.
© David R. Frazier/Photography

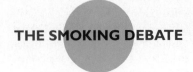

Tobacco is a crop that yields high value. Recent harvesting of tobacco has brought prices of over $3,000 per acre.

THE SMOKING DEBATE

SOME FREQUENTLY ABUSED DRUGS

The intent of the following paragraphs is to provide some basic data about the drugs most frequently abused in this society. This is not intended to be a comprehensive presentation. Not everyone who uses any drug or drugs will suffer addiction. No one plans on abusing drugs or becoming an addict. It is impossible to determine in advance who will and who will not have difficulty with a specific drug or drugs. For this reason, it is important for an individual who chooses to use any of these substances to understand some of their potential hazards.

Tobacco

Tobacco contains the highly addictive drug nicotine.[4] Use of nicotine is associated with a variety of symptoms. Nicotine causes a release of adrenaline, initially stimulates sensory receptors, and increases respiration, heart rate, and blood pressure. Smoking one cigarette has been shown to reduce hunger pangs for up to an hour.[5] Regular smoking of cigarettes leads to continuous constriction of blood vessels, decreased skin temperature, increased blood pressure, and decreased oxygen-carrying capacity. Nicotine actually has toxic effects on humans, as is evidenced by any first-time smoker who reacts with nausea, dizziness, and weakness, which are indications of low-level nicotine poisoning. Long-term damage in habitual smokers is indicated by a much higher incidence of many diseases, including coronary heart disease, peripheral arterial disease, various types of cancer, peptic ulcers, and chronic obstructive pulmonary disease.

Tobacco smoke is harmful to people who do not smoke. (Children of smoking parents have more respiratory infections and problems and poorer lung function than children of nonsmoking parents. Babies born to smokers weigh less and have smaller head circumferences. Smokers have spontaneous abortions more often and experience higher incidence of neonatal deaths. Data increasingly indicate that **passive** (or sidestream or secondhand) **smoke** can have detrimental effects on nonusers.[6]

Other people's smoke (passive, secondhand, or sidestream smoke) is at the root of a profound controversy. Smokers feel that their rights are being taken away from them as smoke-free environments relentlessly invade their terrain. Even as the battle wages, young people, especially young, white females, are the fastest growing group of smokers nationwide. Why the debate over passive smoke? Is it so important?

Experts now rank passive smoke as the third leading cause of preventable deaths (active smoking is in first place). Estimates are that 46,000 to 54,500 nonsmokers will die each year from the effects of passive smoke. The Environmental Protection Agency (EPA) classifies passive smoke as the cause of multiple respiratory disorders in children. Children of smokers have more bronchitis, pneumonia, wheezing, coughing, and middle-ear infections and a higher probability of retarded lung function. While not widely recognized, passive smoke produces heart disease 10 times more often than it does lung cancer.

Living or working with a smoker means that nonsmokers get more than their share of passive smoke and more than their share of illness and premature death.

"Other People's Smoke," *University of California at Berkeley Wellness Letter* 8 (October 1991): 7.

All tobacco use is addicting. Many smokers repeatedly attempt to quit, only to find their craving for nicotine so strong that they soon resume their smoking habit. Few smokers quit the first time they try. Smoking and use of tobacco products serve people differently. Some begin smoking because of peer pressure . Young people may smoke to look older. Many young females begin smoking in an attempt to control their weight (a few pounds are far less harmful than the effects of cigarette smoking), while many young males begin dipping or chewing because the athletes they emulate use smokeless tobacco.

People continue to smoke also for different reasons. Addiction to nicotine is one very powerful reason. The irony of nicotine is that although it increases heart rate, blood pressure, and other bodily functions, smokers often claim that smoking makes them feel calmer and less emotionally stressed. Self-assessment 11.1 in Appendix C is designed to help smokers determine *why* they smoke.

There is no doubt that quitting smoking is extremely difficult. Quitting is, however, extremely beneficial to the smoker. The lungs have the ability to regenerate, and upon quitting, a smoker's lungs can begin to undo the effects of weeks, months, or years of smoking. Lung function can eventually return to the level of a nonsmoker. Stopping a cigarette smoking habit after a malignancy has developed will not cause the tumor to go away. It is important to quit smoking before cancer cells have the opportunity to develop, especially since lung cancer is frequently unrecognized and undiagnosed before it has spread.

Alcohol

Alcohol not only is socially acceptable but also is frequently a social must. In fact, there are many environments where nondrinking is socially unacceptable, such as sorority and fraternity functions, business luncheons, and parties. However, alcohol is associated with over 100,000 deaths every year, and these deaths are frequently among young people. Alcohol-related traffic crashes killed more than 22,000 people in 1990. Forty percent of all Americans will be involved in an alcohol-related traffic accident during their lifetime.[7] Pregnant women who drink run a substantial risk of delivering a baby with **fetal alcohol syndrome,** with symptoms ranging from low birth weight and abnormal facial features to mental retardation and heart abnormalities. Alcohol is second only to tobacco as a leading cause of premature death.

Although many people consider beer a "safe" drink, the pure alcohol content of one 12-ounce beer is the same as for 5 ounces of wine or 1.5 ounces of 80-proof alcohol. The effect of the alcohol, including how rapidly it is absorbed, is influenced by different factors. An empty stomach absorbs alcohol more rapidly than a full one; aspirin ingestion can hasten absorption; body weight and gender affect alcohol absorption. On an average, a 150-pound man can reach a **blood alcohol concentration (BAC)** of 0.10 (the point of legal intoxication) if he consumes two to three beers in one hour.

Once alcohol has been ingested, there is no way to hurry the process of metabolism. This means that drinking coffee or taking a shower or walking or any other activity will not hasten the sobering-up process. One drink takes approximately one hour to metabolize, two drinks would require approximately two hours to metabolize, and so on. Only time will allow the effects of alcohol to diminish.

Every cell in the body can absorb alcohol from the blood, but the central nervous system is the most influenced. While under the influence of alcohol, memory, judgment, and perception are impaired; the degree to which they are impaired is dependent upon the level of BAC. Increased ingestion of alcohol can alter personality, lead to depression or violence, and induce drowsiness, yet it can also disrupt sleeping patterns. The most common effect of overindulgence is a hangover. A hangover is caused only by overdrinking—not by mixing drinks or by drinking inexpensive alcohol. Many young people are not aware that the rapid consumption of large amounts of alcohol—chug-a-lugging or engaging in beer-drinking contests—can anesthetize the brain to the extent that respiration can stop and death can occur. This is in addition to the problems associated with drinking and driving and the interpersonal problems that can develop from excessive drinking.

Quitting tobacco is no easy accomplishment. Surveys indicate that recidivism rates for smoking are comparable to alcohol or heroin. Data from one study revealed that after 2 months 40% of smokers, drinkers and heroin users were still abstaining. After 1 year, 35% of drinkers were still abstaining but only 25% of smokers and heroin users remained clean.

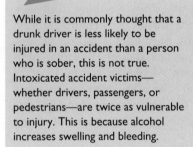

While it is commonly thought that a drunk driver is less likely to be injured in an accident than a person who is sober, this is not true. Intoxicated accident victims—whether drivers, passengers, or pedestrians—are twice as vulnerable to injury. This is because alcohol increases swelling and bleeding.

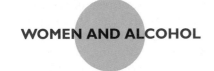
According to the Dietary Guidelines for Americans, moderate drinking for women is one drink a day (12 oz. of beer, 1.5 oz. of 80-proof spirits, 5 oz. of wine), while moderate drinking for males is two drinks a day (24 oz. of beer, 3 oz. of 80-proof spirits, 10 oz. of wine). This disparity is based not on sexist attitudes that females should not drink like males but on data that indicate that males and females react differently to the same amount of alcohol. Partly because women tend to be smaller with more body fat and correspondingly less body water, a female will become more intoxicated than a male on the same amount of alcohol. Indications are that the enzyme in the stomach that breaks down alcohol is less active in women than in men.

Long-term consequences of excessive drinking are more serious for women than for men. Women develop cirrhosis of the liver at lower levels of alcohol intake and are at increased risk for osteoporosis. Pregnant women who drink risk delivering babies with fetal alcohol syndrome—a condition with lifelong consequences.

Adapted from Dietary Guidelines for Americans (3d ed.), U.S. Department of Agriculture/U.S. Department of Health and Human Services, 1990; and "What Controls Alcohol Tolerance?" *The Health Letter* 35, no. 7 (August 19, 1991): 4.8.

Alcoholism   Many people drink alcohol at some time during their lives. Some will use alcohol for a while and quit (35 percent of the adult population are abstainers[8]). Some will drink in moderation throughout their lives. Other people will have severe problems with alcohol. Some people will become alcoholics. An alcoholic is anyone who suffers from the disease of **alcoholism,** defined as "a primary, chronic disease with genetic, psychosocial and environmental factors influencing its development....that is often progressive and fatal."[9] It is characterized by (1) impaired control over drinking, (2) preoccupation with alcohol, and (3) denial that a problem with alcohol exists. The cause or causes of alcoholism are not easily identified. Data indicate that children of heavy drinkers are more likely to become alcoholics even if raised in nonalcoholic families, but no gene for alcoholism has ever been isolated. On an individual basis, it is impossible to predict who will become alcoholic and who will not.

Alcoholism, like all forms of drug abuse, follows a variety of patterns. The most obvious are street drunks who have no home and will drink anything from shoe polish to rubbing alcohol to get their fix. Many alcoholics never reach this position in life. Some are weekend binge drinkers or drink only once a month or less. Often alcoholics hold down successful jobs or professions, though over time, indications of excessive alcohol consumption will occur. Alcoholics can be 13 or 70 years of age.[10] The primary indication of alcoholism is an inability to control one's drinking. Alcoholics differ from social drinkers in that they cannot stop after one or a reasonable number of drinks. They often drink until they pass out or are unable to function.

Although not easily accomplished, alcoholism is treatable. First and foremost, an alcoholic must recognize the problem. A variety of programs are available, but any one program will not suit everyone. The first step is to begin. Self-assessment 11.2 in Appendix C provides a checklist of indications of a problem with alcohol.

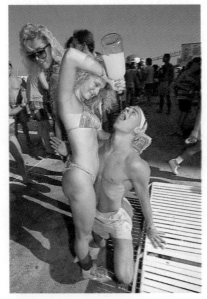

The use of drugs when making decisions about sex may have long-term, undesirable consequences.

© Christopher Brown/Stock Boston

● Cocaine

Cocaine is an extremely fast acting stimulant. Derived from the coca plant in South America, cocaine has been used in various forms by other societies since the 1800s. In the United States, cocaine was at one time the drug of the rich, and few recognized the potentially fatal effects the drug would have.

Cocaine can be administered in a variety of ways. It can be ingested (often in the form of drinks and tonics), snorted, smoked and injected. In the past two decades, smoking cocaine mixed with baking soda or ammonia **(crack)** has taken on gigantic proportions. Crack is relatively inexpensive and provides an immediate and powerful high. The sense of euphoria alone seems capable of creating addicts within weeks of initial use.[11] Use of crack or cocaine is followed by a period of depression. The sense of despair following the high encourages repeated use of the drug to ward off the depression. Chronic users cease to experience the euphoria that beginners find enthralling; for them, the use of crack may be an ongoing effort to fight off the paranoia and horror of not having the drug.

Cocaine increases respiration, heart rate, blood pressure, and body temperature. Rapid, irregular heartbeats often result. Cocaine suppresses appetite, Users report sensations of euphoria, alertness, and awareness and a reduction in fatigue during use. At high doses, convulsions and seizures can occur.

Chronic use of cocaine rapidly leads to tolerance. Chronic use also has a variety of undesirable side effects, including irregular heartbeat, sleep disturbances, nasal burns, and coughing. Over time, psychological disturbances also appear that may involve irritable or violent behavior, depression, anxiety, paranoia, psychosis, hallucination, and suicidal tendencies.[12]

At one time, the addiction to cocaine was thought to be psychological only. Since counselors and medical personnel have observed people withdrawing from cocaine, the evidence increasingly points to a physiological aspect as well. Cocaine abusers tend to develop similar patterns and behaviors while undergoing withdrawal. Current research indicates that abuse of cocaine leads to depletion of certain hormones that contribute to the enjoyment of life. Without cocaine and experiencing the depletion of these hormones, former long-term users undergo extended periods during which they are unable to experience happiness. Depending on a person's history, it could take an individual months to years to again be able to enjoy life without drugs.

 ## OTHER DRUGS OF ABUSE

Drug use and abuse patterns change with social level, cultural affiliation, area of the country, age, gender, and the passing of time. Some drugs go through phases when they are the "in" drug, and others seem to find a consistent group of people so that use remains stable. The following drugs currently have sufficient users to be mentioned briefly.

Hallucinogens

Probably the most universally well known **hallucinogen** is **lysergic acid diethylamide (LSD),** a partially synthetic drug that is extremely potent. A "trip" from LSD may last 12 hours or longer and cannot be ended prematurely. Some plants, such as peyote cactus and certain mushrooms, can also produce hallucinations, as can synthetic amphetamine-like drugs such as "Ecstasy." All hallucinogens produce perceptual and sensory distortions that can be either pleasant or terrifying. Tolerance can rapidly develop, including cross-tolerance to other hallucinogens. Synthetic hallucinogens can also produce fatigue after the effects of the drug have worn off.[13]

Heroin

Heroin is derived from morphine, the primary active ingredient in opium. Heroin, which is faster acting and has more analgesic properties than morphine, is also more addictive. Because of its highly addictive qualities, heroin has no medicinal use.

Heroin addiction has long been part of the drug culture, although heroin has been used less than many other drugs. In recent years, heroin use and addiction have increased, partly because of the use of crack in the form of a speedball—a cocaine and heroin mix designed to reduce the severe depression following a cocaine high.[14] A diluted, cheaper form of heroin suitable for smoking has been used extensively in the speedball. Initial use of heroin can produce nausea and vomiting, but with repeated use, these symptoms vanish.

● Marijuana

Marijuana and its major derivative, hashish (hash) are from the plant *cannabis sativa*. The primary active ingredient is tetrahydrocannabinol (THC). The amount of THC in a given amount of marijuana or hash determines the drug's potency. Modern breeding techniques have increased potency of some plants so that much of the marijuana on the streets today is considerably more powerful than the marijuana available even a few years ago.[15] Long-term effects of recently produced marijuana have yet to be determined.

Marijuana is the most used illegal drug in the country. There have been several controversial attempts to legalize the drug because of claims by proponents that it is less harmful than alcohol or tobacco. Marijuana is usually smoked and is therefore damaging to respiratory system. It contains more carcinogens than cigarette smoke. Use of marijuana is associated with a temporary impaired ability to perform ordinary motor functions. It has not been shown that long-term use results in physical addiction, although there is controversy over the drug's psychological effects. Chronic use of marijuana is associated with **amotivational syndrome,**[16] reproductive impairment, and infant mortality when used by pregnant women.

OINTS TO PONDER

1. Explain the difference between drug use, misuse, and abuse.
2. What is the addictive drug in tobacco, and what are its effects on the human body?
3. Should public areas be declared no-smoking zones? Why or why not?
4. Describe the characteristics of alcoholism.

◢ SEXUALLY TRANSMITTED DISEASES

The average age for first-time sexual intercourse is 16 when conditions such as gender, social class, and race are factored out.[25] Centers for Disease Control in Atlanta, Georgia, estimate that 40 percent of all ninth graders have had sex. By the twelfth grade, that number has risen to 72 percent. This is a conservative

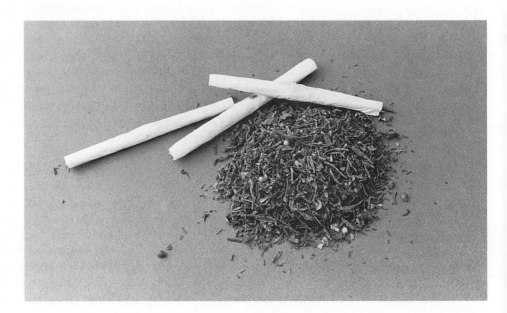

Marijuana is usually rolled and smoked like a cigarette.

© Frank Steinman/Stock Boston

Facts, Fallacies, and Timely Tidbits

1. Since 1967, the cost of soft drinks and milk has quadrupled and the cost of all other consumer goods has tripled, but the cost of alcohol has not even doubled.[17]
2. 500,000,000 people alive today will die from tobacco-related diseases, according to the World Health Organization.[18]
3. The World Health Organization projects that 25 million to 30 million people will become infected with HIV worldwide by the year 2000.[19]
4. People over 50 years of age account for 10% of all AIDS cases in the United States.[20]
5. Approximately 10 million infants will be born HIV-positive by the year 2000.[21]
6. One out of every 10 U.S. adolescent females becomes pregnant every year; half of them will give birth, resulting in 500,000 babies born to teenage mothers.[22]
7. 25%-30% of smokers who use a nicotine patch along with an education and support program quit (about twice the rate using an education/support program alone).[23]
8. AIDS is currently the sixth leading cause of death among 15 to 24-year-olds.[24]
9. Fetal alcohol syndrome is completely preventable, but it is the number one cause of mental retardation and the number three cause of birth defects.

number compared to a recent survey done by *Seventeen* magazine. The survey's data indicated that 75 percent of unmarried females and 86 percent of unmarried males have had sex by the age of 19.[26] An American teenager becomes pregnant every 30 seconds, and 80 percent of the pregnancies are unintentional.[27] Eighty-six percent of all sexually transmitted diseases (STDs) occur among 15 to 29-year-olds.[28] Today, it is the norm to have multiple STDs. While most STDs are curable, some, most notably HIV, are not. Because of the deadly consequences of having multiple sex partners, it is important to have a basic understanding of some of the leading STDs.

Chlamydia

The most common sexually transmitted disease is chlamydia. Estimates are that more than 4 million new cases of chlamydia occur each year.[29] Chlamydia is a frequent silent bacterial infection that can be cured if diagnosed. Symptoms tend to be mild. As with most STDs, males are more likely to have observable symptoms than females. Approximately 50 percent of males develop inflammation of the **urethra,** although inflammation can also occur in the rectum or **epididymis.** Females may experience low-grade infection, with tenderness in the abdomen. Undiagnosed chlamydia is responsible for 50 percent of all pelvic inflammatory disease (PID) in the United States (500,000 cases). Males and females can become sterile, and females can experience **ectopic pregnancies.** Babies born to women with chlamydia can develop chlamydial pneumonia and conjunctivitis.

Diagnosis is usually by laboratory tests using a specimen from the cervical canal or urethra. Diagnosis and treatment for chlamydia and all other STDs are specific. Being treated for gonorrhea will not cure chlamydia and vice versa. Since tests for most STDs are not routine with pap smears, unless there is a reason to test, many females can carry a disease for years.

Gonorrhea

Gonorrhea is a close second to chlamydia in prevalence. Also caused by a bacteria, gonorrhea is treatable with antibiotics when diagnosed. While gonorrhea tends to produce more symptoms than chlamydia, approximately 20 percent of infected males remain asymptomatic. A thick discharge from the penis creates extreme discomfort. Females experience mild, often unnoticeable symptoms that frequently lead to PID. It is also possible to develop rectal and oral gonorrhea that is unnoticed. Without treatment, infections such as arthritis, meningitis, and liver, heart, brain, and spinal cord damage can occur.[30]

Genital Warts

Also vying for the number one STD is a condition caused by the human papillomavirus (HPV)—genital warts. Estimates suggest that as many as one in ten Americans will experience them at some time in their lives.[31] The earlier in life one experiences sexual intercourse, particularly with multiple partners, the greater the likelihood of contracting the virus that causes genital warts. HPV is highly contagious and can be spread regardless of whether warts are visible to the unaided eye. Many small warts cannot be seen without the use of a special magnifying instrument. Since most females with genital warts will have them internally, it is often impossible to detect them without testing.

Warts are soft, flat, and irregularly shaped. They can appear in the mouth, throat, or genital area and increase in number and size over time. They may remain dormant for years. Although the warts are benign, they are closely linked to cancers of the cervix and penis. Treatment involves surgery with a laser or through freezing but does not guarantee an end to the disease. Warts frequently recur. With or without the presence of the warts, it is possible to infect partners.

Hepatitis

Hepatitis is an inflammatory condition of the liver that can be caused by a variety of factors (bacteria, viruses, alcohol, etc.) and is characterized by **jaundice**, enlargement of the liver, and abnormal liver function. Mild forms of hepatitis can lead to temporary inflammation and heal completely. Severe hepatitis can result in chronic (possibly lifetime) liver dysfunction or cirrhosis.

Hepatitis can be caused by lack of sanitation, overcrowding, and reusing of needles, including tattoo needles. The two types of hepatitis most often associated with sexual contact are hepatitis B and C. The primary source of hepatitis C is intravenous (IV) drug use, but approximately 10 percent is due to sexual relations.

Hepatitis B, an extremely contagious form of hepatitis, is the ninth leading cause of death worldwide.[32] Originally known as serum hepatitis, there has been increasing evidence that this form of hepatitis is sexually transmitted. At particular risk are male prisoners and promiscuous males and females as well as IV drug users. Hepatitis B is considerably more contagious than HIV (the virus that causes AIDS) and can survive for extended periods outside the human body. It can be spread through casual contact such as a shared toothbrush, saliva, or cuts in the skin.[33] Health professionals who treat hepatitis patients are at considerable risk of contacting hepatitis B. A vaccine is available to prevent development of the disease and is recommended for individuals in the high-risk category for this condition.

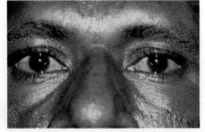

Jaundice can typically be identified when the skin and whites of the eyes take on a yellow cast.

© 1993 NMSB/Custom Medical Stock Photo

Syphilis

Syphilis is an ancient STD that was at one time believed to have originated in sheep. More recent thought is that it was spread to humans through the bite of a bear or contact with infected bear carcasses. Although syphilis declined in the United States during the early 1980s, its incidence has increased steadily since then. Syphilis rose 59 percent between 1986 and 1989.[34] It continues to rise partly because of the increase in drug use and the sex-for-drugs exchange.

Syphilis has the ability to mimic many different diseases; for this reason it can be misdiagnosed. As with other STDs, early symptoms can be slight or unnoticeable. One symptom is a painful-looking yet painless sore (called a chancre) that may appear in the area of the anus, genitals, or mouth. Since a chancre does not hurt, it can easily go unnoticed. Since the chancre contains the bacteria that causes syphilis, contact with it can spread the disease. This contact does not have to be through intercourse but can be through a cut or a wound.

Syphilis is a slow-progressing disease that does irreparable damage to body systems, especially the heart, central nervous system, and brain. Individuals progress through a series of stages with syphilis. The first stage is the *primary*

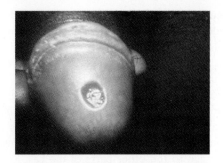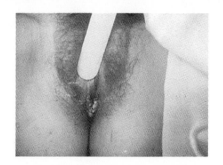

The chancre associated with syphilis may appear on the external genitalia or other parts of the body. Since the chancre is painless, it is often ignored or undetected.

© Centers for Disease Control

stage, when the chancre appears at the site where the bacteria entered the body. *Secondary syphilis* occurs anywhere from a month to a year after the chancre disappears. Secondary syphilis can include such symptoms as headaches, swollen glands, fever, hair loss, arthritis, or sores in the mouth or on the genitals. Though these symptoms will go away if untreated, the disease will continue to flourish. *Latent syphilis* is a period of time where there are no manifestations of clinical symptoms. The person with syphilis is no longer contagious, but the disease can be detected during this time through a blood test. *Late syphilis* is the last stage and can appear anywhere from 10 to 20 years after initial exposure. This is the phase of the disease where the results of the bacteria manifest. The person with syphilis may develop blindness, deafness, paralysis, or psychosis, among other conditions.

● Genital Herpes

Five million to 20 million Americans have genital herpes, and approximately 500,000 new cases develop annually.[35] Genital herpes is caused by either herpes simplex virus 1 (HSV-1) or herpes simplex virus 2 (HSV-2). Herpes causes painful, blisterlike lesions on the **vulva,** rectum, and penis. In some people, these blisters will occur only once, but in 75 percent of documented cases, they do recur. The lesions of genital herpes can be precipitated by trauma, stress, sunlight, fever, diet or menstruation. The virus can be passed on whether or not blisters are present, but the spread of the disease is greatest when the lesions are active.

Herpes is associated with the development of cervical cancer, meningitis, neural damage, and impotence. There is no cure for herpes—it is a lifetime disease—but treatment is available. Medication that can be used orally or topically can reduce the length and pain of an outbreak.

● HIV and AIDS

When AIDS first appeared on the public scene, temporary panic prevailed. This was a completely new and different disease that was killing people within a few months or years after being diagnosed. The extent of the disease was unimagined, but the mistaken belief AIDS could be spread through many forms of casual contact terrified many. Twelve years into the epidemic has reduced fear but not the incidence of the disease. By early 1992, 12 million people worldwide had been infected with HIV. The spread of the virus has not stopped anywhere. New infections continue to increase in countries where it is already present, and it is invading new communities and countries throughout the world.[36] Estimates are that by 1995, another 6.9 million people will become HIV infected.[37] This means that by 1995, nearly 19 million people are expected to be HIV positive.

HIV is a lethal virus that eventually leads to the death of the host through suppression of the immune system. HIV is a **retrovirus.** Estimates are that HIV in its deadly form has been infecting humans for at least 20 years but not more than 100 years.[38]

AIDS cannot be transmitted through mosquitoes or other insects, because HIV cannot survive inside this type of host. HIV requires an appropriate host in order to survive. This is why the virus quickly dies outside a human host and is not readily spread through touch, toilet seats, or saliva.

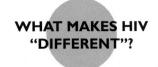

The first discernible difference in HIV and other diseases is the explosive way it suddenly appeared on the American scene in the early 1980s. This is not the only disease that lacks a cure, nor is it the only STD caused by a virus. What really marks the difference between HIV and other diseases, including other viruses, is that it is a retrovirus.

Simply put, viruses take over and exploit cells for their own use. Retroviruses also do this, but they have the added ability to reverse the genetic process. Ordinarily, the DNA in the cell nucleus releases genetic information that is transported by RNA to proteins. A retrovirus uses RNA to change the genetic message to the other parts of the cell. Retroviruses change the RNA and then insert the new pattern into the original DNA, thereby altering cell function.

Retroviruses are not new, but for many years they were found only in animals. Before 1980, many researchers believed that retroviruses would never affect humans. Before HIV, only two other retroviruses had been isolated in humans. Both of these retroviruses caused rare types of cancer. The first retroviruses were isolated in 1980—one year before the symptoms of HIV first appeared.

Adapted from J. Piel (Ed.), *Readings from Scientific American: The Science of AIDS*, New York: Freeman, 1989.

AIDS (acquired immunodeficiency syndrome) is a condition that can eventually result from the immunodeficiency virus (HIV). HIV is associated with the development of immunosuppression that can lead to AIDS, but an HIV-positive person does not automatically have AIDS. AIDS is a condition marked by scientific guidelines (see Table 11.2). Many people die from other diseases before they "have" AIDS.

The origin of the virus has been highly controversial. The most recent is that the virus has been around for a long time but has only recently mutated to its current form.[39] Whatever its reason, AIDS is NOT a homosexual disease. Worldwide, the vast majority of victims are heterosexual, and AIDS is spreading disproportionately among females, African-Americans, and Hispanics.

AIDS is now the sixth leading cause of death among 15- to 24-year-olds.[40] Between 1989 and 1992, the number of cases diagnosed in this age group rose by

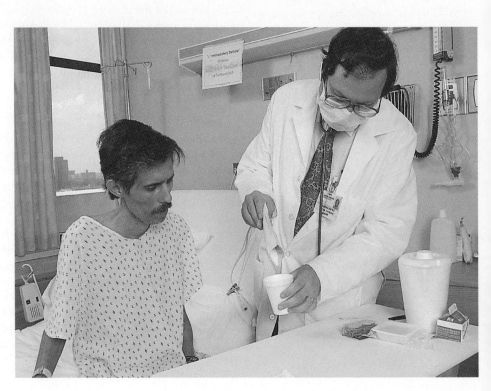

The individual with HIV may become emaciated and require prolonged hospitalization.

© Yoar Levy/Phototake NYC

TABLE 11.2 Current Criteria for HIV and AIDS

As of January 1, 1993, the definition of AIDS was expanded to include certain characteristic diseases while using the CD4+ T-cell count as a marker for progression of the disease. There are now 26 indicator diseases that mark the condition known as AIDS. This table lists the 26 diseases and describes the difference between HIV+ and AIDS.

HIV+ CLASSIFICATION	AIDS CLASSIFICATION
1. CD4+ T-cell count ≥ 500 /μ L and asymptomatic or symptomatic without indicator conditions.	1. CD4+ T-cell count ≥ 500 /μ L with AIDS indicator conditions.*
2. CD4+ T-cell count of 200–499 /μ L and asymptomatic or symptomatic without indicator conditions.	2. CD4+ T-cell count of 200–499 /μ L with AIDS indicator conditions.*
	3. CD4+ T-cell count of < 200 /μ L and asymptomatic or symptomatic or with indicator conditions.*

*AIDS Indicator Conditions

Candidiasis: bronchi, trachea, lung	Lymphoma: immunoblastic
Candidiasis: esophagus	Lymphoma: primary in braid
Cervical cancer: invasive	Mycobacterium avium complex
Coccidioidomycosis	Mycobacterium: tuberculosis (any site)
Cryptococcosis	Myobacterium: other
Cryptosporidiosis (one month or longer)	Pneumocystis carinii pneumonia
Cytomegalovirus: excluding liver, spleen, nodes	Recurrent pneumonia (within 12 mo. period)
Cytomegalovirus retinitis (loss of vision)	Progressive multifocal leukoencephalopathy
HIV encephalopath	Salmonella septicema: recurrent
Herpes simplex (one month or more duration)	Toxoplasmosis: brain
Histoplasmosis	Tuberculosis
Isosporiasis (more than one month)	HIV wasting syndrome
Kaposi's sarcoma	Burkitt's lymphoma

Adapted from Centers for Disease Control, *Morbidity and Mortality Weekly Report* (supplement), December 1992; and L. Wilson (Ed.), *The Messenger*, January 15, 1993, p. 1.

77 percent.[41] HIV is spread through some form of sexual contact (vaginal, rectal, or oral), sharing needles, or exchange of blood or from mother to child while breastfeeding or during the birth process. The virus can remain dormant for weeks to months to years—even 10 years or longer. The first recognizable symptoms of the virus are usually fatigue, loss of weight, fever, and night sweats. These symptoms may be the first indication of the need to get medical attention, but the virus can be spread whether or not symptoms are present.

HIV infection has been cited as the number 1 cause of death among males aged 25-44 years in 5 states and 64 cities in 1990 (see Table 11.3). HIV related deaths rank first for women in 9 cities and no states. These figures do not reflect current figures, which are expected to be higher. This is because 1990 is the last year that mortality rates are available for all states but it is known that HIV related deaths increased in 1991.[42] The ages 25-44 years are often the most productive from a labor force perspective and all the years when parenting usually takes place.

HIV-positive people can look perfectly healthy, clean, and well-kept. There is no way to determine who has the virus just by looking at a person. The virus can be detected with a blood test, usually within two months. Antibodies to the virus usually begin to show up in the blood a few weeks after infection. From that time on, the individual is contagious and can spread the disease. More than 50 percent of people diagnosed with HIV have died, but the period of time from diagnosis until fatal illness can be prolonged through a combination of specific drugs. The course of the disease has always varied in time, with very few people surviving longer than 10 years. Why some people live longer than others is not completely understood but seems related to life habits, attitude, the presence or absence of other diseases, amount of virus originally contacted, and other, unknown factors.

TABLE 11.3 AIDS Killing Men Ages 25–44

In 1990, AIDS and related infections were the leading cause of death among men in the 25–44 age group in California, Florida, Massachusetts, New Jersey and New York. The cities with the highest percentage of deaths in that age group that were AIDS-related.

MALE DEATHS		FEMALE DEATHS[1]	
San Francisco	61%	Newark, N.J.	43%
Ft. Lauderdale, Fla.	51%	Jersey City	38%
Elizabeth, N.J.	51%	Paterson, N.J.	37%
Newark, N.J.	45%	Stamford, Conn.	30%
Miami	43%	New Haven, Conn.	28%
Jersey City	43%	Miami	28%
Paterson, N.J.	39%	New York	24%
Seattle	39%	Ft. Lauderdale, Fla.	22%
Atlanta	38%	Baltimore	15%
Pasadena, Calif.	38%		
Denver	38%		
Arlington, Va.	38%		

[1]AIDS-related illness was the leading cause of death for women in only nine cities

Source: *Journal of the American Medical Association* and USA Today, Wednesday June 16, 1993. Copyright 1993, USA TODAY. Reprinted with permission.

The course of the disease is usually exposure to HIV, development of HIV antibodies (usually within two months), period of latency as the T-cell count begins to lower, early symptoms, the use of medication to prolong the asymptomatic period, the onset of certain HIV-related conditions and/or diseases, and full-blown AIDS.[43] The point at which HIV infection becomes AIDS is determined by the presence of specific diseases and the reduced count of a specific T-cell (CD4+). Table 11.2 outlines the physiological criteria for different stages of the disease. There is no cure, although treatment can prolong one's life. The average time of life expectancy from the development of early symptoms until death is approximately two years, although many people live longer. This is increasingly possible as different medications are mixed in more and more effective "cocktails."

Prevention is the best cure. It is not always the number of sexual partners an individual has but who the individual's partner's previous partners have been. It must be remembered that this and all STDs can have dormant periods where there are no symptoms although the disease is being spread.

SAFE SEX—HOW SAFE IS IT?

The popular "safe sex" slogan has been changed to "safer sex," and wisely so. Just as there are no foolproof methods of birth control, there are no foolproof ways of engaging in sex and remaining disease free. Espoused as being the most effective method of preventing STDs is the condom, of which there is now a female version. There is no doubt that use of the condom can reduce the incidence of STDs, but the failure rate runs 10 percent to 12 percent in the prevention of pregnancy.[46] While the rates of prevention for condoms have been as high as 98 percent, they have also been as low as 80 percent. This means that on the average, every 100 times a condom is used there is a good chance that ten pregnancies will occur.

Most failed condom use is due to human error and not to failure of the product. However, there is *always* a risk of contracting an STD if (1) you have more than one sex partner, (2) your partner has engaged or is currently engaging in sex with other people or (3) you or your partner shares needles.

There is much pressure for people to engage in sex today. This is true for all age groups, and the pressure is put on people by the media as well as by one's

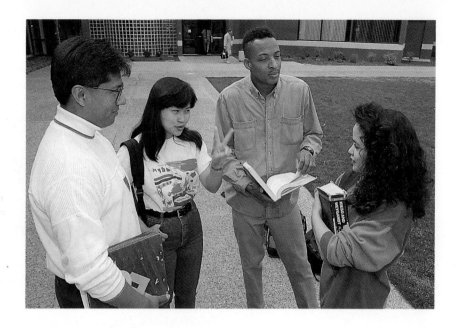

An alternative to unhealthy behavior choices is taking time to talk about problems and to discuss options with friends of both sexes.

© David R. Frazier/Photography

peers. Although abstinence is the safest sex, it may not be the most realistic in today's society. Sex is an enjoyable and important aspect of life when engaged in responsibly. But one needs to carefully consider the consequences of engaging in risky or indiscriminate sex for a few moments of self-gratification, especially when the consequences can be disastrous, or even fatal.

 Safety Tips

SAFE SEXUAL PRACTICES

The media (movies, television, and books) are rife with sexual activity and portray it as wonderful, exciting, fulfilling, and natural. Sexuality is very much the basis of who we are and why we act the way we do and is a natural part of life. However, there are consequences associated with sexual behavior that are not always positive. The following is some information you need to know before you make the life-changing decision to engage in sex.

1. Females who engage in sexual intercourse before age 20 have a higher risk of developing cervical cancer.
2. Females with multiple sex partners or who have a promiscuous male partner are at increased risk for developing cervical cancer.
3. Breakage rates for condoms are affected by type and duration of sexual activity; the more active and the longer the session lasts, the greater the chance that the condom will break.
4. Oil-based lubrications (Vaseline, lotion, mineral oil) can cause a condom to break.
5. Using a condom that feels brittle or gummy or has been stored in a hot area (such as a car) are more likely to break or leak.

6. 50% of all condom failures occur when a condom slips off during withdrawal.
7. Condoms used to prevent the spread of HIV should be made of latex, preferably with nonoxynol-9.
8. Sexual abstinence or permanent mutual monogamy between two uninfected partners is the only sure way to prevent contacting HIV or any other STD.
9. High-risk behavior includes having multiple sex partners, having intercourse with someone who has multiple partners, having intercourse with a prostitute, having intercourse with an IV drug user, or sharing needles.
10. HIV can remain dormant for years, so even if both partners are currently monogamous and not IV drug users, testing needs to be done to ensure that neither person is infected if either has at any time engaged in high-risk behavior.
11. Honesty and care for yourself could mean the difference between life and death.[47]

POINTS TO PONDER

1. Do you think people today are wise in engaging in sex with multiple partners? Under what circumstances do you think it is appropriate for people to have sexual intercourse or to engage in any form of sexual activity?
2. Why is it important to be tested specifically for each STD?
3. List the STDs that are bacterial and those that originate from a virus. How are the two groups different?
4. How do you think HIV will affect the future, especially your future? Would your behavior change if you were HIV positive? If so, how would it change?

▲ CHAPTER HIGHLIGHTS

- Drugs serve a variety of functions, some of which enhance quality of life.
- Drugs are problematic when people abuse them.
- Drug addiction indicates an obsession and compulsion for a drug that can be physiologically and psychologically detrimental.
- Psychoactive drugs are most likely to be abused.
- Tobacco contains the addictive drug nicotine.
- All tobacco use is associated with addiction.
- Tobacco smoke harms not only smokers but also the people who breathe smokers' second-hand smoke.
- Alcohol is a socially acceptable drug that causes problems for many people.
- One's ability to consume alcohol is based on a variety of factors, including gender, stomach contents, body weight, and speed with which the drink is ingested.
- Excessive drinking can result in death.
- Alcoholism is the inability to stop drinking once started.
- Alcoholism can affect anyone and is not limited by social class, income, gender, profession, or intelligence.
- Cocaine is a fast-acting stimulant.
- Cocaine has a number of side effects, both physiological and psychological.
- The "high" of cocaine is followed by a "low" that can be overwhelming.
- Hallucinogens produce sensory and perceptual distortions.
- Heroin is frequently mixed with cocaine to reduce the depression following cocaine use.
- Marijuana is the most used illegal drug in the U.S.
- The average age for first sexual intercourse is 16.
- Most individuals today will have more than one STD simultaneously.
- Chlamydia is the leading STD in the U.S.
- Treatment for each STD is specific; treating one STD will not cure another.
- Laboratory tests are specific for each STD, and each test is different.
- Gonorrhea is the second leading STD.
- STDs that originate from viruses have no cure.
- STDs that are caused by bacteria are curable if they are recognized and treatment completely followed.
- Hepatitis is a highly contagious STD that can be contracted in other ways as well.
- The first symptom of syphilis is a chancre.
- Genital herpes can be spread whether or not the lesions are present.

- Genital herpes and warts tend to recur periodically.
- HIV is the virus that leads to AIDS.
- HIV can be present for years before symptoms appear.
- HIV is a particularly deadly virus that eventually kills its host.
- AIDS is the sixth leading cause of death among 15- to 24-year-olds.
- HIV and AIDS are sexually transmitted diseases that cannot be spread through casual contact.
- HIV can be detected through a blood test.
- A person with the HIV antibodies can spread the disease whether or not symptoms are present.
- Condoms have an average failure rate of 10%–12%.

● REFERENCES

1. C. O. Byer and L.W. Shainberg, *Living Well*, New York: Harper Collins, 1991, p. 324.
2. Ibid. p. 334.
3. O. Ray and C. Ksir, *Drugs, Society and Human Behavior*, St. Louis: Times Mirror/Mosby, 1990, p. 1.
4. Centers for Disease Control, Smoking, Tobacco, and Health "Passive Smoking and Heart Disease," *The health Letter* 40 (February 1993): 4.
5. O. Ray and C. Ksir, *Drugs Society*, 1990.
6. "Other People's Smoke," *University of California Berkeley Wellness Letter*, 8 (October 1991): 1, p. 7.
7. "Alcohol Perspective," *University of California at Berkeley Wellness Letter* 40 (February 1993): 4.
8. Centers for Disease Control, *Smoking, Tobacco and Health* "Passive Smoking and Heart Disease," *The Health Letter* 40 (February 1993): 210.
9. "Alcohol Perspective," February 1993, p. 4.
10. "Alcoholism in the Elderly," *Mayo Clinic Health Letter* (August 1990): 6.
11. "The Men Who Created Crack," *U.S. News & World Report*, August 19, 1991, p. 44.
12. W. Payne, D. Hahn, and R. Pinger, *Drugs: Issues for Today*, St. Louis: Mosby Year Book, 191, p. 217
13. Ibid.
14. "Heroin Comes Back," *Time*, February 19, 1990, p. 63.
15. W. Payne, D. Hahn, and R. Dinger, *Drugs: Issues*, 1991.
16. Ibid.; O. Ray and C. Ksir, *Drugs, Society*, 1990.
17. "Alcohol Perspective," February 1993.
18. "Fascinating Facts," *University of California at Berkeley Wellness Letter* 9 (October 1992): 1.
19. "The Changing Face of AIDS," *University of California at Berkeley Wellness Letter* 7 (May 1991): 6.
20. Ibid.
21. Ibid.
22. "How Much Do You Really Know About Sex?" *University of California at Berkeley Wellness Letter* 7 (April 1991): 4.
23. "Digest," *Workplace Health*, April 1993, p. 12.
24. "Vitality Digest," *Vitality*, March 1993, p. 7.
25. "How Much Do You Really Know?" April 1991.
26. "The Sex Quiz: Who's Doing What?" *Seventeen*, February 1993, p. 40.
27. "How Much Do You Really Know?" April 1991.
28. Ibid.
29. "Most Common Sexually Transmitted Disease," *The Health Letter* 40 (March 1993): 2.
30. D. J. Anspaugh, M. H. Hamrick, and F. D. Rosato, *Wellness Concepts and Applications*, St. Louis: Mosby Year Book, 1991, p. 231.
31. "The Most Common Venereal Disease," *Wellness Letter* 7 (June 1991): 7.
32. "Earning Its Letter," *H.M.S. Health Letter*, October 1990, p. 3.
33. "The Disease That Should Die," *University of California at Berkeley Wellness Letter* 7 (April 1991): 2, 5.
34. "The Most Common Venereal Disease," June 1991.
35. Ibid.
36. J. Mann, D. J. M. Tarantola, and T. W. Netter (Eds.), *A Global Report, AIDS in the World*, Cambridge: Harvard University Press, 1992, p. 3.
37. J. Piel (Ed.) *Readings from Scientific American: The Science of AIDS*, New York: Freeman, 1989, p. 3.
38. Ibid.
39. "The Future of AIDS," *Newsweek*, March 22, 1993, p. 47.
40. "Teenagers and AIDS," *Newsweek*, August 3, 1992, p. 45; "AIDS Update," *American Health*, April 1992, p. 10. "The Disease That Should Die," April 1991. p. K. Haas and A. Haas, *Understanding Sexuality*, St. Louis: Mosby 1993, p. 438.
41.
42. Selik, R. M. et al, "HIV Infection as Leading Cause of Death Among Young Adults in U.S. Cities and States," JAMA, 269(23), June 16, 1993, p. 2991–2994.
43. USA Today
44. "AIDS Update" *American Health*
45. "How Effective Are Condoms?" *University of California at Berkeley Wellness Letter* 9 (December 1992): 6; "A Condom for Women," *University of California at Berkeley Wellness Letter* 8 (August 1992): 6.
46. "How Effective are Condoms?"

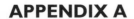

APPENDIX A

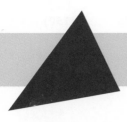

Fast-Food Nutrients

| TABLE A.1 | Main Meal Items in Calories, Fat, and Sodium |

BREAKFAST ITEMS	CALORIES	FAT (TSP)	SODIUM (MG)
Grapefruit or orange juice, 6 oz.	80	0	2
English muffin w/butter (McDonald's)	186	1	310
Arby's butter croissant (Arby's)	220	2	225
Scrambled eggs (McDonald's)	180	3	205
Omelet w/mush., onion, green pepper (Wendy's)	210	3	200
Biscuit (Roy Rogers)	231	3	575
Breakfast Jack (Jack-Box)	307	3	871
Egg McMuffin (McDonald's)	340	4	885
Mushroom & swiss croissant (Arby's)	340	5	630
Crescent roll (Roy Rogers)	287	5	547
Omelet-ham, cheese & mushroom (Wendy's)	290	5	570
French toast, 2 slices (Wendy's)	400	4	850
Biscuit w/egg (Hardee's)	383	5	819
Bacon & egg croissant (Arby's)	420	6	550
Pancake platter w/ham (Roy Rogers)	506	4	1264
Breakfast crescent sandwich (Roy Rogers)	401	6	867
Sausage biscuit (Hardee's)	413	6	864
Sausage McMuffin (McDonald's)	427	6	942
Steak & egg biscuit (Hardee's)	527	7	973
Ham & egg biscuit (Hardee's)	458	6	1585
Sausage & egg croissant (Arby's)	530	10	745
Sausage McMuffin w/egg (McDonald's)	517	7	1044
Biscuit with sausage (McDonald's)	467	7	1147
Sausage & egg biscuit (Hardee's)	521	8	1033
Pancake platter w/sausage (Roy Rogers)	608	7	1167
Biscuit w/bacon, egg, cheese (McDonald's)	483	7	1269
Egg & biscuit platter w/sausage (Roy Rogers)	550	9	1059
Sausage crescent (Jack-Box)	584	10	1012
Biscuit w/sausage and egg (McDonald's)	585	9	1301
Brkfst crescent sandwich w/ham (Roy Rogers)	557	9	1192
Scrambled eggs breakfast (Jack-Box)	720	10	1110

CHICKEN	CALORIES	FAT (TSP)	SODIUM (MG)
Original Recipe drumstick (Ky. Fd. Chkn.)	117	1	207
Litely breaded chicken (D'Lites)	170	2	430
Original Recipe wing (Ky. Fd. Chkn.)	136	2	302
Fried chicken leg (Church's)	147	2	286
Chicken sandwich multi-grain bun (Wendy's)	320	2	500
Roasted chicken breast (Arby's)	254	2	500
Original Recipe breast (Ky. Fd. Chkn.)	199	3	558
Chicken filet sandwich (D'Lites)	280	3	760

CHICKEN	CALORIES	FAT (TSP)	SODIUM (MG)
Original Recipe thigh *(Ky., Fd. Chkn.)*	257	4	566
Chicken breast *(Roy Rogers)*	324	4	601
Fried breast *(Church's)*	278	4	560
Kentucky Nuggets (6) *(Ky. Fd. Chkn.)*	282	4	810
Chicken McNuggets (6) *(McDonald's)*	323	5	512
Fried wing *(Church's)*	303	4	583
Fried thigh *(Church's)*	305	5	448
Chicken filet sandwich *(Hardee's)*	510	6	360
Extra Crispy thigh *(Ky. Fd. Chkn.)*	343	5	549
Turkey club sandwich *(Hardee's)*	426	5	1185
Chicken breast filet sand. *(Ky. Fd. Chkn.)*	436	5	1093
Chicken breast & wing *(Roy Rogers)*	466	6	867
Chicken salad croissant *(Arby's)*	460	8	725
Chicken club sandwich *(Arby's)*	620	7	1300
Chicken Supreme *(Jack- Box)*	601	8	1582
Specialty chicken sandwich *(Burger King)*	690	10	775

FISH	CALORIES	FAT (TSP)	SODIUM (MG)
Chilled shrimp, 1 piece *(L. J. Silver)*	6	0	19
Battered shrimp, 1 piece *(L. J. Silver)*	47	1	154
Baked fish w/sauce *(L. J. Silver)*	151	0	361
Catfish, one 3/4 ounce piece *(Church's)*	67	1	151
1/4-pound fish filet sandwich *(D'Lites)*	390	5	520
Fisherman's filet *(Hardee's)*	469	5	1013
Whaler sandwich *(Burger King)*	540	5	745
Moby Jack *(Jack-Box)*	444	6	820
Filet-o-Fish *(McDonald's)*	435	6	799
Whaler sandwich w/cheese *(Burger King)*	590	6	885

MEAT ITEM	CALORIES	FAT (TSP)	SODIUM (MG)
Burgers			
Jr. D'Lite *(D'Lites)*	200	2	210
Hamburger, kid's meal *(Wendy's)*	200	2	265
Hamburger *(McDonald's)*	263	3	506
Hamburger *(Burger King)*	310	3	560
Hamburger *(Hardee's)*	305	3	682
Happy Star Hamburger *(Carl's Jr.)*	330	3	670
Hamburger, multi-grain bun *(Wendy's)*	340	4	290
Cheeseburger *(McDonald's)*	318	4	743
Cheeseburger *(Burger King)*	360	4	705
Bacon cheeseburger *(D'Lites)*	370	4	730
Whopper Jr. *(Burger King)*	370	4	545
Double D'Lite *(D'Lites)*	450	5	290
Cheeseburger *(Hardee's)*	335	4	789
Double hamburger *(Burger King)*	430	5	585
Whopper Jr. w/cheese *(Burger King)*	410	5	685
Quarter-Pounder *(McDonald's)*	427	5	718
Hamburger *(Roy Rogers)*	456	6	495
Jumbo Jack *(Jack-Box)*	485	6	905
Mushroom 'n' Swiss burger *(Hardee's)*	512	5	1051
Big Deluxe *(Hardee's)*	546	6	1083
Bacon cheeseburger, white bun *(Wendy's)*	460	6	860
Quarter-Pounder w/cheese *(McDonald's)*	525	7	1220
Big Mac *(McDonald's)*	570	8	979
Bacon double-cheeseburger *(Burger King)*	600	8	985
Whopper *(Burger King)*	670	9	975

TABLE A.1 Main Meal Items in Calories, Fat, and Sodium—*Continued*

MEAT ITEM	CALORIES	FAT (TSP)	SODIUM (MG)
Cheeseburger *(Roy Rogers)*	463	8	1404
McD-L-T *(McDonald's)*	680	10	1030
RR-Bar Burger *(Roy Rogers)*	611	9	1826
Whopper w/cheese *(Burger King)*	760	10	1260
Bacon Cheeseburger Supreme *(Jack-Box)*	724	10	1307
Double-beef Whopper *(Burger King)*	890	12	1015
Double-beef Whopper w/cheese *(Burger King)*	980	14	1295
Triple cheeseburger *(Wendy's)*	1040	15	1848
Roast Beef Sandwiches			
Junior roast beef *(Arby's)*	220	2	530
Roast beef sandwich *(Roy Rogers)*	317	2	785
Regular roast beef *(Arby's)*	350	3	880
Roast beef sandwich *(Hardee's)*	377	4	1030
Roast beef sandwich w/cheese *(Roy Rogers)*	424	4	1694
Large roast beef w/cheese *(Roy Rogers)*	467	5	1953
Super roast beef *(Arby's)*	620	6	1420
Bac'n cheddar deluxe *(Arby's)*	561	8	1375
Ham Sandwiches			
Hot ham 'n cheese *(D'Lites)*	280	2	1160
Hot ham 'n cheese *(Hardee's)*	376	3	1067
Hot ham 'n cheese sandwich *(Arby's)*	353	3	1655
Ham biscuit *(Hardee's)*	349	4	1415
Specialty ham 'n cheese *(Burger King)*	550	7	1550

MISCELLANEOUS	CALORIES	FAT (TSP)	SODIUM (MG)
Reduced cal. Italian dressing (1 Tbsp) *(Wendy's)*	25	0	180
Cole slaw *(Ky. Fd. Chkn.)*	121	2	225
Thousand island dressing (1 Tbsp.) *(Wendy's)*	70	1	115
Pick-up window side salad *(Wendy's)*	110	1	540
12" cheese pizza, 2 slices *(Domino's)*	340	1	660
Potato salad *(Roy Rogers)*	107	1	696
Regular taco *(Jack-Box)*	191	2	406
Club Pita *(Jack-Box)*	284	2	953
Chili, 8 oz. *(Wendy's)*	260	2	1070
Macaroni *(Roy Rogers)*	186	2	603
Vegetarian D'Lite *(D'Lites)*	270	3	610
Chef salad *(Hardee's)*	277	4	517
16" pepperoni pizza, 2 slices *(Domino's)*	440	3	1080
Onion rings *(Burger King)*	270	4	450
Taco salad *(Wendy's)*	390	4	1100
Hot dog *(Hardee's)*	346	5	744
Veal parmigiana *(Burger King)*	580	6	805
Pasta seafood salad *(Jack-Box)*	394	5	1570
Shrimp salad *(Hardee's)*	362	7	941
Seafood salad *(L. J. Silver)*	471	7	993

POTATOES	CALORIES	FAT (TSP)	SODIUM (MG)
Baked and others			
Baked potato *(several)*	215	0	10
Mashed potatoes *(Ky. Fd. Chkn.)*	64	0	268
Potato skins, per skin *(D'Lites)*	90	1	174

POTATOES	CALORIES	FAT (TSP)	SODIUM (MG)
Potato with margarine *(Roy Rogers)*	274	2	161
Mexiskins, per skin *(D'Lites)*	99	2	227
Hash brown potatoes *(McDonald's)*	125	2	325
Potato cakes (2) *(Arby's)*	201	3	476
Potato w/chicken a la king *(Wendy's)*	350	1	820
Hash rounds *(Hardee's)*	200	3	310
Potato w/broccoli & cheddar *(D'Lites)*	410	4	820
Potato w/chili & cheese *(Wendy's)*	510	5	610
Potato w/sour cream & chives *(Wendy's)*	460	5	230
Mexican potato *(D'Lites)*	510	4	1000
Broccoli & cheddar potato *(Arby's)*	541	5	475
Mushroom & cheese potato *(Arby's)*	510	5	640
Potato w/taco beef & cheese *(Roy Rogers)*	463	5	726
Potato w/stroganoff & sour cream *(Wendy's)*	490	5	910
Home fries *(Wendy's)*	360	5	745
Taco potato *(Arby's)*	620	6	1060
Potato w/cheese *(Wendy's)*	590	8	450
Potato w/bacon & cheese *(Wendy's)*	570	7	1180
Deluxe potato *(Arby's)*	650	9	480
Fries			
Kentucky fries *(Ky. Fd. Chkn.)*	184	2	174
Fries, regular *(McDonald's)*	220	3	109
Fryes, bigger better *(L. J. Silver)*	247	3	6
French fries, regular *(D'Lites)*	260	3	100
French fries, small *(Hardee's)*	239	3	121
French fries, regular *(Burger King)*	210	3	230
French fries *(Arby's)*	211	2	39
French fries, regular *(Wendy's)*	280	3	95
French fries, large *(Hardee's)*	381	5	192

Adapted from: Center for Science in Public Interest, 1501 16th St., NW, Washington, DC 20036. First Printing 1986.

TABLE A.2   Desserts and Dairy Products by Calories, Fat, Sodium, and Sugar

DESSERTS	CALORIES	FAT (TSP)	SODIUM (MG)	SUGAR (TSP)
Chocolate D'Lite *(D'Lites)*	203	1	70	5
Soft serve with cone *(McDonald's)*	185	1	109	4
Strawberry sundae *(McDonald's)*	320	2	90	9
Caramel sundae *(McDonald's)*	361	2	145	10
Lemon meringue pie *(L. J. Silver)*	200	1	254	5
Brownie *(Roy Rogers)*	264	3	150	5
McDonaldland cookies *(McDonald's)*	308	2	358	6
Hot fudge sundae *(Roy Rogers)*	337	3	186	9
Frosty dairy dessert, 12 oz. *(Wendy's)*	400	3	220	10
Apple turnover *(Hardee's)*	282	3	310	5
Big cookie *(Hardee's)*	278	3	258	5
Apple pie *(Burger King)*	330	3	385	4
Cherry pie *(McDonald's)*	260	3	427	4
Chocolaty chip cookies *(McDonald's)*	342	4	313	5
Danish *(Wendy's)*	360	4	340	2
Blueberry turnover *(Arby's)*	340	5	255	6
Strawberry shortcake *(Roy Rogers)*	447	4	674	7
Pecan pie *(L. J. Silver)*	446	5	435	10
Apple turnover *(Jack-Box)*	410	5	350	7

SHAKES, MILK	CALORIES	FAT (TSP)	SODIUM (MG)	SUGAR (TSP)
Milk, 2.0% butterfat *(McDonald's)*	86	1	125	0
Whole milk *(several)*	150	2	125	0
Milk shake, average *(Jack-Box)*	323	2	147	9
Milk shake *(Hardee's)*	391	2	74	11
Milk shake, average *(McDonald's)*	367	2	236	10
Milk shake, average *(Roy Rogers)*	326	2	278	9
Milk shake, average *(Arby's)*	368	2	275	10
Milk shake, average *(Burger King)*	340	2	300	9

Adapted from: Center for Science in Public Interest, 1501 6th St., NW, Washington, DC 20036. First Printing 1986.

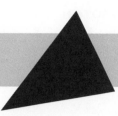

APPENDIX B

Nutrients of Selected Foods

TABLE B.1 Selected Foods by kcal, Protein, Fat, and Carbohydrates

FOOD	WEIGHT g	oz	APPROXIMATE MEASURE AND DESCRIPTION	kcal	PROTEIN g	FAT g	CARBO-HYDRATE g
Alcoholic beverages (located in Table B.2)							
Apples, raw	150	5.3	1 apple, about 3 per lb.	70	tr	tr	18
Apple, baked	130	4.6	1 medium apple, 2½ in dia.	120	tr	tr	30
Apple brown betty	115	4.0	½ cup	175	2	4	34
Apple juice (sweet cider)	124	4.3	½ cup, bottled or canned	60	tr	tr	15
Apple pie (see pies)							
Applesauce, canned sweetened	128	4.5	½ cup	115	tr	tr	31
Apricots, fresh, raw (as purchased)	114	4.0	3 apricots, about 12 per lb.	55	1	tr	29
Apricots, canned	130	4.6	½ cup or 4 medium halves, 2 tbsp. juice (syrup pack)	110	1	tr	29
Apricots, dried, stewed	108	3.8	½ cup (scant) or 8 halves, 2 tbsp. juice, sweetened	135	2	tr	34
Apricot nectar (peach and pear nectar have similar values)	125	4.4	½ cup	70	1	tr	19
Asparagus, cooked, green	73	2.6	½ cup, 1½-to 2-in. lengths	15	2	tr	3
Avocado, raw (as purchased)	142	5.0	½ cup avocado, 3⅛ in. dia., pitted and peeled	185	3	19	7
Bacon, broiled or fried	15	0.5	2 slices, cooked crisp (20 slices per lb., raw)	90	5	8	1
Bacon, Canadian, cooked	43	1.5	3 slices, cooked crisp	100	18	12	tr
Bananas, raw (as purchased)	175	6.1	1 medium banana	100	1	tr	26
Bavarian cream, orange	99	3.5	½ cup	210	2	10	30
Bean sprouts, mung, cooked	63	2.2	½ cup, drained	18	2	tr	4
Beans, green snap, cooked	63	2.2	½ cup	15	1	tr	4
Beans, dry, green lima, cooked	144	5.0	¾ cup	195	12	1	37
Beans, immature, green lima, cooked	85	2.8	½ cup	95	7	1	17
Beans, dry, red kidney, canned	191	6.7	¾ cup	173	11	1	32
Beans, dry, white, canned with tomato sauce, without pork	196	6.9	¾ cup	233	12	1	45
Beans, dry, white, canned with tomato sauce and pork	191	6.7	¾ cup	233	12	5	37
Beef, corned, canned	85	3.0	3 slices, 3 × 2 × ¼ in.	185	22	10	0
Beef, corned hash, canned	85	3.0	½ cup (approx.)	155	7	10	9
Beef, dried or chipped	57	2.0	4 thin slices, 4 × 5 in.	115	19	4	0
Beef, hamburger, broiled	85	3.0	1 patty, 3 in. dia. (regular ground beef)	245	21	17	0
Beef, heart, braised	85	3.0	2 round slices, 2½ in. dia., ½ in. thick	160	27	5	1
Beef liver (see liver)							
Beef loaf (see meat loaf)							
Beef potpie, baked	227	7.9	1 pie, 4¼ in. dia.	560	23	33	43
Beef, pot roast, cooked	85	3.0	1 piece, 4 × 3¾ × ½ in.	245	23	16	0
Beef roast, oven-cooked	85	3.0	2 slices, 6 × 3¼ × ⅛ in., relatively lean	165	25	7	0
Beef steak, broiled	85	3.0	1 piece, 3½ × 2 × ¾ in., relatively fat, no bone	330	20	27	0

FOOD	WEIGHT g	WEIGHT oz	APPROXIMATE MEASURE AND DESCRIPTION	kcal	PROTEIN g	FAT g	CARBO-HYDRATE g
Beef stroganoff, cooked	130	4.6	½ cup	250	17	18	6
Beef tongue, braised	85	3.0	7 slices, 2¼ × 2¼ × ⅛ in.	210	18	14	tr
Beets, cooked	85	3.0	½ cup, diced	28	1	tr	6
Beverages, alcoholic (see p. 316)							
Beverages, cola-type	185	6.5	about ¾ cup	75	0	0	19
Beverages, ginger ale	240	8.4	1 cup	75	0	0	19
Biscuits, baking powder	28	1.0	1 biscuit, 2 in. dia. (enriched flour)	105	2	5	13
Blackberries, raw	72	2.5	½ cup	45	1	1	10
Blueberries, raw	70	2.5	½ cup	45	1	1	11
Bluefish cooked	85	3.0	1 piece, 3½ × 2 × ½ in.	135	22	4	0
Bologna (see sausage)							
Bouillon cubes	4	0.1	1 cube, ⅝ in.	5	1	tr	tr
Bran flakes	26	0.9	¾ cup, 40% bran, (thiamin and iron added)	80	3	1	21
Bread, Boston brown	48	1.7	1 slice, 3 × ¾ in.	100	3	1	22
Bread, cracked wheat	25	0.9	1 slice, 18 slices per lb. loaf	65	2	1	13
Bread, French or Vienna	20	0.7	1 slice, 3¼ × 2 × 1 in. (enriched flour)	60	2	1	11
Bread, Italian	20	0.7	1 slice, 3¼ × 2 × 1 in. (enriched flour)	55	2	tr	11
Bread, light rye	25	0.9	1 slice, 18 slices per lb. loaf (⅓ rye, ⅔ wheat)	60	2	tr	13
Bread, pumpernickel	34	1.2	1 slice, 3¼ × 2 × 1 in. (dark rye flour)	85	3	0	19
Bread, raisin	25	0.9	1 slice, 18 slices per lb. loaf	65	2	1	13
Bread, white firm crumb (enriched)	23	0.8	1 slice, 20 slices per lb. loaf	65	2	1	12
Bread, white soft crumb (enriched)	25	0.9	1 slice, 18 slices per lb. loaf	70	2	1	13
Bread, white soft crumb (enriched), toasted	22	0.8	1 slice, 18 slices per lb. loaf	70	2	1	13
Bread, white soft crumb (unenriched)	25	0.9	1 slice, 18 slices per lb. loaf	70	2	1	13
Bread, whole wheat firm crumb	25	0.9	1 slice, 18 slices per lb. loaf	60	3	1	12
Bread crumbs	25	0.9	¼ cup, dry grated	98	3	1	18
Broccoli, cooked	78	2.7	½ cup, stalks cut into ½-in. pieces	20	3	1	4
Brussels sprouts, cooked	78	2.7	½ cup or 5 medium sprouts	28	4	1	5
Buns (see rolls)							
Butter	14	0.5	1 tbsp or ⅛ stick	100	tr	12	tr
Cabbage, cooked	73	2.6	½ cup, cooked short time in little water	15	1	tr	3
Cabbage, raw	45	1.6	½ cup, finely shredded	10	1	tr	3
Cabbage, raw, Chinese	38	1.3	½ cup, 1-in. pieces	5	1	tr	1
Cake, angel food (from mix)	53	1.9	1 piece, 1/12 of 10-in.-dia. cake	135	3	tr	32
Cake, Boston cream pie	69	2.4	1 piece, 1/12 of 8-in.-dia. pie (unenriched flour)	210	4	6	34
Cake, plain, chocolate-iced cupcake (from mix)	36	1.3	1 cupcake, 2½ in. dia.	130	2	5	21
Cake, plain uniced cupcakes (from mix)	25	0.9	1 cupcake, 2½ in. dia.	90	1	3	14
Cake, 2-layer devil's food with chocolate icing (from mix)	69	2.4	1 piece (mix), 1/16 of 9-in.-dia. cake	235	3	9	40
Cake, fruit, dark	15	0.5	1 slice, 1/30 of 8-in.-long loaf (enriched flour)	55	1	2	9
Cake, pound	30	1.1	1 slice, 2¾ × 3 × ⅝ in.	140	2	9	14
Cake, sponge	66	1.4	1 piece, 1/12 of 10-in.-dia. cake (unenriched)	195	5	4	36
Cake, 2-layer white with chocolate icing	71	2.5	1 piece, 1/16 of 9-in.-dia. cake	250	3	8	45
Candy, caramels	28	1.0	4 small	115	1	3	22

TABLE B.1 Selected Foods by kcal, Protein, Fat, and Carbohydrates—*Continued*

FOOD	WEIGHT g	oz	APPROXIMATE MEASURE AND DESCRIPTION	kcal	PROTEIN g	FAT g	CARBO-HYDRATE g
Candy, plain chocolate	28	1.0	1 bar, 3¾ × 1½ × ¼ in.	145	2	9	16
Candy, chocolate with almonds	51	1.8	1 bar, 5⅓ × 1⅞ × ⅓ in.	265	4	19	25
Candy, chocolate creams	28	1.0	2 pieces, 1¼ in dia. (base), ⅝ in. thick	110	1	4	20
Candy, chocolate fudge	28	1.0	1 piece, 1¼ × 1¼ × 1 in.	115	1	4	21
Candy, hard	28	1.0	6 pieces, 1 in. dia., ¼ in. thick	110	0	tr	28
Candy, peanut brittle	28	1.0	1 piece, 3¼ × 2½ × ¼ in.	125	2	4	21
Cantaloupes	385	13.5	½ melon, 5 in. dia.	60	1	tr	14
Carrots, raw grated	55	1.9	½ cup grated	23	1	tr	6
Carrots, raw whole or strips	50	1.8	1 carrot, 5½ in. long or 25 thin strips	20	1	tr	5
Carrots, cooked	73	2.6	½ cup diced	23	1	tr	5
Catsup, tomato (see tomato)							
Cauliflower, cooked	60	2.1	½ cup flowerets	13	2	tr	3
Celery, raw diced	50	1.8	½ cup	8	1	tr	2
Celery, raw whole	40	1.4	1 stalk, large outer, 8 in. long	5	tr	tr	2
Cheese, blue (Roquefort type)	28	1.0	¾-in. sector or 3 tbsp.	105	6	9	1
Cheese, cheddar (American), cubed	28	1.0	1 cube, 1⅛ in.	115	6	10	2
Cheese, cheddar (American), grated	7	0.3	1 tbsp	30	2	2	tr
Cheese, creamed cottage	61	2.1	¼ cup (made from skim milk)	65	8	3	2
Cheese, uncreamed cottage	28	1.0	2 tbsp (made from skim milk)	25	5	tr	1
Cheese, cream	16	0.5	1 tbsp	60	1	6	tr
Cheese, Swiss (domestic)	28	1.0	1 slice, 7 × 4 × ⅛ in.	105	8	8	1
Cheese foods, cheddar	28	1.0	2 round slices, 1⅝ in. dia., ¼ in. thick or 2 tbsp	90	6	6	2
Cheese sauce	60	2.1	¼ cup	110	5	9	4
Cheese soufflé	79	2.8	¾ cup	200	10	16	7
Cheesecake	162	5.7	⅒ of 9-in.-dia. cake	400	15	23	35
Cherries, raw sweet	130	4.6	1 cup with stems	80	2	tr	20
Cherries, raw West Indian (acerola)	11	0.4	2 medium cherries	3	—	—	1
Chick peas, dry raw (garbanzos)	105	3.7	½ cup	380	22	5	64
Chicken, broiled	85	3.0	3 slices, flesh only	115	20	2	0
Chicken, canned	85	3.0	⅓ cup boned meat	170	18	10	0
Chicken, creamed	99	3.5	½ cup	222	20	12	6
Chicken breast, fried	94	3.3	½ breast with bone	155	25	5	1
Chicken drumstick, fried	59	2.1	1 drumstick with bone	90	12	4	tr
Chicken pie (see poultry potpie)							
Chili con carne with beans, canned	188	6.5	¾ cup	250	14	11	23
Chili con carne without beans, canned	191	6.7	¾ cup	383	20	29	11
Chili powder	15	0.5	1 tbsp hot red peppers, dried and ground	50	2	2	8
Chili sauce	17	0.6	1 tbsp, mainly tomatoes	20	tr	tr	4
Chocolate, bitter (baking chocolate)	28	1.0	1 square	145	3	15	8
Chocolate candy (see candy)							
Chocolate-flavored milk drink	250	8.8	1 cup (made with skim milk)	190	8	6	27
Chocolate morsels	15	0.5	30 morsels or 1½ tbsp	80	1	4	10
Chocolate syrup	40	1.4	2 tbsp	80	tr	tr	22
Chop suey, cooked	122	4.3	¾ cup	325	19	20	16
Clams, canned	85	3.0	½ cup or 3 medium clams	45	7	1	2
Cocoa, beverage	182	6.3	¾ cup (made with milk)	176	7	8	20
Coconut, dried, shredded, sweetened	16	0.6	¼ cup	85	1	6	8
Coconut, fresh shredded	33	1.2	¼ cup	113	1	12	3
Codfish, dried	51	1.8	½ cup	190	41	2	0
Coffee cake, frosted	79	2.8	1 piece, 3 × 3 × 1¼ in.	260	4	11	37

FOOD	WEIGHT g	WEIGHT oz	APPROXIMATE MEASURE AND DESCRIPTION	kcal	PROTEIN g	FAT g	CARBO-HYDRATE g
Cole slaw	60	2.1	½ cup	50	1	4	5
Cookies, brownies	26	0.9	1 piece, 1⅞ × 1⅞ × ⅞ in.	145	2	9	17
Cookies, chocolate chip	11	0.4	1 cookie, 2¼ in. dia.	60	1	3	7
Cookies, coconut bar chews	11	0.4	1 cookie, 3 × ⅞ × ⅓ in.	55	tr	2	9
Cookies, oatmeal with raisins and nuts	11	0.4	1 cookie, 2⅝ in. dia.	65	4	4	6
Cookies, sugar, plain	9	0.3	1 cookie, 2½ in. dia.	40	1	2	6
Corn, sweet, cooked	140	4.9	1 ear, 5 in. long	70	3	1	16
Corn, sweet, canned	128	4.5	½ cup, solids and liquid	85	3	1	20
Corn grits, cooked	163	5.7	⅔ cup, enriched and degermed	85	2	tr	18
Corn muffins	40	1.4	1 muffin, 2⅜ in. dia., enriched flour and enriched degermed meal	125	3	4	19
Corned beef (*see* beef)							
Corned beef hash (*see* beef)							
Cornflakes	33	1.2	1⅓ cup (added nutrients)	133	3	tr	28
Cornmeal, dry	138	4.8	1 cup, white or yellow, enriched and degermed	500	11	2	108
Cow peas (*see* peas)							
Crabmeat, canned	85	3.0	½ cup flakes	85	15	2	1
Crackers, graham, plain	14	0.6	2 medium or 4 small	55	1	1	10
Crackers, saltines	8	0.3	2 crackers, 2 in. square	35	1	1	6
Cranberry juice, canned	125	4.4	½ cup or 1 small glass, ascorbic acid added	85	tr	tr	21
Cranberry sauce, canned	69	2.4	¼ cup, strained and sweetened	85	tr	tr	21
Cream, coffee (light cream)	15	0.5	1 tbsp	30	1	3	1
Cream, half-and-half	15	0.5	1 tbsp	20	1	2	1
Cream, heavy, whipping	15	0.5	1 tbsp, unwhipped (volume doubled when whipped)	55	tr	6	1
Creamer, coffee (imitation cream)	2	—	1 tsp powder	10	tr	1	1
Cucumber, raw	50	1.8	6 slices, pared, ⅛ in. thick	5	tr	tr	2
Custard, baked	124	4.3	½ cup	143	7	7	14
Dates, pitted	45	1.6	¼ cup or 8 dates	123	1	tr	33
Dessert topping, whipped	11	0.4	2 tbsp (low-calorie, with nonfat dry milk)	17	1	—	3
Doughnuts, cake-type	32	1.1	1 (enriched flour)	125	1	6	16
Egg, raw, boiled, or poached	50	1.8	1 whole egg	80	6	6	tr
Egg white, raw	33	1.2	1 egg white	15	4	tr	tr
Egg yolk, raw	17	0.6	1 egg yolk	60	3	5	tr
Eggs, creamed	113	4.0	½ cup (1 egg in ¼ cup white sauce)	190	9	14	7
Eggs, fried	54	1.9	1 egg, cooked in 1 tsp. fat	115	6	10	tr
Eggs, scrambled	64	2.2	1 egg, with milk and fat	110	7	8	1
Endive, curly, raw	57	2.0	3 leaves (includes escarole)	10	1	tr	2
Farina, cooked	163	5.7	⅔ cup (quick, enriched)	70	2	tr	14
Fats, cooking, lard	13	0.5	1 tbsp solid fat	115	0	13	0
Fats, cooking, vegetable	13	0.5	1 tbsp solid fat	110	0	13	0
Figs, dried	21	0.7	1 large fig, 1 × 2 in.	60	1	tr	15
Figs, fresh raw	114	4.0	3 small, 1½ in. dia.	90	1	tr	23
Fish (*see* various kinds of fish)							
Fish, creamed (tuna, salmon, or other, in white sauce)	136	4.8	½ cup	220	20	13	8
Fish sticks, breaded, cooked	114	4.0	5 sticks, each 3.8 × 1.0 × 0.5 in.	200	19	10	8
Frankfurter, heated	56	2.0	1 frankfurter	170	7	15	1
French toast, fried	79	2.8	1 slice (enriched bread)	180	6	12	14
Fruit balls, raw (dried apricots, dates, nuts)	11	0.4	1 ball, 1 in. dia.	45	1	1	8
Fruit cocktail, canned	128	4.5	½ cup, with heavy syrup	98	1	tr	25
Gelatin, plain, dry	7	0.3	1 tbsp (1 envelope)	25	6	tr	0
Gelatin dessert, plain	120	4.2	½ cup, ready to eat	70	2	0	17
Gingerbread	63	2.2	1 piece (mix), ⅑ of 8-in. square	175	2	4	32
Grapefruit, white, raw (as purchased)	241	8.4	½ medium, 3¾ in. dia.	45	1	tr	12

TABLE B.1 Selected Foods by kcal, Protein, Fat, and Carbohydrates—*Continued*

FOOD	WEIGHT g	oz	APPROXIMATE MEASURE AND DESCRIPTION	kcal	PROTEIN g	FAT g	CARBO-HYDRATE g
Grapefruit, white, canned	125	4.4	½ cup, syrup pack	88	1	tr	22
Grapefruit juice, canned	124	4.3	½ cup, unsweetened	50	1	tr	12
Grapefruit juice, dehyrated crystals	124	4.3	½ cup or 1 small glass, prepared, ready to serve	50	1	tr	12
Grapes, raw American-type	153	5.4	1 cup or 1 medium bunch (slip skin, as Concord)	65	1	1	15
Grapes, raw European-type	160	5.6	1 cup or 40 grapes (adherent skin, as Tokay)	95	1	tr	25
Grape juice, canned	127	4.4	½ cup	83	1	tr	21
Greens, collards, cooked	95	3.3	½ cup	28	3	1	5
Greens, dandelion, cooked	90	3.2	½ cup	30	2	1	6
Greens, kale, cooked	55	1.9	½ cup, leaves and stems	15	2	1	2
Greens, mustard, cooked	70	2.5	½ cup	18	2	1	3
Greens, spinach, cooked	90	3.2	½ cup	20	3	1	3
Greens, turnip, cooked	73	2.6	½ cup	15	2	tr	3
Guavas, raw	82	2.8	1 guava	50	1	tr	12
Haddock, fried	85	3.0	1 fillet, 4 × 2½ × ½ in.	140	17	5	5
Ham, boiled	57	2.0	1 slice, 6¼ × 3¾ × ⅛ in.	135	11	10	0
Ham, cured, roasted	85	3.0	2 slices, 5½ × 3¾ × ⅛ in.	245	18	19	0
Hamburger (see beef, hamburger)							
Honey, strained	21	0.7	1 tbsp	65	tr	0	17
Hot dog (see frankfurter)							
Ice cream, plain	50	1.8	1 container, 3 fluid oz (factory packed)	95	2	5	10
Ice cream, plain brick	71	2.5	1 slice, ⅛ of qt brick	145	3	9	15
Ice milk	66	2.3	½ cup	100	3	4	15
Jams, jellies, preserves	20	0.7	1 tbsp	55	tr	tr	14
Kale (see greens)							
Lamb chop, cooked	137	4.8	1 thick chop with bone	400	25	33	0
Lamb, leg roasted	85	3.0	2 slices, 3 × 3¼ × ⅛ in., lean and fat, no bone	235	22	16	0
Lard (see fats, cooking)							
Lemon juice, fresh	15	0.5	1 tbsp	5	tr	tr	1
Lemonade	248	8.7	1 cup (made from frozen, sweetened concentrate)	110	tr	tr	28
Lentils, dry, cooled	100	3.5	½ cup	120	9	tr	22
Lettuce, headed, raw,	454	16.0	1 head (compact, as iceberg), 4 ¾ in. dia.	60	4	tr	13
Lettuce, loose leaf, raw	50	1.8	2 large leaves or 4 small leaves	10	1	tr	2
Lime juice, canned	62	2.2	¼ cup	15	tr	tr	6
Liver, beef, fried	57	2.0	1 slice, 5 × 2 × ⅓ in.	130	15	6	3
Liver, calf, fried	74	2.6	1 slice, 5 × 2 × ½ in.	230	15	15	4
Liver, chicken, fried	85	3.0	3 medium livers	235	20	15	5
Liver, pork, fried	70	2.5	1 slice, 3¾ × 1¾ × ½ in.	225	17	15	3
Macaroni, cooked	105	3.7	¾ cup (enriched)	115	4	1	24
Macaroni and cheese, baked	150	5.3	¾ cup (enriched macaroni)	325	13	17	30
Mackerel, broiled	85	3.0	1 piece	200	19	13	0
Mangoes, raw	198	7.0	1 medium mango	90	1	—	23
Margarine	14	0.5	1 tbsp or ⅛ stick (fortified with vitamin A)	100	tr	12	tr
Marshmallows	9	0.3	1, 1¼ in. dia.	25	tr	0	8
Meat loaf, beef, baked	77	2.7	1 slice, 3¾ × 2¼ × ¾ in.	240	19	17	3
Milk, dry skim (nonfat)	17	0.6	¼ cup powder, instant	61	6	tr	9
Milk, dry whole	26	0.9	¼ cup powder	129	7	7	10
Milk, evaporated, canned	126	4.4	½ cup, undiluted and unsweetened	173	9	10	12
Milk, fluid, skim or buttermilk	245	8.6	1 cup (½ pt)	90	9	tr	12
Milk, fluid, whole	244	8.5	1 cup (½ pt), 3.5% fat	160	9	9	12
Milk, malted, plain	353	12.4	1 fountain size glass (about 1½ cup)	368	17	15	42
Milkshake, chocolate	342	12.0	1 fountain size glass	420	11	18	58
Molasses, cane, black-strap	20	0.7	1 tbsp, 3rd extraction	45	—	—	11

FOOD	WEIGHT g	WEIGHT oz	APPROXIMATE MEASURE AND DESCRIPTION	kcal	PROTEIN g	FAT g	CARBO-HYDRATE g
Molasses, cane, light	20	0.7	1 tbsp, 1st extraction	50	—	—	13
Muffins, plain	40	1.4	1 muffin, 2¾ in. dia. (enriched white flour)	120	3	4	17
Mushrooms, canned	122	4.3	½ cup, solids and liquid	20	3	tr	3
Noodles, egg, cooked	120	4.2	¾ cup (enriched)	150	5	2	28
Nuts, almonds	36	1.3	¼ cup shelled	213	7	19	7
Nuts, cashew, roasted	35	1.2	¼ cup	196	6	16	10
Nuts, peanuts (see peanuts, roasted)							
Nuts, pecan halves	27	0.9	¼ cup	185	3	19	4
Nuts, walnut halves	25	0.9	¼ cup, English or Persian	163	4	16	4
Oatmeal or rolled oats, cooked	160	5.6	⅔ cup (regular or quick-cooking)	87	3	1	15
Oils, salad or cooking	14	0.5	1 tbsp	125	0	14	0
Okra, cooked	43	1.5	4 pods, 3 × ⅝ in.	13	1	tr	3
Olives, green	16	0.6	4 medium or 3 large	15	tr	2	tr
Olives, ripe	10	0.4	3 small or 2 large	15	tr	2	tr
Onions, raw	110	3.9	1 onion, 2½ in. dia.	40	2	tr	10
Onions, cooked	105	3.7	½ cup or 5 onions, 1¼ in. dia.	30	2	tr	7
Onions, young green	50	1.8	6 small, without tops	20	1	tr	5
Oranges	180	6.3	1 orange, 2⅝ in. dia. (all commercial varieties)	65	1	tr	16
Orange juice, canned unsweetened	125	4.4	½ cup or 1 small glass	60	1	1	13
Orange juice, dehydrated crystals	124	4.3	½ cup or 1 small glass prepared, ready to serve	60	1	tr	14
Orange juice, fresh	124	4.3	½ cup or 1 small glass (all varieties)	55	1	tr	15
Orange juice, frozen concentrate	125	4.4	½ cup or 1 small glass, diluted ready to serve	60	1	tr	14
Oysters, raw	120	4.2	½ cup or 8-10 oysters	80	10	2	4
Oyster stew, milk	230	8.1	1 cup with 3-4 oysters	200	11	12	11
Pancakes, wheat	27	0.9	1 griddle cake, 4 in. dia. (enriched flour)	60	2	2	9
Papayas, raw	91	3.2	½ cup in ½-in. cubes	35	1	tr	9
Parsley, raw	4	0.1	1 tbsp chopped	tr	tr	tr	tr
Parsnips, cooked	77	2.7	½ cup	50	1	1	12
Peaches, canned halves or slices	129	4.5	½ cup, solids and liquid, syrup-pack	100	1	tr	26
Peaches, canned whole	123	4.3	½ cup, solids liquid (water pack)	38	1	tr	10
Peaches, raw sliced	84	2.9	½ cup fresh or frozen	33	1	tr	8
Peaches, raw whole	114	4.0	1 peach, 2 in. dia.	35	1	tr	10
Peanuts, roasted	36	1.3	¼ cup halves, salted	210	9	18	7
Peanut butter	32	1.1	2 tbsp	190	8	16	6
Pears, canned	117	4.1	2 medium halves with 2 tbsp	90	tr	tr	23
Pears, raw (as purchased)	182	6.3	1 pear, 3 × 2½ in. dia.	100	1	1	25
Peas, cowpeas, dry, cooked (blackeye peas or frijoles)	124	4.3	½ cup	95	7	1	17
Peas, green, cooked	80	2.8	½ cup	58	5	1	10
Peas, pigeon, dry raw (gandules)	99	3.5	6 tbsp	310	22	2	50
Peas, split, dry cooked	125	4.4	½ cup	145	10	1	26
Peppers, green, stuffed	113	4.0	1 medium pepper, cooked with meat stuffing	200	12	14	12
Peppers, hot red (see chili powder)							
Peppers, pimentos, canned	38	1.3	1 medium pod	10	tr	tr	2
Peppers, raw sweet green	74	2.6	1 medium pod without stem	15	1	tr	4
Peppers, raw sweet red	60	2.1	1 medium pod without stem and seeds	20	1	tr	4
Perch, ocean, fried	85	3.0	1 piece, 4 × 3 × ½ in.	195	16	11	6
Persimmons, raw (Japanese)	125	4.4	1 fruit, 2½ in. dia.	75	1	tr	20
Pickle relish	15	0.5	1 tbsp	20	tr	tr	5

FOOD	WEIGHT g	WEIGHT oz	APPROXIMATE MEASURE AND DESCRIPTION	kcal	PROTEIN g	FAT g	CARBO-HYDRATE g
Pickles, cucumber, bread and butter	42	1.5	6 slices ¼ × 1½ in. dia.	30	tr	tr	7
Pickles, cucumber, dill	65	2.3	1 large pickle, 3¼ × 1½ in.	10	1	tr	1
Pickles, cucumber, sweet	15	0.5	1 pickle, 2½ × ¾ in. dia.	20	tr	tr	6
Pie, apple	135	4.7	4-in. sector of ⅐ of 9-in.-dia. pie (unenriched flour)	350	3	15	51
Pie, cherry	135	4.7	4-in. sector of ⅐ of 9-in.-dia. pie	350	4	15	52
Pie, custard	130	4.6	4-in. sector or ⅐ of 9-in.-dia. pie (unenriched flour)	285	8	14	30
Pie, lemon meringue	120	4.2	4-in. sector or ⅐ of 9-in.-dia. pie (unenriched flour)	305	4	12	45
Pie, mince	135	4.7	4-in. sector or ⅐ of 9-in.-dia. pie (unenriched flour)	365	3	16	56
Pie, pumpkin	130	4.6	4-in. sector or ⅐ of 9-in.-dia. pie (unenriched flour)	275	5	15	32
Pineapple, canned crushed	130	4.6	½ cup (syrup packed)	100	1	tr	25
Pineapple, canned slices	122	4.3	1 large or 2 small slices, 2 tbsp juice (syrup pack)	90	tr	tr	24
Pineapple, raw	70	2.5	½ cup, diced	38	1	tr	10
Pineapple juice, canned	125	4.4	½ cup or 1 small glass	68	1	tr	17
Pizza (cheese)	75	2.6	5½-in. sector or ⅛ of 14-in.-dia. pie	185	7	6	27
Plantain, raw, green	100	3.5	1 baking banana, 6 in.	135	1	—	32
Plums, canned	128	4.5	½ cup or 3 plums with 2 tbsp juice (syrup pack)	100	1	tr	27
Plums, raw	60	2.1	1 plum, 2 in. diameter	25	tr	tr	7
Popcorn, popped	9	0.3	1 cup (oil and salt) added	40	1	2	5
Pork chop, cooked	99	3.5	1 thick chop, trimmed, with bone	260	16	21	0
Pork roast, cooked	85	3.0	2 slices, 5 × 4 × ⅛ in.	310	21	24	0
Potato chips	20	0.7	10 medium chips, 2 in. dia.	115	1	8	10
Potatoes, baked	99	3.5	1 medium potato, about 3 per pound raw	90	3	tr	21
Potatoes, boiled	122	4.3	1 potato, peeled before boiling	80	2	tr	18
Potatoes, French fried	57	2.0	10 pieces, 2 × ½ × ½ in. cooked in deep fat	155	2	7	20
Potatoes, mashed	98	3.4	½ cup (milk and butter added)	95	2	4	12
Poultry (chicken or turkey potpie	227	7.9	1 indiv. pie, 4½ in. dia.	535	23	31	42
Pretzels	3	0.1	5, 3⅛-in. sticks	10	tr	tr	2
Prunes, dried, cooked	105	3.7	5 medium prunes with 2 tbsp	160	1	tr	25
Prune juice, canned	128	4.5	½ cup or 1 small glass	100	1	tr	25
Pudding, chocolate blanc mange	130	4.6	½ cup	190	6	8	26
Pudding, cornstarch (plain, blanc mange)	124	4.3	½ cup	140	5	5	20
Pudding, rice with raisins (old fashioned)	136	4.8	½ cup	300	8	8	52
Pudding, tapioca	74	2.6	½ cup	140	5	5	12
Radishes, raw	40	1.4	4 small	5	tr	tr	1
Raisins, seedless	10	0.4	1 tbsp pressed down	30	tr	tr	8
Raspberries, raw, red	62	2.2	½ cup	35	1	1	9
Rhubarb, cooked	136	4.8	½ cup (sugar added)	190	1	tr	50
Rice, parboiled, cooked	131	4.6	¾ cup (enriched)	140	3	tr	31
Rice, puffed	15	0.5	1 cup (nutrients added)	60	1	tr	13
Rice flakes	30	1.1	1 cup (nutrients added)	115	2	tr	26
Rolls, bagel (egg)	55	1.9	1 roll, 3 in. dia.	165	6	2	28
Rolls, barbecue bun	40	1.3	1 bun, 3½ in dia. (enriched)	120	3	2	21
Rolls, hard	52	1.8	1 round roll	160	5	2	31
Rolls, plain, white	28	1.0	1 commercial pan roll (enriched flour)	85	2	2	15
Rolls, sweet, pan	43	1.5	1 roll	135	4	4	21

FOOD	WEIGHT g	oz	APPROXIMATE MEASURE AND DESCRIPTION	kcal	PROTEIN g	FAT g	CARBO-HYDRATE g
Rutabagas, cooked	77	2.7	½ cup	25	1	tr	6
Salad, chicken	125	4.4	½ cup, with mayonnaise	280	25	19	1
Salad, egg	128	4.5	½ cup, with mayonnaise	190	6	18	1
Salad, fresh fruit (orange, apple, banana, grapes)	125	4.4	½ cup, with French dressing	130	—	6	21
Salad, jellied, vegetable	122	4.3	½ cup, no dressing	70	3	—	16
Salad, lettuce	130	4.6	½ solid head, with French dressing	80	1	6	5
Salad, potato	139	4.9	½ cup, with mayonnaise	185	2	12	17
Salad, tomato aspic	119	4.2	½ cup, no dressing	45	5	0	7
Salad, tuna fish	102	3.6	½ cup, with mayonnaise	250	21	18	1
Salad dressing, blue cheese	15	0.5	1 tbsp	75	1	8	1
Salad dressing, boiled	16	0.6	1 tbsp, home-made	25	1	2	2
Salad dressing, commercial	15	0.5	1 tbsp, mayonnaise-type	65	tr	6	2
Salad dressing, French	16	0.6	1 tbsp	65	tr	6	3
Salad dressing, low-calorie	26	0.9	2 tbsp (cottage cheese, nonfat dry milk, no oil)	17	2	0	2
Salad dressing, mayonnaise	14	0.5	1 tbsp	100	tr	11	tr
Salad dressing, Thousand Island	16	0.6	1 tbsp	80	tr	8	3
Salmon, boiled or baked	119	4.2	1 steak, 4 × 3 × ¼ × ½ in.	200	34	7	tr
Salmon, pink, canned	85	3.0	½ cup	120	17	5	0
Salmon loaf	113	4.0	½ cup or 1 slice, 4 × 1½ in.	235	29	10	5
Sardines, canned oil	57	2.0	5 small fish, 3 × 1 × ¼ in.	120	13	6	0
Sauce, chocolate	40	1.4	2 tbsp	75	1	4	9
Sauce, custard	31	1.1	2 tbsp (low calorie, with nonfat dry milk)	45	2	1	7
Sauce, hard	17	0.6	1 tbsp	90	—	6	11
Sauce, hollandaise (mock)	26	0.9	2 tbsp	75	2	7	3
Sauce, lemon	28	1.0	2 tbsp	40	0	1	8
Sauerkraut, canned	118	4.1	½ cup, solids and liquid	25	1	tr	5
Sausage, bologna	57	2.0	2 slices, 4.1 × 0.1 in.	173	7	16	1
Sausage, Frankfurters (see frankfurters)							
Sausage, liverwurst	57	2.0	3 slices, 2½ in. dia. ¼ in. thick	150	10	12	1
Sausage, pork, cooked	26	0.9	2 small patties or links	125	5	11	tr
Sausage, Vienna	16	0.6	1 canned sausage, about 2 in. long	40	2	3	tr
Shad, baked	85	3.0	1 piece, 4 × 3 × ½ in.	170	20	10	0
Sherbet, orange	97	3.4	½ cup	130	1	1	30
Shrimp, canned	85	3.0	½ cup, meat only	100	21	1	30
Syrup, table blends	21	0.7	1 tbsp, light and dark	60	0	0	15
Soup, bean with port, canned	250	8.8	1 cup, ready to serve	170	8	6	22
Soup, beef broth, bouillon, consommé, canned	240	8.4	1 cup, ready to serve	30	5	0	3
Soup, chicken noodle, canned	250	8.8	1 cup, ready to serve	65	4	2	8
Soup, clam chowder, canned	255	8.9	1 cup, ready to serve	85	2	3	13
Soup, cream of vegetable(e.g., tomato, mushroom), canned	240	8.4	1 cup, ready to serve	135	2	10	10
Soup, minestrone, canned	245	8.6	1 cup, ready to serve	105	5	3	14
Soup, tomato, canned	245	8.6	1 cup, ready to serve	90	2	3	16
Soup, vegetable, canned	250	8.8	1 cup, ready to serve	80	3	2	14
Spaghetti, cooked	105	3.7	¾ cup (enriched)	115	4	1	24
Spaghetti, in tomato sauce, with cheese	188	6.5	¾ cup	200	7	7	28
Spaghetti, in tomato sauce, with meat balls	186	6.5	¾ cup	250	15	9	30
Spinach (see greens)							
Squash, summer, cooked	105	3.7	½ cup, diced	15	1	tr	4
Squash, winter, baked	103	3.6	½ cup, mashed	65	2	1	16
Stew, beef and vegetable	176	6.2	¾ cup	160	11	8	11
Strawberries, raw	75	2.6	½ cup, capped	30	1	1	7

FOOD	WEIGHT g	WEIGHT oz	APPROXIMATE MEASURE AND DESCRIPTION	kcal	PROTEIN g	FAT g	CARBO-HYDRATE g
Sugar, brown	14	0.5	1 tbsp firmly packed	50	0	0	13
Sugar, granulated	11	0.4	1 tbsp (beef or cane)	40	0	0	11
Sugar, lump	6	0.2	1 domino, 1⅛ × ¾ × ⅜ in.	25	0	0	6
Sugar, powdered	8	0.3	1 tbsp	30	0	0	8
Sweet potatoes, baked	110	3.9	1 medium potato, about 6 oz raw	155	2	1	36
Sweet potatoes, candied	175	6.1	1 potato, 3½ × 2¼ in.	295	2	6	60
Tangerine	116	4.1	1 medium tangerine, 2⅜ in. dia.	40	1	tr	10
Tarter sauce (see salad dressing, mayonnaise)							
Toast, melba	6	0.2	1 slice, 3¾ × 1¾ in.	20	1	tr	4
Tomato catsup	15	0.5	1 tbsp	15	tr	tr	4
Tomato juice, canned	122	4.3	½ cup or 1 small glass	23	1	tr	5
Tomatoes, canned	121	4.2	½ cup	25	1	1	5
Tomatoes, raw	200	7.0	1 tomato, about 3 in. dia., 2⅛ in. high	40	2	tr	9
Topping, whipped	4	0.1	1 tbsp, pressurized	10	tr	1	tr
Tortillas	20	0.7	1 tortilla, 5 in. dia.	50	1	1	10
Tuna fish, canned in oil	85	3.0	½ cup, drained solids	170	24	7	0
Tuna salad (see salad, tuna fish)							
Turnip greens (see greens)							
Turnips, cooked	78	2.7	½ cup, diced	18	1	tr	4
Veal cutlet, breaded (wiener schnitzel)	136	4.8	2 slices, 2½ × 2½ × ¾ in.	315	26	21	5
Veal cutlet, broiled	85	3.0	1 cutlet, 3¾ × 3 × ½ in.	185	23	9	—
Veal roast, cooked	85	3.0	2 slices, 3 × 2½ × ¼ in.	230	23	14	0
Vinegar	15	0.5	1 tbsp	2	0	—	1
Waffles	75	2.6	1 waffle, 7 in. dia. (enriched flour)	210	7	7	28
Watermelon, raw	925	32.4	1 wedge, 4 × 8 in., with rind	115	2	1	27
Welsh rarebit	125	4.4	½ cup	330	19	26	6
Wheat flour, white enriched	115	4.0	1 cup, sifted	420	12	1	88
Wheat flour, white unenriched	110	3.9	1 cup, sifted	400	12	1	84
Wheat flour, whole wheat	120	4.2	1 cup, hard wheat	400	16	2	85
Wheat germ	9	0.3	2 tbsp	30	2	1	4
Wheat flakes	30	1.1	1 cup (nutrients added)	105	3	tr	24
Wheat, shredded	25	0.9	1 biscuit, 4 × 2¼ in.	90	2	1	20
White sauce (medium)	65	2.3	¼ cup	110	3	8	6
Yeast, brewers, dry	8	0.3	1 tbsp	25	3	tr	3
Yeast, compressed	28	1.0	one 1-oz cake	25	3	tr	3
Yeast, dry active	28	1.0	four ¼-oz packages	80	12	tr	12
Yogurt, plain	245	8.6	1 cup (made from partially skimmed milk)	125	8	4	13

Adapted from C.F. Adams, *Nutritive Value of American Foods* (Washington, D.C.: U.S. Dept. of Agriculture, 1975).

TABLE B.2 Caloric Content of Selected Alcoholic Beverages

BEVERAGE	AMOUNT	NUMBER OF CALORIES
Beer	8-oz glass	100
Eggnog, holiday variety, made with whiskey and rum	½ cup	225
Whiskey, gin, rum, and vodka		
100 proof	1 jigger (1½ oz)	125
90 proof	1 jigger (1½ oz)	110
86 proof	1 jigger (1½ oz)	105
80 proof	1 jigger (1½ oz)	100
70 proof	1 jigger (1½ oz)	85
Wines		
table wines (such as chablis, claret, Rhine wine, and sauterne)	1 wine glass (about 3 oz)	75
dessert wines (such as muscatel, port, sherry, or Tokay)	1 wine glass (about 3 oz)	125

Adapted from C.F. Adams, *Nutritive Value of American Foods* (Washington, D.C.: U.S. Dept. of Agriculture, 1975).

APPENDIX C

Self-Assessments

ASSESSMENT OF WELLNESS

The attainment of wellness through a physically active life is the essence of this text. Assessment 1.1 will help you identify objectively your current lifestyle behaviors, while Assessment 1.2 will help you clarify your attitudes about exercise.

1.1 Health/Wellness Inventory

Directions

For each statement in the Assessment Personal Inventory, circle the number that most closely applies to your behavior according to the following:

5 if the statement is ALWAYS true
4 if the statement is FREQUENTLY true
3 if the statement is OCCASIONALLY true
2 if the statement is SELDOM true
1 if the statement is NEVER true

After completing the inventory, enter the numbers you have circled next to the statement numbers in Table 1.1 and total your score for each category. Refer to the section entitled "Wellness Status" to determine your degree of wellness.

Wellness Status

To assess your status in each of the six categories, compare your total score in each to the following key:

0–34 In need of substantial improvement.
35–44 Good, but some improvement is desirable.
45–50 Excellent. You are doing very well.

Those who are in need of improvement should carefully examine their scores in each category and target one or two areas for improvement and work on those. Do not become overly ambitious and try to change everything at once, because this strategy will not work.

The Assessment Personal Inventory

Situation		*Score*			
1. I am able to identify the situations and factors that overstress me.	5	4	3	2	1
2. I eat only when I am hungry.	5	4	3	2	1
3. I don't take tranquilizers or other drugs to relax.	5	4	3	2	1
4. I support efforts in my community to reduce environmental pollution.	5	4	3	2	1
5. I avoid buying foods with artificial colors and flavors.	5	4	3	2	1
6. I rarely have a problem concentrating on what I'm doing because of worrying about other things.	5	4	3	2	1
7. My employer (school) takes measures to ensure that my work (study) place is safe.	5	4	3	2	1
8. I try not to use medications when I feel unwell.	5	4	3	2	1
9. I am able to identify certain bodily responses and illnesses as my reactions to stress.	5	4	3	2	1
10. I question the use of diagnostic x-rays.	5	4	3	2	1
11. I try to alter personal living habits that are risk factors for heart disease, cancer, and other lifestyle diseases.	5	4	3	2	1
12. I avoid taking sleeping pills to help me sleep.	5	4	3	2	1
13. I try not to eat foods with refined sugar or corn sugar ingredients.	5	4	3	2	1
14. I accomplish goals I set for myself.	5	4	3	2	1
15. I stretch or bend for several minutes each day to keep my body flexible.	5	4	3	2	1
16. I support immunization of all children for common childhood diseases.	5	4	3	2	1
17. I try to prevent friends from driving after they drink alcohol.	5	4	3	2	1
18. I minimize extra salt intake.	5	4	3	2	1
19. I don't mind when other people and situations make me wait or lose time.	5	4	3	2	1
20. I walk four or fewer flights of stairs rather than take the elevator.	5	4	3	2	1
21. I eat fresh fruit and vegetables.	5	4	3	2	1
22. I use dental floss at least once a day.	5	4	3	2	1
23. I read product labels on foods to determine their ingredients.	5	4	3	2	1
24. I try to maintain a normal body weight.	5	4	3	2	1
25. I record my feelings and thoughts in a journal or diary.	5	4	3	2	1

Continued

26. I have no difficulty falling asleep.	5	4	3	2	I
27. I engage in some form of vigorous physical activity at least three times a week.	5	4	3	2	I
28. I take time each day to quiet my mind and relax.	5	4	3	2	I
29. I am willing to make and sustain close friendships and intimate relationships.	5	4	3	2	I
30. I obtain an adequate daily supply of vitamins from my food or vitamin supplements.	5	4	3	2	I
31. I rarely have tension or migraine headaches or pain in the neck or shoulders.	5	4	3	2	I
32. I wear a seat belt when driving or riding in a car.	5	4	3	2	I
33. I am aware of the emotional and situational factors that lead me to overeat.	5	4	3	2	I
34. I avoid driving my car after drinking alcohol.	5	4	3	2	I
35. I am aware of the side effects of the medicines I take.	5	4	3	2	I
36. I am able to accept feelings of sadness, depression, and anxiety, knowing that they are almost always transient.	5	4	3	2	I
37. I would seek several additional professional opinions if my doctor recommended surgery for me.	5	4	3	2	I
38. I agree that nonsmokers should not have to breathe the smoke from cigarettes in public places.	5	4	3	2	I
39. I agree that pregnant women who smoke are harming their babies.	5	4	3	2	I
40. I feel I get enough sleep.	5	4	3	2	I
41. I ask my doctor why a certain medication is being prescribed and inquire about alternatives.	5	4	3	2	I
42. I am aware of the calories expended in my activities.	5	4	3	2	I
43. I am willing to give priority to my own needs for time and psychological space by saying no to others' requests of me.	5	4	3	2	I
44. I walk instead of drive whenever feasible.	5	4	3	2	I
45. I eat a breakfast that contains about one third of my daily need for calories, proteins, and vitamins.	5	4	3	2	I
46. I prohibit smoking in my home.	5	4	3	2	I
47. I remember and think about my dreams.	5	4	3	2	I
48. I seek medical attention only when I have symptoms or feel that some (potential) condition needs checking rather than have routine yearly checkups.	5	4	3	2	I
49. I endeavor to make my home accident free.	5	4	3	2	I
50. I ask my doctor to explain the diagnosis of my problem until I understand all that I care to.	5	4	3	2	I
51. I try to include fiber or roughage (whole grains, fresh fruits and vegetables, or bran) in my diet.	5	4	3	2	I
52. I can deal with my emotional problems without alcohol or other mood-altering drugs.	5	4	3	2	I
53. I am satisfied with my school/work.	5	4	3	2	I
54. I require children riding in my car to be in infant seats or in shoulder harnesses.	5	4	3	2	I
55. I try to associate with people who have a positive attitude about life.	5	4	3	2	I
56. I try not to eat snacks of candy, pastries, and other junk food.	5	4	3	2	I
57. I avoid people who are down all the time and bring down those around them.	5	4	3	2	I
58. I am aware of the calorie content of the foods I eat.	5	4	3	2	I
59. I brush my teeth after meals.	5	4	3	2	I
60. (for women only) I routinely examine my breasts.	5	4	3	2	I
(for men only) I am aware of the signs of testicular cancer.	5	4	3	2	I

TABLE 1.1 Wellness Category Scores

EMOTIONAL	FITNESS AND BODY CARE	ENVIRONMENTAL HEALTH	STRESS	NUTRITION	MEDICAL SELF-RESPONSIBILITY
6.____	15.____	4.____	I.____	2.____	8.____
12.____	20.____	7.____	3.____	5.____	10.____
25.____	22.____	17.____	9.____	13.____	11.____
26.____	24.____	32.____	14.____	18.____	16.____
36.____	27.____	34.____	19.____	21.____	35.____
40.____	33.____	38.____	28.____	23.____	37.____
47.____	42.____	39.____	29.____	30.____	41.____
52.____	44.____	46.____	31.____	45.____	48.____
55.____	58.____	49.____	43.____	51.____	50.____
57.____	59.____	54.____	53.____	56.____	60.____
Total ____	____	____	____	____	____

1.2 Your Fitness Attitudes

Directions

Respond to each of the following statements by checking the appropriate column. This assessment should help to clarify your attitudes and tendencies about participation in physical fitness activities.

Statements	Agree	Disagree
1. I enjoy exercising.	_____	_____
2. I enjoy active sports and fitness activities.	_____	_____
3. I am inclined toward leading an active rather than a sedentary life.	_____	_____
4. I want to be in good physical condition.	_____	_____
5. I feel that exercising is productive use of leisure time.	_____	_____
6. I find exercise to be invigorating.	_____	_____
7. I feel better after a vigorous workout.	_____	_____
8. I feel that being fit improves my appearance.	_____	_____
9. I feel relaxed after I exercise.	_____	_____
10. I feel that exercise improves my energy level.	_____	_____
11. I do not feel guilty if I miss a day of exercise.	_____	_____
12. I feel guilty if I miss three consecutive days of exercise.	_____	_____
13. I am at the proper weight for my body type.	_____	_____
14. I believe that exercising regularly improves my health status.	_____	_____

My score is _____.

My score indicates _____.

Scoring

1. If you agree with all statements, you have a positive attitude about exercise; and if you begin to exercise, you have a very good chance to continue successfully.
2. If you disagree with one to four statements, your attitude is primarily positive; and if you begin to exercise, you have a good chance to continue successfully.
3. If you disagree with more than four statements, your attitude is less than positive, and you may have difficulty adhering to exercise.

MOTIVATION

Fitness goals are achieved through motivated behavior. Assessment 2.1 will help you determine your likelihood of sticking with an exercise program; Assessment 2.2 will help you quantify your exercise goals and habits; and Assessment 2.3 is a personal fitness contract between you and an important person in your life. This may be the incentive that you need to begin and continue exercising as a way of life.

2.1 Exercise Adherence Scale

Directions

Evaluate yourself using the scale in Table 2.1 by circling the number under the letter that most closely approximates your behavior for each of the seven statements. The key to each letter is as follows:

A very atypical of me
B more or less atypical of me
C neither typical nor atypical of me
D more or less typical of me
E very typical of me

TABLE 2.1 Assessing Exercise Adherence

| SCALE | | | | | |
A	B	C	D	E	ADHERENCE ISSUE
5	4	3	2	1	1. I get discouraged easily.
5	4	3	2	1	2. I don't work any harder than I have to.
1	2	3	4	5	3. I seldom if ever let myself down.
5	4	3	2	1	4. I'm just not the goal-setting type.
1	2	3	4	5	5. I'm good at keeping promises, especially the ones I make to myself.
5	4	3	2	1	6. I don't impose much structure on my activities.
1	2	3	4	5	7. I have a very hard-driving, aggressive personality.

Scoring Procedure

Add the numbers that you have circled for the seven statements to get a total score. Dropout-prone behavior is suggested by a score equal to or less than 24. If your score falls in this category, make a special effort to employ some of the motivational techniques presented in this chapter. Remember, each time you drop out before completing a task, the easier it becomes to drop out of the next one.

SOURCE: Adapted from R. K. Dishman and W. J. Ickes, in B. Falls et al., *Essentials of Fitness*, Philadelphia: Saunders College, 1980.

2.2 The Physical Activity Questionnaire

Your answers to the following questions should help to (1) quantify the amount of of exercise that you are doing currently, (2) point out the types of exercise in which you are interested, (3) underline your reasons for participation, and (4) clarify your attitude regarding exercise.

1. Do you exercise regularly:
   a. 3 to 5 times per week _____
   b. 30 minutes or more per session _____
   c. at 65% of maximum heart rate or greater _____
2. Do you participate regularly in aerobic exercise (walking, jogging, cycling, swimming, and so on)? _____
3. Do you participate regularly in lifetime sports (racquetball, handball, tennis, badminton, and so on)? _____
4. Do you participate primarily in one activity or a combination of activities? _____
5. Do you participate regularly (at least twice a week) in resistance exercises (weight training, calisthenics, and so on)? _____
6. Do you compete in your event(s), or do you exercise for reasons other than competition? _____
7. Is competition, including competing with yourself, an important element of your exercise program? _____
8. Do you prefer to exercise with other people or by yourself? _____
9. Rank the following from the most important to the least important as a motive for you to exercise, with 1 being the most important and 5 being the least important. If your most important is not listed, add it at the bottom of the list and rank it #1.
   a. health _____
   b. physical appearance _____
   c. stress reduction _____
   d. fun and enjoyment _____
   e. competition _____
   f. other _____
10. Which of the following components is most important and which is least important as an outcome of your exercise program?
    a. muscular development _____
    b. cardiorespiratory endurance _____
    c. flexibility _____
11. Is becoming fit and maintaining physical fitness important to you? _____ If so, reflect on the reasons.
12. Do you feel that one can achieve high-level wellness without being physically fit? _____ Think about why you feel the way you do.

2.3 Personal Fitness Contract

Directions

1. State with whom you are contracting (for example: yourself or mother, father, spouse, boyfriend, girlfriend).
2. List specific goals in priority order.
3. Place a check under the fitness component that you are seeking to achieve with each objective. The abbreviations for the fitness components are CRE—cardiorespiratory endurance; MS—muscular strength; ME—muscular endurance, FL—flexibility; and BC—body composition.
4. Fill in the activities that you have selected for the achievement of your objectives.
5. Place a check under each of the fitness components that you believe each of the activities may develop.
6. Fill in the intensity and duration and place a check for the frequency of exercise.

7. Sign and date the contract in the presence of a witness.
8. Have the witness sign the contract.
9. You will find a completed sample contract plus a blank contract for your convenience.

Personal Fitness Contract

I, <u>Lisa Lane</u> am contracting with <u>Dorothy Lane (mother)</u> to develop and participate in a physical fitness program for the purposes listed below
(your name)   (name of significant other)
beginning on the date listed below.

SPECIFIC FITNESS GOALS	FITNESS COMPONENTS				
	CRE	MS	ME	FL	BC
1. Lose 15 lbs—one lb/wk					✓
2. Increase energy level	✓				
3. Gain strength and muscle tissue		✓	✓		✓
4. To increase flexibility				✓	

Activities and Exercise Principles

ACTIVITIES	INTENSITY	DURATION	FREQUENCY							FITNESS COMPONENTS				
			M	T	W	TH	F	SA	SUN	CRE	MS	ME	FL	BC
1. Walk/Jog	Moderate	30–40 min	✓		✓		✓	✓		✓				✓
2. Weight training	8–12 reps	2–3 Sets		✓		✓					✓	✓		✓
3. Stretching	Moderate	8–10 min	✓	✓	✓	✓	✓						✓	
4.														

My program will begin <u>April 1, 1994</u>. I will abide by the conditions of this contract.
Signed Lisa Lane   Date March 21, 1994
Witness Sam Lane   Date March 21, 1994

I, _____ am contracting with _____ to develop and participate in a physical fitness program for the purposes listed below
(your name)   (name of significant other)

beginning on the date listed below.

SPECIFIC FITNESS GOALS	FITNESS COMPONENTS				
	CRE	MS	ME	FL	BC
1.					
2.					
3.					
4.					

Activities and Exercise Principles

ACTIVITIES	INTENSITY	DURATION	FREQUENCY							FITNESS COMPONENTS				
			M	T	W	TH	F	SA	SUN	CRE	MS	ME	FL	BC
1.														
2.														
3.														
4.														

My program will begin _____. I will abide by the conditions of this contract.
Signed _____ Date _____
Witness _____ Date _____

GUIDELINES FOR EXERCISE

Assessments 3.1 and 3.2 provide you with an opportunity to design an exercise program based upon your specific objectives in accordance with accepted exercise guidelines.

3.1 The Karvonen Formula

Use the Karvonen formula to calculate your target heart rate in beats per minute (bpm) during exercise:

THR = target heart rate bpm

Cardiac reserve = maximum heart rate (MHR) minus resting heart rate (RHR)

TI% = training intensity

A. $220 - \underset{\text{your age}}{\underline{\hspace{1.5cm}}} = \underset{\text{your MHR}}{\underline{\hspace{1.5cm}}}$

B. THR = (MHR − RHR) × TI% + RHR

$\text{THR} = (\underset{\text{your MHR}}{\underline{\hspace{1.5cm}}} - \underset{\text{your RHR}}{\underline{\hspace{1.5cm}}}) \times \underset{\text{training level}}{\underline{\hspace{1.5cm}}} + \underset{\text{your RHR}}{\underline{\hspace{1.5cm}}}$

$\text{THR} = \underset{\text{MHR} - \text{RHR}}{\underline{\hspace{1.5cm}}} \times \underset{\text{training level}}{\underline{\hspace{1.5cm}}} + \underset{\text{RHR}}{\underline{\hspace{1cm}}}$

THR = _____ bpm

*See Table 3.2 (Chapter 3, p. 52) for the appropriate exercise intensity for your fitness level.

3.2 Your Personal Exercise Program

Directions

Design your personal exercise program by supplying the following information:

1. What are your reasons for beginning or continuing an exercise program? List your objectives and be as specific as possible.
   1. _____
   2. _____
   3. _____
2. What physical activities will you select to meet your objectives?
   1. _____
   2. _____
   3. _____
   4. _____
3. How often per week do you plan to exercise (frequency)?
   _____
4. How long will each exercise session last (duration)?
   _____
5. How hard do you plan to exercise (intensity)?
   _____

FIELD TEST FLEXIBILITY MEASUREMENTS

It is important to maintain full range of motion throughout life. Loss of flexibility is caused by inactivity rather than aging. You may wish to quantify your current level of flexibility by performing each of the three field tests presented in this chapter. Be sure to warm up before doing each test. Warming up should include light to moderate aerobic activities to heat the muscles, followed by gentle stretches of the muscles and joints to be tested.

4.1 Sit-and-Reach

The sit-and-reach test is primarily a measure of hamstring flexibility, but it also provides some measure of hip and low-back flexibility. The testing device consists of a ruler attached to the top of a wooden box (Figure 4.1). The ruler extends 9 inches (23 centimeters) over the edge of the box facing the subject, who sits on the floor with both legs extended and both feet flat against the box. The subject places one hand on top of the other and, without bending the knees, slowly leans forward, sliding the hands along the ruler as far as possible. The scores are read from the ruler, and the best of three trials is recorded. Bouncing is not permitted, and the knees must not bend at any time during this test. Perform three trials and compare your best score to the standards in Table 4.1

4.2 Back Extension

In this test, the subject lies face down with the hands placed under the shoulders palms down as if getting ready to do a push-up. The subject then extends the arms as shown in Figure 4.2 while keeping the pelvis in contact with the floor. A partner may be needed to help keep the pelvis down. The subject elevates the chest by pushing up with the arms. The muscles of

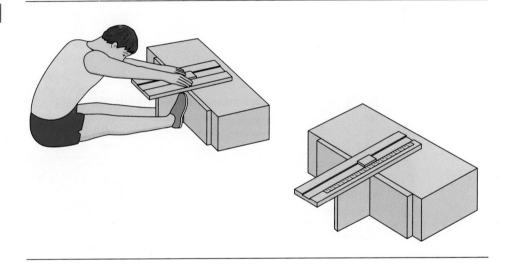

FIGURE 4.1

Sit-and-Reach Test

TABLE 4.1	Sit-and-Reach Test Standards*		
MEN	**WOMEN**	**CLASSIFICATION**	
17.5 or above	18 or above	Excellent	
15.75–17.4	16.5–17.9	Good	
13.5–15.74	14.5–16.4	Average	
10.5–13.4	12.25–14.4	Fair	
Less than 10.5	Less than 12.25	Poor	

*All scores are in inches. An individual's score is the best of three trials.

From R. R. Pate, *Norms for College Students: Health Related Physical Fitness Test,* American Alliance for Health, Physical Education, Recreation and Dance, 1985.

the back are not to be used to assist the lifting action. The score is the distance from the suprasternal notch (the groove at the top of the breastbone) to the floor. Two trials are given, and the best score is compared to the standards in Table 4.2.

4.3 Shoulder Flexion

The shoulder flexion test provides a measure of the elasticity of the deltoids and shoulder girdle. The subject lies in the prone position, arms fully extended, with the chin in contact with the floor (Figure 4.3). From this position, a straight edge held at shoulder width with both hands is raised as high as possible. The distance between the floor and the straight edge is measured, and the best of three trials is recorded and compared to the standards in Table 4.3.

Record your data for the three flexibility tests in the summary box on page 315. How well did you do?

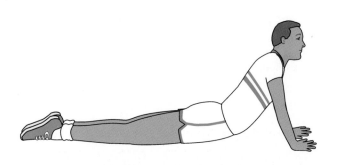

FIGURE 4.2

Back Extension Test

TABLE 4.2 Back Extension Test Standards

| RATING | BACK EXTENSION | |
	cm	in.
Excellent	>30	>11.8
Good	20–29	7.87–11.4
Marginal	10–19	3.9–7.48
Needs Work	<9	<3.9

Adapted from D. Imrie and L. Barbuto, "The Back Power Program," in S. N. Blair et al. (Eds.), *Resource Manual for Exercise Testing and Prescription*, Philadelphia: Lea and Febiger, 1988.

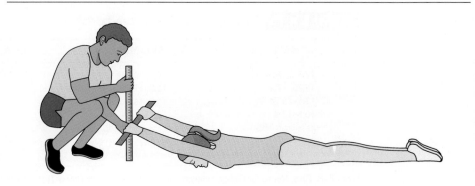

FIGURE 4.3

Shoulder Flexion Test

TABLE 4.3 Shoulder Flexion Test Standards*

MEN	WOMEN	CLASSIFICATION
26 or above	27 or above	Excellent
23–25	24–26	Good
18–22	19–23	Average
13–17	14–18	Fair
12 or below	13 or below	Poor

*All scores are in inches. An individual's score is the best of three trials.

Adapted from W. E. Prentice and C. A. Bucher, *Fitness for College and Life,* St. Louis: Times/Mirror Mosby, 1988; and F. D. Rosato, *Fitness and Wellness: The Physical Connection,* St. Paul: West, 1986.

Summary of Your Flexibility Test Scores

Name _____   Date _____

Complete the following table with your flexibility test scores.

TEST	YOUR SCORE	CLASSIFICATION
Sit-and-Reach		
Back Extension		
Shoulder Flexion		

STRENGTH AND ENDURANCE TESTS

The measurement of muscular strength and endurance requires that several of the major muscle groups be tested. Assessments 5.1, 5.2, and 5.3 comprise a battery of tests that meet strength and endurance testing criteria.

5.1 Muscular Strength Test

Gauging relative muscular strength is not merely measuring the ability to manipulate a weight. A heavier individual may lift more weight than a lighter individual, but the weight may be proportionately less than the lighter person lifted relative to the person's body weight. To be more specific, a 150-pound subject bench presses 200 pounds, while a 250-pound subject bench presses 275 pounds. Who is stronger pound for pound?

The answer is figured by dividing the body weight into the weight lifted. The calculations are as follows.
For 150-lb subject:

$$\frac{200}{150} = 1.33$$

For 250 lb subject:

$$\frac{275}{250} = 1.10$$

You can see that the lighter individual can exert more strength per unit of body weight than can the heavier person.

To determine your own strength per pound of body weight, test yourself in a one-trial maximum effort on the biceps curl, overhead press, bench press, half-squat, and hamstring curl (Figures 5.9, 5.10, 5.11, 5.16, and 5.18 in Chapter 5, pp. 117–121)

TABLE 5.1 Strength-to-Body-Weight Ratio for Men

BICEPS CURL	OVERHEAD PRESS	BENCH PRESS	HALF-SQUAT	HAMSTRING CURL	STRENGTH CATEGORY
.65 and above	1.0 and above	1.30 and above	1.85 and above	.65 and above	Excellent
.55–.64	.90–.99	1.15–1.129	1.65–1.84	.55–.64	Good
.45–.54	.75–.89	1.0–1.14	1.30–1.64	.45–.54	Average
.35–.44	.60–.74	.85–.99	1.0–1.29	.35–.44	Fair
.34 and below	.59 and below	.84 and below	Less than 1.0	.34 and below	Poor

Values adapted from B. L. Johnson and J. K. Nelson, *Practical Measurement for Evaluation in Physical Education*, Minneapolis: Burgess, 1986; and W. W. K. Hoeger, *Lifetime Physical Fitness and Wellness*, Englewood, Colo.: Morton, 1989.

TABLE 5.2 Strength-to-Body-Weight Ratio for Women

BICEPS CURL	OVERHEAD PRESS	BENCH PRESS	HALF-SQUAT	HAMSTRING CURL	STRENGTH CATEGORY
.45 and above	.50 and above	.85 and above	1.45 and above	.55 and above	Excellent
.38–.44	.42–.49	.70–.84	1.30–1.44	.50–.54	Good
.32–.37	.32–.41	.60–.69	1.0–1.29	.40–.49	Average
.25–.31	.25–.31	.50–.59	.80–.99	.30–.39	Fair
.24 and below	.24 and below	.49 and below	.79 and below	.29 and below	Poor

Values adapted from B. L. Johnson and J. K. Nelson, *Practical Measurement for Evaluation in Physical Education*, Minneapolis: Burgess, 1986; and W. W. K. Hoeger, *Lifetime Physical Fitness and Wellness*, Englewood, Colo.: Morton, 1989.

Summary of Your Strength Test Scores

Name _____ Date _____

Complete the following table with your flexibility test scores.

TEST	YOUR SCORES	STRENGTH CATEGORY
Biceps curl		
Overhead press		
Bench press		
Half-squat		
Hamstring curl		

and calculate the ratio by dividing the weight lifted by your body weight. To assess yourself in terms of averages, consult Tables 5.1 and 5.2, which present strength-to-body-weight standards for men and women, respectively.

Note: Do not attempt to lift maximum amounts of weight until you have been in training for at least two months. It is not necessary to test yourself to achieve the health benefits of strength training.

5.2 Muscular Endurance Test

This assessment analyzes muscular endurance of the arm flexors (chin-ups for men—Figure 5.25, p. 125; flexed-arm hang for women—Figure 5.30, p. 127) and the abdominals (bent-knee sit-ups—Figure 5.28, p. 126). Gauge your abdominal endurance by the number of repetitions in 60 seconds. Arm flexor endurance should be measured by repetitions for men and hang time for women.

Table 5.1 presents standards for these muscle endurance categories. Compare your results to the norms in the table to assess your muscular endurance status.

5.3 Canadian Trunk Strength Test

All sit-ups, including the bent-knee type, utilize ancillary muscle groups (the quadriceps and hip flexors) to raise the trunk. The muscle groups, particularly the hip flexors, can be nullified by a partial sit-up or curl-up. It is not necessary nor is it desirable to raise the trunk more than 30 degrees (attained when the shoulder blades clear the mat) for the development of abdominal strength. Sit-ups beyond 30 degrees cause the abdominals

to contract isometrically, while the hip flexors raise the trunk the remainder of the way. The sit-up test in Figure 5.28 (Chapter 5, p. 128) has received a great deal of support and has been administered to literally millions of youths and adults. It is an accepted test and has therefore been included in this Self-Assessment. But I recommend, for the reasons given regarding sitting up beyond 30 degrees, that an adaptation of the Canadian trunk strength test be substituted for the conventional bent-knee sit-up.* Figure 5.1 (p. 319) illustrates this test, which is done in the following manner:

1. Lie on your back with knees bent 90 degrees.
2. Extend your arms so that the fingertips of both hands touch a strip of tape perpendicular to the body on each side (Figure 5.1a).
3. Two additional strips of tape are located parallel to the first two, 8 centimeters apart (approximately 3.15 inches).
4. Curl up, sliding your fingertips along the mat until they touch the second set of tape strips (Figure 5.1b) and then return to the starting position. The tester's hands are placed on the mat below the point where the back of the subject's head would contact the mat. The curl-up is completed when the subject's head touches the tester's hands.
5. The curl-up is slow, controlled, and continuous, with a cadence of 20 curl-ups per minute (three seconds per curl-up).
6. A metronome provides the speed of movement. It is set at 40 beats per minute (curl up on one beat, down on the second).
7. Subjects perform as many curl-ups as they can up to a maximum of 75 without missing a beat. See Table 5.4 for interpretation of your score.

SOURCE: R. A. Faulkner et al., "Partial Curl-up Research Project Final Report," submitted to the Canadian Fitness and Lifestyle Research Institute, 1988.

TABLE 5.3   **Muscle Endurance Standards for Men and Women**

MEN			WOMEN		
Bent-knee Sit-ups (60 sec)	Chin-ups	Endurance Classification	Bent-knee Sit-ups (60 sec)	Flexed-arm Hang (sec)	Endurance Classification
60 or more	20 or more	Excellent	52 or more	30 or more	Excellent
52–59	15–19	Good	44–51	24–29	Good
40–51	10–14	Average	35–43	15–23	Average
35–39	6–9	Fair	30–34	9–14	Fair
34 or fewer	5 or fewer	Poor	29 or fewer	8 or fewer	Poor

Values adapted from R. R. Pate, *Norms for College Students: Health Related Physical Fitness Test,* Reston, Va.: AAHPERD, 1985; and B. L. Johnson and J. K. Nelson, *Practical Measurement for Evaluation in Physical Education,* Minneapolis: Burgess, 1989.

Summary of Your Muscle Endurance Test Scores

Name _____   Date _____

Complete the following table with your flexibility test scores.

TEST	YOUR SCORES	ENDURANCE CLASSIFICATION
Bent-knee sit-up		
Chin-ups		
Flexed-arm hang		

FIGURE 5.1

Canadian Trunk Strength Test

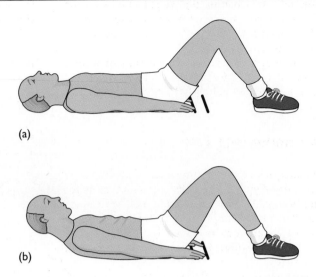

(a)

(b)

TABLE 5.4 **Standards for Partial Curl-up Test**

	NUMBER OF CURL-UPS COMPLETED					
	MEN/AGE			**WOMEN/AGE**		
RATING	**<35**	**35–44**	**>45**	**<35**	**35–44**	**>45**
Excellent	60	50	40	50	40	30
Good	45	40	25	40	25	15
Marginal	30	25	15	25	15	10
Needs Work	15	10	5	10	6	4

Adapted from R. A. Faulkner et al., "Partial Curl-up Research Project Final Report," submitted to the Canadian Fitness and Lifestyle Research Institute, 1988.

ASSESSING CARDIORESPIRATORY FITNESS

The field tests for measuring aerobic capacity are performed outside of the laboratory setting. Using simple equipment, these tests, which estimate VO_2 max, have been validated by comparing their results to those achieved through conventional laboratory techniques. Although not as accurate as laboratory methods, these tests offer a convenient and inexpensive way to estimate cardiorespiratory endurance.

6.1 Rockport Fitness Walking Test

This field test was developed to evaluate aerobic capacity (VO_2 max) without expensive equipment or test technicians. This walking test was validated by testing 343 men and women between the ages of 30 and 69 in the laboratory with a maximum exercise tolerance test. This was followed by two brisk one-mile walks on a measured track on separate days. The results of the walks and the exercise tolerance test were correlated to determine the degree of relationship between the two. There was a high-positive correlation that led the researchers to conclude that aerobic fitness could be predicted quite accurately with the one-mile walking test. The researchers calculated that this test has an estimated error of less than 12 percent.

This walking test has several advantages over the field tests for determining aerobic capacity, including the following: (1) it employs a natural form of locomotion (walking) with which we are all familiar, (2) it is a low-impact activity, (3) it is appropriate for all ages and both sexes, and (4) minimal risk is associated with taking this test.

Since there is some risk associated with virtually all physical activity, it is important before taking this test to review the guidelines established by the American College of Sports Medicine in Chapter 3 regarding medical clearance for exercise.

The Rockport Fitness Walking Test estimates aerobic capacity based upon the variables of age, sex, time needed to walk one mile, and the heart rate achieved at the end of the test. The directions for taking the test are as follows:

1. Heart rate is counted for 15 seconds and multiplied by four to get beats per minute.
2. The course should be flat and measured, preferably a 440-yard track.
3. Be sure to have a stopwatch or a watch with a second hand.
4. Warm up for 5 to 10 minutes before taking the test. Warmup should include a ¼-mile walk followed by the stretching exercises in Chapter 4.
5. When you take the test, walk at a brisk, even pace and cover the distance as rapidly as possible.
6. Take your pulse rate immediately after the test and enter it in the appropriate graph (based upon your age and sex) in Figure 6.1.
7. Draw a vertical line through your time and a horizontal line through your heart rate. The point where the lines intersect will determine your fitness level. (See Figure 6.1).

Rockport provides a series of 20-week walking programs based on the results of the walking test. The programs are available for a nominal fee ($1.00 at this writing) by sending a request to Rockport Fitness Walking Test, 72 Howe St., Marlboro, MA 01752.

6.2 Running Tests

Running tests have become a very popular means for estimating cardiorespiratory endurance. A measured course, preferably a 440-yard track, and a stopwatch are required. Many people can be tested simultaneously. Running tests of sufficient length correlate quite well with treadmill values when subjects are allowed to practice running the course. Practice promotes familiarization with the test and provides an opportunity to develop the sense of pacing needed for optimum performance.

This writer recommends the Balke 1.5-mile run test for adults and older teenagers. This is an adequate distance for the measurement of aerobic capacity. Children and young teenagers should be tested over a shorter distance, such as a one-mile or a nine-minute run. the Balke test covers a fixed distance, making it easy to administer on a track because participants begin and end the tests at the same place. The time taken to run/walk this test represents the score earned. Table 6.1 (p. 324) translates the time spent to cover the distance into estimated VO_2 max in O_2/kg/min. Table 6.2 (p. 324) places the obtained VO_2 max value into a fitness category.

6.3 Bench Step Test

For mass testing, the YMCA utilizes a three-minute bench step test. This test is easy to administer and interpret. The equipment needed includes a sturdy 12-inch high bench, a metronome set at 96 beats per minute (24 cycles per minute—one cycle consists of four steps as follows: up left foot, up right foot, down left foot, down right foot), and preferably a stethoscope to count the heart rate. (If a stethoscope is unavailable, palpation of the wrist or carotid pulse will do.

The subect should step up and down in cadence with the metronome for three minutes. Every beat of the metronome is accompanied by a step by the subject. At the end of the three minutes of stepping, the subject immediately sits down. The pulse count must be started within the first five seconds and continued for one full minute. This one-minute post-exercise heart rate is the score for the test. Turn to Table 6.3 (p. 324) for scoring.

Turn to page 325 and record your data for the cardiorespiratory endurance tests in the summary box. How did your performances on the three tests compare?

FIGURE 6.1

Relative Fitness Level Charts

These charts are designed to tell you how fit you are compared to other individuals of your age and sex. For example, if your coordinates place you in the above-average section of the chart, you're in better shape than the average person in your category. The charts are based on weights of 170 lbs for men and 125 for women. If you weigh substantially more, your relative cardiorespiratory fitness level will be slightly overestimated. If you weigh substantially less, your relative cardiorespiratory fitness level will be slightly underestimated.

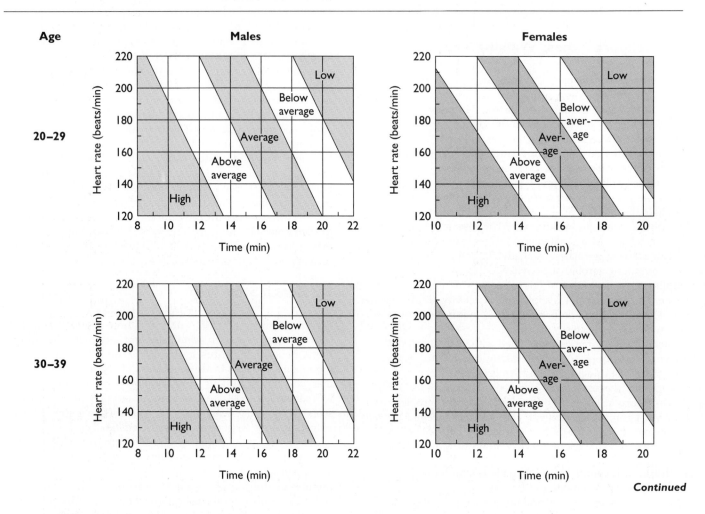

Continued

FIGURE 6.1

Relative Fitness Level Charts—*Continued*

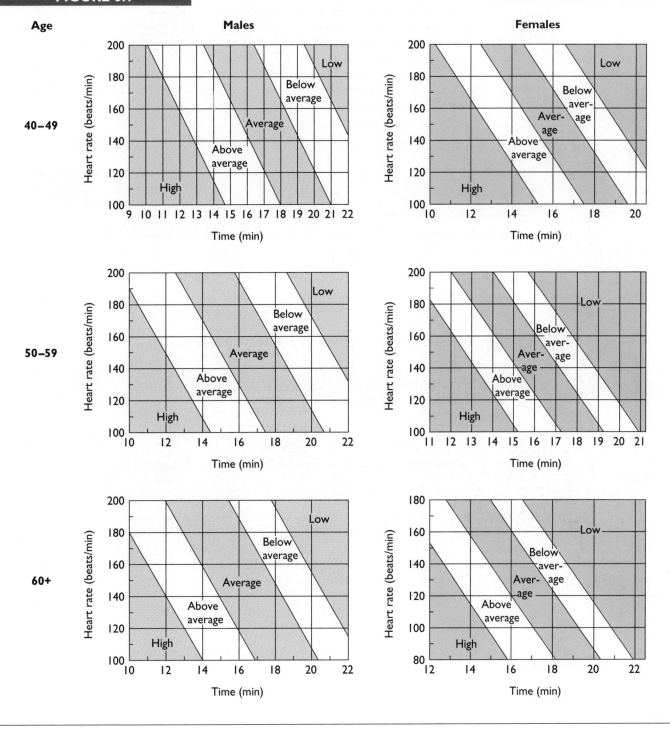

TABLE 6.1   1.5-Mile Run Test—Estimated VO$_2$ Max

TIME IN MINUTES AND SECONDS	ESTIMATED VO$_2$ MAX (ML/KG/MIN)	TIME IN MINUTES AND SECONDS	ESTIMATED VO$_2$ MAX (ML/KG/MIN)
7:30 or less	75	12:31–13:00	39
7:31–8:00	72	13:01–13:30	37
8:01–8:30	67	13:31–14:00	36
8:31–9:00	62	14:01–14:30	34
9:01–9:30	58	14:31–15:00	33
9:31–10:00	55	15:01–15:30	31
10:01–10:30	52	15:31–16:00	30
10:31–11:00	49	16:01–16:30	28
11:01–11:30	46	16:31–17:00	27
11:31–12:00	44	17:01–17:30	26
12:01–12:30	41	17:31–18:00	25

Adapted from K. H. Cooper, "A Means of Assessing Maximal Oxygen Intake," *Journal of the American Medical Association* 203 (1968): 201.

TABLE 6.2   1.5-Mile Run Test—Estimated VO$_2$ Max Fitness Category

AGE GROUP (YR) MALES*	HIGH	GOOD	AVERAGE	FAIR	POOR
10–19	Above 66	57–66	47–56	38–46	Below 38
20–29	Above 62	53–62	43–52	33–42	Below 33
30–39	Above 58	49–58	39–48	30–38	Below 30
40–49	Above 54	45–54	36–44	26–35	Below 26
50–59	Above 50	42–50	34–41	24–33	Below 24
60–69	Above 46	39–46	31–38	22–30	Below 22
70–79	Above 42	36–42	28–35	20–27	Below 20

*The average maximum oxygen uptake of females is 15% to 20% lower than that of males. To find the appropriate category for females, locate the score in the table and shift one category to the left; e.g., the Average category for males is the Good category for females.

Adapted from J. H. Wilmore, *Training for Sport and Activity*, Boston: Allyn and Bacon, 1982.

TABLE 6.3   YMCA 3-Minute Bench Step Test Post-Exercise 1-Minute Heart Rate (beats/minute)

AGE (YRS)	18–25		26–35		36–45	
Gender	M	F	M	F	M	F
Excellent	70–78	72–83	73–79	72–86	72–81	74–87
Good	82–88	88–97	83–88	91–97	86–94	93–101
Above Average	91–97	100–106	91–97	103–110	98–102	104–109
Average	101–104	110–116	101–106	112–118	105–111	111–117
Below Average	107–114	118–124	109–116	121–127	113–118	120–127
Poor	118–126	128–137	119–126	129–135	120–128	130–138
Very Poor	131–164	141–155	130–164	141–154	132–168	143–152

Adapted from L. A. Golding et al., *The Y's Way to Physical Fitness*, Champaign, Ill.: Human Kinetics, 1989. For age ranges above those listed in the table, refer to the preceding source. *Note:* Pusle is to be counted for one full minute following 3 minutes of stepping at 24 cycles per minute on a 12-inch bench.

Summary of Cardiorespiratory Endurance Tests

Name _____ Date _____

Complete the following table with your cardiorespiratory endurance scores.

	H. R.	TIME	VO$_2$ MAX	FITNESS CATEGORY
Rockport Test				
1 ½-Mile Run Test				
Bench Step Test				

CARDIOVASCULAR RISKS: IDENTIFICATION AND APPLICATION

You can identify your risk factors for heart disease in Assessment 7.1. Assessment 7.2 gives the opportunity to apply your knowledge of the risk factors to the case study provided.

7.1 Cardiac Risk

Now that you have a better understanding of the risk factors associated with heart disease, you are ready to take and appreciate the Cardiac Risk Assessment test in Table 7.1. Carefully examine each category of risk factors and select the description and accompanying score that applies to you. If you don't know your blood cholesterol level, examine the fat content of your diet and answer accordingly. If you still cannot decide, select the box that contains 20 percent animal fat for your answer. Total your score for all 8 categories and determine your degree of risk by comparing your score with the Risk Keyat the bottom of the table (You will note that stress is momitted as one of the risks, because it is unimportant, but because it is difficult to quantify.)

7.2 Case Study—Robert S.

Directions
Apply your knowledge of cardiovascular health and wellness to the case below. Use the Cardiac Risk Assessment to assist you in evaluating the risk of Robert S.

Robert S., a 54-year-old male who is 5'9" tall and weighs 210 lbs, has the following history:

1. Father died of a heart attack at age 61, and grandfather died of a heart attack at age 52.
2. Cholesterol level is 268 mg/dL; LDL is 182 mg/dL; HDL is 37 mg/dL.
3. Blood pressure is consistently in the 155/95 range.
4. Smoked two packs of cigarettes per day for 30 years but quit three months ago.
5. Drinks six to eight brewed cups of coffee daily.
6. Occasionally plays a set of tennis on Sunday afternoons.
7. Self-employed—often works 60 to 65 hours per week.

Answer the following:

1. His total risk according to the Cardiac Risk Assessment is

_____.

TABLE 7.1 Cardiac Risk Assessment

FACTOR	SCORE	FACTOR	SCORE
Age		**Exercise**	
10–20	1	Intensive occupational and recreational exertion	1
21–30	2	Moderate occupational and recreational exercise.	2
31–40	3	Sedentary work and intense recreational exertion.	3
41–50	4	Sedentary work and moderate recreational exertion.	5
51–60	6	Sedentary work and light recreational exertion.	6
61–70	8	Complete lack of exercise.	8
Weight		**Cholesterol**	
More than 5 lb below standard weight.	0	Below 180 mg. Diet contains no animal or solid fats.	1
Standard weight.	1	181–205 mg. Diet contains 10% animal or solid fats.	2
5–20 lb overweight.	2	206–230 mg. Diet contains 20% animal or solid fats.	3
21–35 lb overweight.	3	231–255 mg. Diet contains 30% animal or solid fats.	4
36–50 lb overweight.	5	256–280 mg. Diet contains 40% animal or solid fats.	5
51–65 lb overweight.	7	281–330 mg. Diet contains 50% animal or solid fats.	7
Blood pressure		**Heredity**	
100 upper reading.	1	No known history of heart disease.	1
120 upper reading.	2	One relative with cardiovascular disease over 60.	2
140 upper reading.	4	Two relatives with cardiovascular disease over 60.	3
160 upper reading.	4	One relative with cardiovascular disease under 60.	4
180 upper reading.	6	Two relatives with cardiovascular disease under 60.	6
200 or over upper reading.	8	Three relatives with cardiovascular disease under 60.	8
Tobacco Usage		**Gender**	
Nonuser.	0	Female.	1
Cigar and/or pipe.	1	Female over 45.	2
10 or fewer cigarettes a day.	2	Male.	3
20 cigarettes a day.	3	Bald Male.	4
30 cigarettes a day.	5	Bald, short male.	6
40 more more cigarettes a day.	8	Bald, short, stocky male.	7

RISK KEY		
Very low risk = 6–11	Average risk = 18–25	Dangerous risk = 33–42
Low risk = 12–17	High risk = 26–32	Extremely dangerous risk = 42–60

G. Edlin and E. Golanty, *Health and Wellness*, Boston: Jones & Bartlett, 1988. Adapted from an instrument developed by John Boyer.

2. Identify his risk factors for cardiovascular disease: _____

_____

3. Which of these risk factors can he change? _____

_____

4. What suggestions can you give him regarding his need for exercise? _____

_____

5. How might exercise affect his coronary risk profile? _____

_____

_____

7.3 Distribution of Body Fat

Fat that accumulates in the upper half of the body is a risk factor for heart attack, stroke, diabetes, and some forms of cancer. To assess your risk, take the following steps:

1. Use a flexible tape measure and be sure that it is parallel to the floor when taking your hip and waist measurements.
2. Make both measurements in the standing position.
3. Measure the circumference of your waist at about the level of your navel and record that value:_____
4. Measure the circumference of your hips at the greatest protuberance of your buttocks and record that value:_____
5. Divide your waist measurement by your hip measurement:

$$\frac{\text{Waist}}{\text{Hip}} = \text{_____}$$

6. Interpretation:

   Females If your waist-to-hip ratio is 80% or greater, you have a higher than normal risk.

   Males If your waist-to-hip ratio is 1.0 or greater, you are at a higher than normal risk.

7.4 Diabetes Check

Directions

Check the appropriate response for each of the items in this inventory. If you checked five more more of these items, see your physician.

	Yes	No
1. Is there a history of diabetes in your family?	_____	_____
2. Do you tire quickly or seem to always be fatigued?	_____	_____
3. Do you urinate frequently?	_____	_____
4. Are you constantly thirsty?	_____	_____
5. Is your vision blurry?	_____	_____
6. Have you suddenly lost weight?	_____	_____
7. Are you overweight?	_____	_____
8. Do you eat excessively?	_____	_____
9. Do wounds heal slowly?	_____	_____
10. Is your skin frequently itchy?	_____	_____

OTHER CHRONIC CONDITIONS: DETRACTORS TO QUANTITY AND QUALITY OF LIFE

Assessment 8.1 exposes you to the risk factors and warning signs of cancer; Assessment 8.2 describes the impact of cigarette smoking on longevity; Assessment 8.3 shows that life change events may effect your health; and Assessment 8.4 makes you aware of how you react to stressful events.

8.1 Cancer Awareness

Directions

This inventory presents the major symptoms for some common forms of cancer. Check only those symptoms that you are currently experiencing. If you have more than one, check for a specific form of cancer and consult your physician. The likelihood of having cancer is minimal, but it is better to be safe.

Symptoms	Check each that applies to you
1. *Bladder*	
a. blood in urine	_____
b. change in bladder habits	_____
c. uncomfortable urination	_____
d. less forceful stream	_____
e. urge to urinate more frequently	_____
2. *Breast*	
a. thickening or lump in the breast	_____
b. lump under the arm	_____
c. thickening or reddening of breast skin	_____
d. puckering or dimpling of breast skin	_____
e. discharge from nipple(s)	_____
f. inverted nipple if previously erect	_____
g. persistent pain and/or tenderness of breast(s)	_____
h. lumps in the breast(s)	_____
3. *Colon/Rectum*	
a. continuous constipation or diarrhea	_____
b. rectal bleeding	_____
c. change in bowel habits	_____
d. increase in intestinal gas	_____
e. abdominal discomfort	_____
4. *Lung*	
a. unusual and persistent cough	_____
b. shortness of breath	_____
c. blood-streaked sputum	_____
d. chest pain	_____
e. recurrent attacks of pneumonia or bronchitis	_____
5. *Oral*	
a. a sore in the mouth that does not heal	_____
b. lump or thickening that bleeds easily	_____
c. difficulty in chewing or swallowing food	_____
d. the sensation of something in the throat	_____
e. restricted movement of the tongue or jaw	_____
6. *Skin*	
a. obvious change in a wart or mole	_____
b. unusual skin condition	_____
c. chronic swelling, redness, or warmth of the skin	_____
d. unexplained itching	_____

Continued

7. *Testicular*
   a. an enlargement or lump _____
   b. change in testicular consistency _____
   c. dull ache in lower abdomen or groin _____
   d. sensation of dragging or heaviness _____
   e. difficult ejaculation _____
8. *Uterine/Cervical*
   a. irregular bleeding _____
   b. unusual vaginal discharge _____
   c. positive Pap smear _____
   d. recurring herpes _____
   e. fibroid tumors of the uterus _____
9. *Leukemia*
   a. fatigue (general and persistent) _____
   b. paleness _____
   c. unexplained weight loss _____
   d. repeated infections _____
   e. easily bruised _____
   f. nosebleeds or other hemorrhages _____
Interpretation _____
1. Number of symptoms checked _____
2. What action should I take _____

*If the symptom(s) you have checked persist for two weeks, see your physician. Bear in mind that these symptoms are associated with many ailments. Let your physician make the diagnosis.

Adapted from several sources from The American Cancer Society.

8.2 Years of Life Lost from Smoking

Directions
Calculate the number of years lost for an individual who has smoked a pack of cigarettes every day for 30 years. Use the figure that 3½ hours of life are lost for every pack of cigarettes smoked.

a. 24 hrs/day × 365 days/yr = _____
b. 3.5 hours × 365 packs/yr = _____ hours of life lost per year
c. 1277.5 hrs lost/yr × 30 yrs = _____ hrs of life lost in 30 years
d. *Divide the answer for (c) by the answer in (a): $\frac{c}{a}$ = _____ years of life lost to cigarette smoking

*The answer to this problem is 4.38 years of life lost.

8.3 Life Events Scale–Student Version

The scale in Table 8.1 is an adaptation of the Holmes-Rahe Life Events Scale. This scale focuses on those events that typically affect college-age people. Respond to the changes in your life by checking those items that you have experienced during the past year. Total the points and interpret the results as follows:

1. 300 points or more—high risk of developing a health problem or experiencing a negative health change in the following year.

2. 150–300 points—you have a 50-50 chance of experiencing a negative health change within two years.
3. Less than 150 points—you have a one-in-three chance of experiencing a negative health change in the next couple of years.

Note: Remember, it is your reaction to life changes rather than the change itself that produces the seriousness of the stress. Deal with life changes constructively by doing the following:

1. Consider what the change means to you personally.
2. Consider the change's meaning in your life and focus on your feelings about it.
3. Examine and explore alternatives for adjusting to the change.
4. Think it through before acting—a measured response is usually better than an impulsive one.
5. Pace yourself. Frenetic activity leads to ineffectiveness, and it is a drain on one's energy reserve.
6. Engage in relaxation activities such as exercise, voluntary relaxation techniques, or other enjoyable activities such as a movie, a concert, a picnic, an outing.
7. Follow a regular daily routine as closely as possible.
8. Talk to family and friends who can be a source of support as well as objective observers who may be able to offer alternative solutions.

TABLE 8.1 Life Events Scale—Student Version

EVENT	LIFE CHANGE UNITS	EVENT	LIFE CHANGE UNITS	EVENT	LIFE CHANGE UNITS
Death of close family member	100	Serious argument with close friend	40	Change in sleeping habits	29
Death of a close friend	73	Change in financial status	39	Change in social activities	29
Divorce between parents	65	Trouble with parents	39	Change in eating habits	28
Jail term	63	Change of major	39	Chronic car trouble	26
Major personal injury or illness	63	New girlfriend or boyfriend	38	Change in number of family get-togethers	26
Marriage	58	Increased workload at school	37	Too many missed classes	25
Fired from job	50	Outstanding personal achievement	36	Change of college/change of work	24
Failed important course	47	First quarter/semester in college	35	Dropped more than one class	23
Change in health of family member	45	Change in living conditions	31	Minor traffic violations	20
Pregnancy	45	Serious argument with instructor	30		
Sex problems	44	Lower grades than expected	29		

Your Score _____

How do you interpret your score? _____

8.4 Manifestation of Stress—Mind, Body, Combination of Both

Directions

Imagine that your turn has come to make a speech to your class on a topic chosen for you by the instructor. You must deliver this presentation without notes. As you walk from your seat to the front of the room to face the class, what emotions are you feeling? What behaviors are produced by this event? Mark only the following items that apply to your feelings in this or another equally stressful situation.

1. _____ My heart beats fast, and I feel that it might explode.
2. _____ I feel anxious, jittery, and tense.
3. _____ I worry too much about things that don't really matter, some of which might never occur. I worry for nothing.
4. _____ I feel that I'm losing out because I can't make decisions quickly enough.
5. _____ I can't stop thinking troublesome thoughts.
6. _____ I perspire, and it often carries a pungent odor.
7. _____ I experience diarrhea in stressful situations.

8. _____ I imagine unpleasant thoughts, such as, "I know I'm going to freeze up and won't be able to talk."
9. _____ I can't sit still—I'm nervous and fidgety, and I pace back and forth.
10. _____ My stomach has butterflies.
11. _____ I experience extraneous and unimportant thoughts.
12. _____ I am reluctant to take action; I become immobilized.
13. _____ I can't keep anxiety-provoking images out of my mind.
14. _____ I find it difficult to concentrate on the important components of the task.

Interpretation

1. Items that I have checked are numbers _____
2. If you checked items 1, 2, 6, 7, 9, 10, and 12, your stress level is primarily manifested in bodily reactions.
3. If you checked items 3, 4, 5, 8, 11, 13, and 14, you manifest your stress level in mental worries.
4. If you have checked more body items, your stress is manifested mainly by physical reactions; if you checked more mind items, you are a mental stress type; if you checked about the same number of each (±1), you are mixed reactor.

THE BASICS OF NUTRITION

Assessment 9.1 lets you examine your current dietary habits; Assessment 9.2 helps you to quantify daily protein requirements; and Assessment 9.3 helps you to develop a two-day food plan based on the recommendations of the Food Guide Pyramid.

9.1 Nutrition Inventory

Directions

We have presented what you should be doing nutritionally, and now you will have the opportunity to examine your eating patterns in the assessment quiz presented in Table 9.1. Answer each of the questions as accurately as possible. Note the number of yes answers at the end of each section and transfer these figures into the appropriate blank in Table 9.2. This will show you how well or how poorly you are doing in each area of nutrition. Finally, total the section scores for an overall score and compare it to the key given in Table 9.2. If your score is in the "poor" or "fair" category, it is time to start making some changes in your nutritional patterns.

9.2 Assessing Protein Requirements

What is the protein requirement for a moderately active 120-lb adult female who consumes 1,900 kCals/day? Assume that 15% of her total kCals comes from protein.

1. Convert body weight in lbs. to kilograms (kg): _____ kg
   1 kg = 2.2 lbs.
   $\dfrac{120}{2.2} =$
2. kCals of protein consumed: _____ kCals
   $1,900 \times .15 =$
3. Grams (gms) of protein consumed: _____ gms
   $\dfrac{285}{4} =$
4. Grams of protein required: _____ gms
   $54.8 \times .8 =$
5. Difference between protein consumed and that which is needed: _____ gms
   (gms consumed) – (gms needed) =

Answers

1. 54.5 kg
2. 285 kCals
3. 71.25 gms
4. 43.6 gms
5. 27.65 gms

9.3 Two-day Food Plan

Using the chart on pages 335 and 336, devise a two day food plan for yourself based on the recommendations of the food guide pyramid. Each day will consist of three meals and one snack. Maintain the proportions suggested in the pyramid.

TABLE 9.1 **Nutrition Quiz**

SECTION 1–MEAT, MEAT ALTERNATES

Do I:	Response	
1. Limit consumption of meat, fish, poultry or egg to once or twice a day?	yes	no
2. Eat red meats (beef, ham, lamb, or pork) three or fewer times per week?	yes	no
3. Remove all visible fat from meat prior to cooking?	yes	no
4. Limit consumption of eggs to three or four per week, including those cooked in other foods?	yes	no
5. Occasionally have meatless days by substituting legumes and nuts for protein?	yes	no
6. Usually broil, bake, roast, or boil meat, fish or poultry and abstain from frying?	yes	no
Total "Yes" Answers _____		

SECTION 2–DAIRY

Do I:	Response	
1. Have two or more cups of milk or the equivalent in milk products daily?	yes	no
2. Drink or use low-fat or skim milk (2% or less butterfat)?	yes	no
3. Limit ice cream or ice milk to twice per week or less?	yes	no
4. Generally consume less than 3 tsp. of margarine or butter per day?	yes	no
Total "Yes" Answers _____		

SECTION 3—FRUIT, VEGETABLES

Do I:	Response	
1. Usually consume at least one-half cup of citrus fruit or juice (oranges, grapefruit, etc.) daily?	yes	no

Continued

TABLE 9.1 Nutrition Quiz—Continued

SECTION 3—FRUIT, VEGETABLES

Do I:	Response	
2. Have at least one serving of dark green or deep orange vegetables daily?	yes	no
3. Eat fresh fruit and vegetables daily?	yes	no
4. Cook vegetables without fat, such as bacon drippings or ham hock?	yes	no
5. Eat fresh fruit for desert more often than cakes, cookies, and other pastries?	yes	no

Total "Yes" Answers _____

SECTION 4—GRAINS

Do I:	Response	
1. Usually eat whole grain breads?	yes	no
2. Usually eat whole grain cereals that are good sources of fiber?	yes	no
3. Eat cereals that have no sugar or are low in sugar?	yes	no
4. Substitute brown rice for white rice?	yes	no
5. Consume at least four servings of bread or cereal grain products each day?	yes	no

SECTION 5–POTPOURRI

Do I:	Response	
1. Remain within 5 to 10 lbs of my optimal weight for my height?	yes	no
2. Drink less than 1 ½ oz of alcohol (one to two drinks) per day?	yes	no
3. Abstain from adding salt to food after it is served and prefer foods that are lightly salted or not salted at all?	yes	no
4. Try to avoid foods high in refined sugar?	yes	no
5. Always eat a breakfast of at least cereal and milk, egg and toast, or other protein carbohydrate combination with fruit or fruit juice?	yes	no

Total "Yes" Answers _____

TABLE 9.2 Nutrition Quiz Score Evaluation

SECTION	EXCELLENT	GOOD	FAIR	POOR	SCORE
1. Meat/meat alternate choices	5–6	4	3	2–0	_____
2. Dairy choices	4	3	2	1–0	_____
3. Fruit/vegetable choices	5	4	3	2–0	_____
4. Grain choice	5	4	3	2–0	_____
5. Potpourri	5	4	3	2–0	_____
				Total Score	_____

Key: Excellent 24–25
Good 19–23
Fair 14–18
Poor 13 or less

Adapted from M. A. Boyle and E. N. Whitney, *Personal Nutrition,* St. Paul: West, 1989.

Meal	Food Selections	Portion
Breakfast		
Snack		
Lunch		
Supper		

Meal	Food Selections	Portion
Breakfast		
Snack		
Lunch		
Supper		

THE REDUCTION EQUATION: EXERCISE + SENSIBLE EATING = FAT CONTROL

Assessment 10.1 provides a method for determining the energy expenditure for various physical activities; Assessment 10.2 allows you to assess your cardiovascular risk with BMI measurements; Assessment 10.3 provides you with a method for determining desirable body weight from BMI measurements; Assessment 10.4 helps you to estimate both resting metabolic rate and total energy expenditure; and Assessment 10.5 helps you to calculate your resting metabolic rate.

10.1 Estimating the Caloric Cost of Exercise

Directions
Refer to Table 10.1 (p. 246) to solve this problem. Select your favorite physical activity or an activity in which you would like to participate. Calculate the energy that you would expend.

1. a. Per workout _____ kCals
   (multiply cal/min/lb × body weight × minutes spent exercising)
   b. Per week _____ kCals
   (multiply kCals per workout × 5)
   c. Per year _____ kCals
   (multiply kCals/wk × 52)
2. At this level of exercise, how much energy in lbs would you expend:
   b. Per week _____ lbs
   (divide kCals per week × 3,500)
   c. Per year _____ lbs
   (divide kCals expended per year by 3,500)

10.2 Estimating Cardiovascular Risk with BMI

Directions
Calculate your BMI using the following procedure:

1. Convert your body weight (BW) in lbs to kilograms (kg):
   $$\frac{BW}{2.2} = \text{_____} \text{ kg}$$
2. Convert height (ht) in inches to meters (m):
   Ht × .0254 = _____ m
3. Insert the preceding conversions into the formula
   $$BMI = \frac{Wt\ (kg)}{Ht\ (m^2)}$$
4. Your BMI is _____ kg/m²
5. Interpretation:
   a. Males
      1. desirable = 22 to 24 kg/m²
      2. cardiovascular risk ≥ 27.8 kg/m²
   a. Females
      1. desirable = 21 to 23 kg/m²
      2. cardiovascular risk ≥ 27.3 kg/m²
6. Does your BMI put you at risk for cardiovascular disease?
   Yes _____ No _____

10.3 Estimating Desirable Body Weight from BMI

Directions
Use the data from Self-Assessment 10.2 to determine your optimal body weight using BMI calculations. If your BMI is in the desirable range of 21 to 23 kg/m² for females and 22 to 24 kg/m² for males, it won't be necessary for you to make a change. Instead, assume that a male friend has asked you to help him attain a desirable body weight. His data are as follows: He is 5'10" tall and weighs 210 lbs. His current BMI is 30.1 kg/m². His goal is to attain a BMI of 22 kg/m². How much weight does he need to lose, and how much would he weigh at a BMI of 22 kg/m²?

If your BMI is outside the acceptable range, use your own data in the following calculations:

1. Your current BMI is _____ kg/m².
2. Your weight in kg is _____ kg.
3. Your height in m² is _____ m².
4. Your desired BMI is _____ (choose this value from Table 10.6 (p. 258).
5. Your desirable body weight in kg is found by multiplying desired BMI times height m²:

   DBW = desired BMI × height m²
   = _____ × _____
6. Convert DBW from kg to lbs by multiplying DBW (kg) times 2.2:

   DBW kg   DBW (lbs)
   _____ × 2.2 = _____
7. Subtract DBW (lbs) from current body weight (lbs) to find out the target weight.
   Current BW (lbs) minus DBW (lbs) = amount of weight to lose in lbs _____

10.4 Calculating Resting Metabolic Rate (RMR) and Total Energy Expenditure

Calculate your resting metabolic rate (RMR). Use the factor 1.0 kCal per kilogram of body weight per hour for males (1 kCal/kg/hr) and 0.9 kCals per kilogram of body weight per hour for females (0.9 kCals/kg/hr). (The lb/kg conversion is 2.2 lb per 1 kg.) Using an example of a 160-lb male, the calculations are as follows:

1. Change body weight in pounds to kilograms:
   $$\frac{160\ lbs}{2.2\ kg} = 72.7\ kg$$
2. Multiply weight in kilograms × the RMR factor:
   72.7 kg × 1 kCal/kg/hr = 72.7 kCals/hr
3. Multiply kCals/hr × 24 hours:
   72.7 kCals/hr × 24 hrs = 1,744.8 kCals/day
4. The RMR is 1,744.8 kCals/day.

Next, you need to approximate the number of kCals expended in daily activities as estimated by the amount of muscular movement you do during the course of a day. This is a rough approximation, but you should be in the ballpark if you use the following guidelines and select the category that fits you best.

- *Sedentary*. Student; desk job; etc; mostly sitting in your occupation and leisure time. Add 40 percent to 50 percent of the RMR.
- *Light Activity*. Teacher; assembly-line worker; walk two miles regularly. Add 55 percent to 65 percent of the RMR.
- *Moderate Activity*. Waitress; waiter; aerobic exercise at about 75 percent of maximum heart rate. Add 65 percent to 70 percent of the RMR.
- *Heavy Activity*. Construction worker; aerobic exercise above 75 percent of maximum heart rate. Add 75 percent to 100 percent of RMR.

Next, determine the kCals expended in daily activities. This 160-lb male 20-year-old is essentially sedentary both occupationally and in his leisure time, so we will multiply the RMR by 45 percent and then add this value back to the RMR.

$1,744.8 \times .45 = 785.2$ kCals burned in daily activities
Add the RMR kCals to the kCals burned for daily activities to get the total energy expenditure for one day.
$1,744.8 + 785.2 = 2,530$ total kCals/day

10.5 Calculating Your RMR

Directions

Following the example in Self-Assessment 10.4, calculate your RMR and complete the following:

1. RMR is _____ kCals.
2. kCals expended in daily activities: _____.
3. Total kCals needed per day: _____.

THE CONSEQUENCE OF NEGATIVE CHOICES: SMOKING AND ALCOHOL

Assessment 11.1 provides smokers with insight as to why they smoke, while Assessment 11.2 helps you recognize behaviors associated with problem drinking.

11.1 Why Do You Smoke?

People frequently use the following statements to describe the benefits they associate with smoking. Think carefully about how you feel when you smoke; then read the statements. Circle the number for each statement that most closely corresponds to your feelings about that statement. Be sure to mark an answer for every statement. When you are finished, follow the directions for scoring your responses.

After completing the above assessment, complete the spaces below with the numbers you circled above. For example, if the answer you circled in A is a numeral 3, place the 3 on the line above the A.

	Never	Seldom	Sometimes	Often	Never
A. I smoke to keep from slowing down.	1	2	3	4	5
B. Handling a cigarette is part of my enjoyment in smoking it.	1	2	3	4	5
C. Smoking is pleasant and relaxing.	1	2	3	4	5
D. I light up when I feel angry about something.	1	2	3	4	5
E. When I run out of something to smoke, I find it unbearable until I can get something.	1	2	3	4	5
F. I smoke automatically, without even being aware of it.	1	2	3	4	5
G. I smoke to stimulate me, to perk me up.	1	2	3	4	5
H. Part of my enjoyment in smoking comes from the steps I take to light up.	1	2	3	4	5
I. I find smoking pleasurable.	1	2	3	4	5
J. When I feel uncomfortable or upset, I light up a smoke.	1	2	3	4	5
K. When I am not smoking, I am very much aware of it.	1	2	3	4	5
L. I light up without realizing I still have a cigarette burning in the ashtray.	1	2	3	4	5
M. I smoke to give me a lift.	1	2	3	4	5
N. When I smoke, part of my enjoyment is watching the smoke I exhale.	1	2	3	4	5
O. I want to smoke most when I am comfortable and relaxed.	1	2	3	4	5
P. When I feel down or want to take my mind off my cares and worries, I smoke.	1	2	3	4	5
Q. I get a real gnawing hunger to smoke when I haven't smoked for a while.	1	2	3	4	5
R. I have found myself smoking and not remembered putting the cigarette in my mouth.	1	2	3	4	5

When you have filled in all the spaces, add the numbers across for a total score. Each line across provides you with a number that indicates how important that aspect of smoking is for you. Knowing *why* you smoke can be important in quitting. If you smoke for pleasurable relaxation, this is the area in which you need to find a substitute. If you score higher than 11 in any area, it indicates that this is an important part of your continued smoking. Explanations of each category are provided on page 340.

				Your Totals
____ + ____ + ____ =				
A	G	M		Stimulation
____ + ____ + ____ =				
B	H	N		Handling
____ + ____ + ____ =				
C	I	O		Pleasurable Relaxation
____ + ____ + ____ =				
D	J	P		Crutch: Tensions Relaxation
____ + ____ + ____ =				
E	K	Q		Craving: Psychological Addiction
____ + ____ + ____ =				
F	L	R		Habit

Stimulation

If you score high in this category, it indicates that you find smoking to be energizing and stimulating. To successfully abstain, you should find alternative sources of providing you with energy.

Handling

For you, cigarettes provide you with something to do with your hands. Abstinence strategies require your finding something to do with your hands.

Relaxation

You feel more relaxed when you are smoking. To quit smoking, you will need to develop new relaxation habits and rewards that are healthy.

Stress

Many smokers find cigarettes a way to comfort themselves when they feel tense from stress. You will need to find different strategies to manage stress.

Craving

This is another category where many smokers score high. The craving you experience indicates that you feel hooked on cigarettes. Since each cigarette you smoke provides a stimulus for the next, total abstinence is required.

Habit

Smoking is an automatic event for you and not necessarily a source of satisfaction. Pay careful attention to your smoking pattern and then attempt to find alternative ways of completing your daily tasks. A change of routine may be the major impetus for you to quit.

SOURCE: Adapted from D. H. Horn, National Clearinghouse for Smoking and Health, DHEW.

11.2 Indications of a Problem with Alcohol

The purposes of this assessment is to help you recognize behaviors associated with problem drinking. The behaviors listed on page 341 are associated with abuse of alcohol. For each question, check either "yes" or "no". Answer each question as honestly as possible.

Look over your questions carefully. The more "yes" answers that you have, the more likely you are to have a problem with alcohol. If you answer yes to more than 5 questions, you may need to consider seeking help.

1. Do you ever drink more than other people yet seem to be less drunk?
2. Do you frequently drink before you attend a party where you know there will be alcohol?
3. Do you drink to stop yourself from worrying or calm your nerves?
4. Has your drinking led to problems or arguments with your family or friends?
5. Do you ever lie about any aspect of your drinking, such as how much or how often?
6. Do you find yourself driving under the influence of alcohol?
7. Once you start drinking, do you find it difficult to stop?
8. Do you sometimes drink to boost your self-confidence?
9. Do you find that you want a drink at a certain time every day?
10. Does the thought of never drinking again make life seem boring and unexciting?
11. Are your grades, work, or social life being affected by your alcohol intake?
12. After drinking, do you ever wake up in the morning and can't remember what you said or did?
13. Have you said things that you were later ashamed of or that embarrassed others when you were drinking?
14. Have you ever told yourself or promised others that you would not drink for a while but found that you could not or did not keep your promise?
15. Do you find yourself drinking enough to get high when you are alone?

Glossary

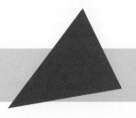

Abuse (of drugs)   Use of any drug, whether legal or illegal, that results in behavior or action that is detrimental to the user's health or the health of others. (Ch. 11)

Active Warmup   Dynamic movements for the purpose of readying the body for physical activity. (Ch. 3)

Acute (or communicable) Disease   A severe disease of short duration. (Ch. 1)

Adenosine Diphosphate (ADP)   A complex, high-energy compound from which ATP is resynthesized. (Ch. 3)

Adenosine Triphosphate (ATP)   A complex, high-energy compound stored in the cells from which the body derives its energy. (Ch. 3)

Adherence   Long-term participation. (Ch. 2)

Adipose Tissue   Fat cells. (Ch. 10)

Aerobic   Literally means "with oxygen." (Ch. 3)

Aerobic Capacity   The maximal ability to take in, deliver, and use oxygen; also referred to as cardiorespiratory endurance, or VO_2 max. (Ch. 6)

Agility   The ability to rapidly change direction while maintaining dynamic balance. (Ch. 1)

Agonist   The muscle that contracts to produce a specific movement; the prime mover. (Ch. 5)

Alcoholism   Abusive use of alcohol characterized by emotional and physical dependence and a loss of control over its use. (Ch. 11)

Alveoli   Tiny air sacs in the lungs that are richly perfused with blood. Gaseous exchange between the lungs and blood occurs at these sites. (Ch. 6)

Amenorrhea   Failure to menstruate. (Ch. 10)

Amino Acids   The building blocks of proteins. (Ch. 9)

Amotivational Syndrome   A collection of symptoms/behavior patterns associated with chronic use of marijuana where the user displays apathy towards life and a passive, introverted personality. (Ch. 11)

Anabolic Steroid   A drug with tissue-building or growth-simulating properties. (Ch. 5)

Anaerobic   Literally means "without oxygen." (Ch. 3)

Anaerobic Threshold   That point where exercise cannot be totally sustained by the aerobic processes. Anaerobic processes contribute to the production of ATP and lactic acid begins to accumulate in the blood. (Chs. 3, 6)

Androgen   Male sex hormone produced in the testes and, to a limited extent, from the adrenal cortex. (Ch. 5)

Android Obesity   Male pattern of fat deposition in the abdominal region. (Ch. 10)

Anorexia Nervosa   A psychological and emotional disorder characterized by excessive underweight. (Ch. 10)

Antagonist   The muscle that stretches in response to the contraction of the agonist muscle. (Ch. 5)

Aorta   Largest artery in the body. (Ch. 5)

Arterial-venous Oxygen Difference (a-vO_2 diff)   The difference between the oxygen (O_2) content of arterial and mixed venous blood. (Chs. 6, 7)

Asthma   Widespread narrowing of the airways of the lungs because of varying degrees of contraction or spasm of smooth muscle, edema of the mucosa, and mucus in the bronchi and bronchioles. (Ch. 8)

Atherosclerosis   A progressive disease that results in the narrowing of arterial channels caused by the buildup of plaque. (Ch. 7)

Autonomic Nervous System   That portion of the nervous system that controls involuntary activity, such as the smooth muscle of the digestive and the cardiac muscle of the myocardium. It includes both sympathetic and parasympathetic nerves. (Ch. 5)

Balance   Involves the maintenance of a desired body position either statically or dynamically. Also referred to as equilibrium. (Ch. 1)

Ballistic Stretching   Also known as dynamic stretching, ballistic stretching employs repetitive contractions of agonist muscles to produce rapid stretches of antagonist muscles. (Ch. 4)

Basal Metabolic Rate (BMR)   The energy required to sustain life while in a fasted and rested state. (Ch. 10)

Bioelectrical Impedance   A noninvasive method for estimating body fat by measuring the speed that an electrical current travels through the body. (Ch. 10)

Blood Alcohol Concentration (BAC)   The concentration of alcohol in a specific amount of blood; a BAC of 0.10% is illegal intoxication in most states, although some states use a BAC of 0.08%. (Ch. 11)

Blood Lactate   A metabolite that produces fatigue and results from incomplete breakdown of sugar. (Ch. 2)

Blood Platelets   Blood cells involved in preventing blood loss. Platelets are important components in clot formation. (Ch. 7)

Blood Pressure   The force that the blood exerts against the walls of the blood vessels. (Ch. 7)

Body composition   The amount of lean versus fat tissue in the body. (Chs. 6, 10)

Body Mass Index (BMI)   A method of estimating body composition by dividing body weight in kilograms by body height in meters squared. (Ch. 10)

Bulimarexia Nervosa   An eating disorder characterized by episodes of secretive binge eating followed by purging. (Ch. 10)

Burnout   A loss of energy, creativity, and direction. (Ch. 2)

Cancer   A large group of disorders characterized by abnormal cellular growth. (Ch. 8)

Carbon Monoxide   A colorless, odorless gas formed by the incomplete oxidation of carbon and highly poisonous when inhaled. (Ch. 7)

Carbohydrate   An organic compound composed of one or more sugars that are derived from plant sources. (Ch. 9)

Cardiac Muscle   Specialized muscle tissue found only in the heart. (Ch. 5)

Cardiac Output   The amount of blood pumped by the heart in one minute. (Ch. 6)

Cardiovascular Disease   A complex of diseases of the heart and circulatory system. (Chs. 1, 7)

Cardiorespiratory Endurance   The ability to take in, deliver, and extract oxygen for physical work. (Ch. 1)

Cerebrovascular Accidents   Diseases of the blood vessels to the brain or in the brain that result in a stroke. (Chs. 2, 7)

Cholesterol   An organic substance—the most abundant steroid in animal tissues, especially in bile and gallstones. Elevated blood cholesterol is a primary risk factor for heart disease. (Ch. 7)

Chronic Disease   A long-lasting and/or frequently occurring disease. (Ch. 1)

Chronological Age   An individual's calendar age. (Ch. 1)

Chylomicrons   Large, buoyant particles that are the primary transporters of triglycerides in the fasting state. (Ch. 7)

Circuit Training   A series of six to ten exercises performed in sequence and as rapidly as one's fitness level allows. (Ch. 5)

Concentric Muscular Contraction   That phase of muscular contraction in which the muscle shortens. (Ch. 5)

Conduction   Transference of heat from one object to another by physical contact. (Ch. 3)

Congenital Heart Disease   Heart defects that exist at birth and occur when the heart or its structures or the blood vessels near the heart fail to develop normally before birth. (Ch. 7)

Convection   Transfer of heat from the body to a moving gas or liquid. (Ch. 3)

Coordination   The integration of body parts resulting in smooth, fluid motion. (Ch. 1)

Cortical Bone   The dense, hard outer layer of bone such as that which appears in the shafts of the long bones of the arms and legs. (Ch. 8)

Crack   A solid form of cocaine, usually mixed with baking soda, that provides a strong, temporary sense of euphoria. (Ch. 11)

Creatine Phosphate (CP)   A chemical that donates its phosphate to ADP for the resynthesis of ATP. (Ch. 3)

Cross-training   Selection and participation in more than one physical activity on a consistent basis. (Ch. 3)

Crude Fiber   The fiber that remains in food after it has been treated with harsh chemicals during laboratory analysis. (Ch. 9)

Dehydration   Excessive loss of body fluids. (Ch. 3)

Depression   Prolonged sadness that persists beyond a reasonable length of time. (Ch. 8)

Diabetes Mellitus   A metabolic disorder in which the ability to oxidize carbohydrates is more or less completely lost because of faulty pancreatic activity and consequent disturbance of normal insulin mechanisms. It is often accompanied by resistance of receptor cells to insulin. (Ch. 7)

Diastolic Blood Pressure   The lowest pressure of arterial blood against the walls of the vessels or heart during diastole. (Ch. 7)

Dietary Fiber   The fiber that remains after food is digested in the human body. (Ch. 9)

Disaccharide   A combination of two simple sugars. (Ch. 9)

Distress   Normal stress that has become chronic. (Ch. 8)

Distressor   Negative or bad stress. (Ch. 8)

Double Product or Rate Pressure Product (RPP)   Heart rate multiplied by systolic blood pressure. It is an estimate of the oxygen required by the heart during aerobic exercise. (Ch. 6)

Drug   Other than food, any substance that enters the body and changes its usual function. (Ch. 11)

Drug Use   The wise, discriminate use of drugs. (Ch. 11)

Dynamic Stretching   (see ballistic stretching)

Eccentric Muscular Contraction   That phase of a muscular contraction in which the muscle lengthens. (Ch. 5)

Ectopic Pregnancy   An abnormal pregnancy where the embryo is implanted outside the uterus. (Ch. 11)

Electrolyte   Any solution that conducts an electrical current through its ions. (Chs. 3, 9)

Endogenous Cholesterol   Cholesterol manufactured within the body. (Ch. 7)

Epididymus   Long, coiled ducts in the male that carry sperm. (Ch. 11)

Erythrocytes   The red blood cells that transport oxygen from the lungs to the various tissues of the body and carbon dioxide from the tissues to the lungs. (Ch. 7)

Eustress   Good stress—occurs when one accepts and successfully handles a challenge. (Ch. 8)

Eustressor   Positive or good stress. (Ch. 8)

Evaporation   The loss of heat by changing a liquid to a vapor. (Ch. 3)

Exogenous Cholesterol   Cholesterol received through the diet. (Ch. 7)

Extrinsic (external) Reward   Any positive reinforcement emanating from an outside source—e.g., friends, coaches—that increases the strength of a response. (Ch. 2)

Fast-twitch Muscle Fiber   A type of muscle fiber that contracts rapidly but fatigues rapidly. Also referred to as white muscle fibers. (Ch. 5)

Fats   Organic compounds that are composed of glycerol and fatty acids. (Ch. 9)

Fetal Alcohol Syndrome (FAS)   Birth defects associated with the consumption of alcohol by the mother during pregnancy. (Ch. 11)

Fiber   The indigestible polysaccharides that are found in the stems, leaves, and seeds of plants. (Ch. 9)

Flexibility   The range of motion about a joint or series of joints. (Chs. 1, 4)

Flexometer   An instrument for measuring static flexibility. (Ch. 4)

Glycogen   The stored form of sugar. (Ch. 3)

Goal   Something toward which effort or movement is directed; an end or objective to be achieved. (Ch. 2)

Golgi Tendon Organ   A specialized receptor located in the muscles that responds to changes in muscles length and tension. (Ch. 4)

Goniometer   A protractorlike device used to measure the flexibility of various joints. (Ch. 4)

Gynoid Obesity   Female pattern of fat deposition in the thighs and gluteal areas. (Ch. 10)

Hallucinogen   Any drug that affects the user's sense of reality, alters visual and auditory perceptions, and causes hallucinations. (Ch. 11)

Health Age   An individual's biological age. (Ch. 1)

Health-related Fitness   A type of fitness that enhances one's health. (Ch. 1)

Heat Exhaustion   A condition characterized by a buildup of body heat. Symptoms include dizziness, fainting, rapid pulse, and cool skin. (Ch. 3)

Heat Stroke   The most dangerous of the heat-stress illnesses. Symptoms include a temperature of 106 degrees F and above, absence of sweating, dry skin, and often delirium, convulsions, and loss of consciousness. (Ch. 3)

Hemoglobin   Iron pigment of the red cells that combines with oxygen. (Chs. 3, 7)

HDL   A lipoprotein that transports cholesterol from the blood to the liver for degradation and removal (good cholesterol). (Ch. 7)

Hydrostatic Weighing   A method for determining specific gravity and percent body fat by underwater weighing. (Ch. 10)

Hyperplasia   An increase in size caused by an increase in the number of cells. (Ch. 5)

Hypertension   Medical term for high blood pressure. (Ch. 7)

Hyperthermia   Overheating; abnormally high body temperature. (Ch. 3)

Hypertrophy   An increase in size caused by an increase in the thickness of fibers. (Ch. 5)

Hypokinesis   Lack of physical activity. (Ch. 7)

Hypothermia   Abnormally low body temperature. (Ch. 3)

Insoluble Fiber   Cellulose, lignin, and hemicellulose that add bulk to the contents of the intestine, accelerating the passage of food rem-

nants through the digestive tract. They reduce the risk of colon cancer as well as other diseases of the digestive tract. (Ch. 9)

Intrinsic (internal) Reward   Reinforcement coming from within; the degree of satisfaction derived from participation in the absence of some visible reward. (Ch. 2)

Isokinetic Muscular Contraction   A dynamic contraction in which the muscles generate force against a variable resistance that moves at a constant rate of speed. (Ch. 5)

Isometric Muscular Contraction   A static concentration in which the muscles generate force against an immovable object with no observable shortening. (Ch. 5)

Isotonic Muscular Contraction   A dynamic contraction in which the muscles generate force against a constant resistance. Movement occurs as the muscles shorten and lengthen with each repetition. (Ch. 5)

Jaundice   Yellow coloring of the skin, mucus membrane, and whites of the eyes. (Ch. 11)

Kilocalories   The amount of energy found in food, it is the quantity of heat needed to raise the temperature of one kilogram of water one degree centigrade. (Ch. 9)

Kyphosis   Abnormal curvature of the thoracic region of the spine. (Ch. 8)

Lactic Acid   A fatiguing metabolite resulting from the incomplete breakdown of sugar. (Ch. 3)

LDL   A lipoprotein that transports cholesterol to the tissues. It is involved in the atherosclerotic process (bad cholesterol). (Ch. 7)

Leukocytes   White blood cells that protect the body against invading microorganisms and remove dead cells and debris from the body. (Ch. 7)

Locomotor Movement   Movements which bring about a change in location, including walking, jogging, climbing, cycling, and swimming, to name but a few. (Ch. 5)

Lordosis   Swayback; abnormal curvature of the low back. (Chs. 5, 8)

Metabolism   The sum of the chemical reactions and processes that supply the energy used by the body. (Ch. 6)

Metastasis The spread of cancer from the original site to other sites in the body. (Ch. 8)

Minerals Inorganic substances that exist freely in nature. (Ch. 9)

Misuse (of drugs) The using of any prescription or nonprescription drug for any reason other than that for which it was intended. (Ch. 11)

Mitochondria The cells power house in which ATP is produced aerobically. (Ch. 6)

Monosaccharide Simple sugars such as table sugar, honey, and molasses. (Ch. 9)

Motivation The internal mechanisms and external stimuli that arouse and direct behavior. (Ch. 2)

Motor Unit A motor nerve and all of the muscle fibers that it innervates. (Ch. 5)

Muscle Spindle A specialized receptor located in the muscles that is sensitive to changes in muscle length. (Ch. 4)

Muscular Endurance The ability of a muscle to sustain repeated contractions or to apply a constant force for a period of time. (Chs. 1, 5)

Muscular Strength The maximum amount of force that a muscle can exert in a single contraction. (Ch. 1)

Myocardial Infarction A heart attack. The term literally means "death of heart muscle tissue." (Ch. 7)

Myocardium Heart muscle. (Ch. 7)

Myotatic Reflex Stretch reflex. (Ch. 4)

Neoplasm Growth of new tissue (tumor). (Ch. 8)

Neurotransmitters Chemical messengers within a nerve cell. (Ch. 11)

Nicotine A stimulant and poisonous drug found in tobacco products. (Ch. 7)

Nonlocomotor Movement Movements that take place around the axis of the body. The subject remains in one place creating dynamic movement by means of stretching, bending, stopping, pushing, pulling, and twisting, among numerous other motions. (Ch. 5)

Obesity Excessive body fat—23 percent to 24 percent or greater for males; 30 percent or greater for females. (Chs. 7, 10)

Oncogene A cancer-causing gene. (Ch. 8)

Osteoarthritis Degenerative joint disease characterized by the deterioration of articular cartilage, particularly in the weight-bearing joints. Often referred to as the wear-and-tear disease. (Ch. 8)

Osteoblast Bone-forming cells. (Ch. 8)

Osteoclast Cells that break down and absorb bone. (Ch. 8)

Osteoporosis Reduction in the quantity of bone as a result of demineralization and atrophy of skeletal tissue. (Ch. 8)

Overload Periodically stressing the body with greater loads than those usually experienced. (Ch. 5)

Overweight Excess weight for one's height regardless of body composition . (Ch. 10)

Oxygen Debt The amount of oxygen needed in recovery from exercise above that normally required during rest. (Ch. 6)

Oxygen Deficit The period of time when exercise begins during which the body does not supply all of the oxygen needed to support exercise. (Ch. 6)

Passive Smoke Also called sidestream or secondhand smoke, the smoke emitted from the end of a burning cigarette. (Ch. 11)

Passive Warmup Inactive means of preparing for physical activity that may include massage and dry and wet heat. (Ch. 3)

Performance-related Fitness A type of fitness that allows one to perform physical skills with a high degree of proficiency. (Ch. 1)

Periodization A way to provide variety in training. The training period is divided into different cycles in which the volume is periodically reduced and the intensity is concomitantly increased. (Ch. 5)

Phospholipids Similar to a triglyceride, except that one of the fatty acids is replaced by a phosphorous-containing acid. (Ch. 9)

Polysaccharides The joining of three or more simple sugars to form starch and glycogen. (Ch. 2)

Positive Reinforcement A reward; increases the strength of a response or responses. (Ch. 2)

Power A function of work divided by the time that it takes to perform the work. (Ch. 1)

Proprioceptive Neuromuscular Facilitation (PNF) A group of stretching techniques involving the alternation of contraction and relaxation of various muscles. (Ch. 4)

Protein A food substance formed from amino acids. (Ch. 9)

Psychoneuroimmunology Branch of medical science that studies how the mind affects the endocrine, neural, and immune systems. (Ch. 1)

Radiation Transfer of heat from the body to the atmosphere by electromagnetic waves. (Ch. 3)

Reaction Time The elapsed time between the presentation of a stimulus and the stimulus's response. Also called response latency. (Ch. 1)

Residual Volume The air remaining in the lungs following a maximum exhalation.

Resting Metabolic Rate (RMR) The conditions for measuring BMR are difficult to achieve, and when they are approximated, the term resting metabolic rate is used. It is an approximation of the energy required to sustain life while in the resting state. (Ch. 10)

Retrovirus Viruses with the ability to interrupt the ordinary flow of genetic material. (Ch. 11)

Risk Factor Genetic tendencies and learned behaviors that increase the probability of premature illness and death. (Ch. 1)

Saturated Fats Found primarily in animal flesh and dairy products. Chemically, they carry the maximum number of hydrogen atoms. (Ch. 9)

Scoliosis   Abnormal lateral curvature of the spine. (Ch. 8)

Self-concept   The set of peoples' beliefs about and evaluations of themselves as persons. (Ch. 2)

Skeletal Muscle   Voluntary muscles whose attachments to the bones of the skeletal system provide the basis for human movement. (Ch. 5)

Skinfold Measurement   A method for determining percent body fat by measuring a pinch of skin at selected sites with a skinfold caliper. (Ch. 10)

Slow-twitch Muscle Fiber   A type of muscle fiber that contracts slowly but is difficult to fatigue. Also referred to as red muscle fibers. (Ch. 5)

Smooth Muscle   Muscle located in the blood vessels and digestive system; not under conscious or voluntary control. (Ch. 5)

Soluble Fiber   Pectin, gums, and other substances that add bulk to the contents of the stomach. They lower blood cholesterol levels. (Ch. 9)

Speed   Performance of a movement in the shortest amount of time. Also known as velocity. (Ch. 1)

Static Stretching   Stretching that employs slow movements and positions that are held for 15 to 30 seconds. (Ch. 4)

Sterol   One of the three major fats with a structure similar to cholesterol. (Ch. 9)

Stimulus   Any energy impinging upon an organism that results in a response. (Ch. 2)

Strength   The force exerted by a muscle or muscle group in a single maximal contraction. (Ch. 5)

Stressor   Any event, condition, or situation that results in change, threat, or loss. (Ch. 8)

Stretch Reflex   The myotatic reflex that responds to stretching of the muscle tissues. (Ch. 4)

Stroke Volume   The amount of blood pumped by the heart with each beat. (Ch. 6)

Systolic Blood Pressure   The greatest pressure in the blood vessels or heart during a cardiac cycle as the result of systole. (Ch. 7)

Testosterone   A sex hormone appearing in much higher concentrations in males than females. (Ch. 5)

Thermogenic Effect of Food (TEF)   The energy required to digest and absorb food. (Ch. 10)

Tidal Volume   The amount of air inhaled and exhaled with each breath. (Ch. 6)

Trabecular Bone   Spongy bone; not as dense as cortical bone. (Ch. 8)

Triglycerides   Consist of three fatty acids attached to a glycerol molecule. (Chs. 7, 9)

Unsaturated fats   Fatty acids in which one or more points is free of hydrogen atoms. (Ch. 9)

Urethra   Small, tubular structure that drains urine from the bladder in males and females. (Ch. 11)

Valsalva Maneuver   Occurs when individuals lift heavy weights and hold their breath. The glottis closes and intrathoriacic pressure increases, hindering the flow of blood to the heart. (Ch. 5)

Ventilation   The amount of air inhaled and exhaled per minute. (Ch. 6)

Very-low Calorie Diet   Diet that contains 800 or fewer kCals per day. (Ch. 10)

Vital Capacity   The amount of air that can be expired after a maximum inhalation. (Ch. 6)

Vitamins   Organic compounds found in food that are essential to normal metabolism. (Ch. 9)

VLDL   Lipoproteins that are the primary transporters of endogenous triglycerides in the fasting state. (Ch. 7)

Vulva   The external female genitalia. (Ch. 11)

W

Weight Cycling   Repeated cycles of weight loss followed by weight gain. (Ch. 10)

Wellness   A dynamic approach to optimal health that emphasizes positive health behaviors and preventive practices. (Ch. 1)

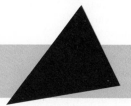

Index

frequency, intensity, duration and rest,
114–115
overload, progression and maintenance,
112–114
tests for
Canadian trunk strength test, 318, 319*f*
endurance, 318
strength, 317*t*–318
summary of, 318
training for
circuit, 111–112, 112*t*
isokinetic, 110–111
isometric, 106–108
isotonic, 108–110
Muscular system, 114*f*, 116*f*
Music, effect of, on exercise, 37–38
Myocardial infarction, 156
Myocardium, 151
Myotatic reflex, 75

National Academy of Sciences, 187
National Cancer Institute, 200
National Heart, Lung, and Blood Institute, 166
National Institute of Mental Health, 32
National Institutes of Health (NIH), 177, 241
National Sporting Goods Association, 15
Natural killer cells, 200–201
Nautilus Diet, 251*t*
Nautilus equipment, exercises performed on,
117*f*, 118*f*, 119*f*, 120*f*, 121*f*
Neck, stretching exercises for, 78*f*–79*f*, 87*f*, 90*f*
Neoplasm, 196
Neurotransmitters, 273
Never-Say-Diet Diet (Simmons), 250
New vegetarian diet, 226
Nicotine
toxic effects of, 160, 274–275
withdrawal symptoms for, 160
Nicotine patch, 279
Nonlocomotor movements, 97
Nonprescription drugs, 273
Norepinephrine, 56
Nutrament, 251*t*
NutriSystems, 250
Nutrition
carbohydrates, 215–218
fats, 219–221, 220*t*
fiber, 218–219
food guide pyramid, 214*f*–215
food labeling, 215, 217*f*
medical school courses in, 12
minerals, 230
protein, 222–223
role of, in death, 243
safety tips for, 232
vegetarianism, 225–226
vitamins, 227–230
Nutritional assessment
inventory for, 333*t*–334*t*
protein requirements, 333
two-day food plan, 333, 335–336

Nutrition Research Center on Aging at Tufts
University, 225

Obesity
android, 241
in children and adolescents, 240
definition of, 240
gynoid, 241
heredity as cause of, 244–245
as risk factor for cardiovascular disease,
175–176
and wellness, 241–243
O'Bryant, H., 109
Obsessiveness, avoiding, about exercise, 39–40
Oligomenorrhea, 238
Oncogenes, 197
Optifast, 251*t*
Osteoarthritis, 190, 194–195, 200
Osteoblasts, 184
Osteoclasts, 184
Osteoporosis, 100, 184
effects of, 185*f*
prevention and treatment of, 186, 187–188
risk factors for, 184–186
types of, 184
Overeaters Anonymous, 251*t*
Overhead press using free and machine
weights, 117*f*
Overload, 112, 114
and progression, 54–55
Over-the-counter drugs, 273
Overtraining, recognizing signs of, 53
Overweight, 240
Oxidation, 213
Oxygen
body mass and utilization of, 135
partial pressure of, at various altitudes, 67*t*
Oxygen debt, 136*f*
Oxygen deficit, 136*f*
Oxygen demand, 48*f*, 142
Ozone, 68

Parallel-bar dips, 125*f*
Passive smoke, 274
Passive warm-up, 49
Pelvic tilt, 192*f*
Perceived exertion, 52, 53*f*
Performance-related fitness, 14, 228–229
Personal exercise program, 311
Personal fitness contract, 309–310
Personality types, 207–208
Pesticides, synthetic, 223
Phospholipids, 219–220
Physical activity
and osteoarthritis, 194–195
in prevention and treatment of osteoporo-
sis, 187

questionnaire for assessing, 309
Physical fitness
attitudes assessment for, 307
in business and industry, 17–19
of children and adolescents, 16
exercise for, 14
as fad, 15–16
objectives of, 12–14, 13*t*
prototype fitness and wellness center, 28*f*
Physical inactivity
effects of, on body composition, 249*t*
most sedentary state in US, 12
as risk factor for cardiovascular disease,
170–175, 172*f*
as risk factor for osteoporosis, 186
Physicians Weight Loss Center, 250
Pole walking, 96
Polysaccharides, 216
Popcorn Plus Diet, 251*t*
Positive attitude as exercise motivator, 39, 40
Positive reinforcements, 30
Posture, 100, 191*f*
Potassium loss during exercise, 64
Potatoes, consumption of, 223
Power, 14
Pregnancy, exercise during, 57–60
Prescription drugs, 273
President's Commission on Mental Health, 205
President's Council on Physical Fitness and
Sports, 21
Press-ups, 193*f*
"Prevention Index," 11
Pritkin Permanent Weight Loss Manual, 251*t*
Progress chart as exercise motivator, 37, 38*t*
Progression, 54–55, 114
Progressive extension with pillows, 193*f*
Progressive relaxation for managing stress, 207
Progressive resistance exercises, 100, 106
Proprioceptive neuromuscular facilitation
(PNF), 76–77
contract-relax technique, 77*f*
hold-relax technique, 77
limitations of, 78
slow-reversal-hold-relax technique, 77*f*–78
Proteins, 222–223
assessing requirements for, 333
daily requirements for, 224*t*–225
energy yield from, 220*t*
as fuel source, 46
recommended consumption of, 216*t*
in selected foods, 295*t*–303*t*
sources of, 223–224*t*
Psychoactive drugs, 273*t*
Psychoneuroimmunology, 5
Pulse meters, 17
Pulse rates, sites for taking, 51, 52*f*
Push-ups, 125*f*
modified version of, 126*f*
risks with arched-back, 86*f*
straight-back, 86*f*

Quadriceps
isometric strength measurement for, 124*f*

stretching exercises for, 82f–83f
risks with, 89f

terol, 169*t*
Total energy expenditure, calculating, 337–338
Trabecular bone, 184
Trace minerals, 231*t*
Training effect, loss of, 142–143
Treadmill, 55*f*
Treatment costs for preventable conditions, 9*t*
Triceps skinfold measurement, 260*f*
Triglycerides, 177–178, 220
Trunk flexion, 192*f*
Trunk rolls, 88*f*
Twins and obesity studies, 244–245
Type A personality, 207
Type B personality, 207

Underweight and exercise, 255–256
Universal equipment, exercises performed on, 118*f*
Unsaturated fats, 221
Upper back, stretching exercises for, 80*f*–81*f*
Urethra, 279

Variety, need for, in exercise program, 39
Vegan diet, 226
Vegetables
    consumption of, by high school students, 223
    most popular, 12
Vegetarianism, 225–226
Ventilation, 134

Very low density lipoprotein (VLDL), 166–168, 167*f*
Very-low kCal diets, 253
Vital capacity, 139
Vitamins, 227-230
    antioxidants, 229-230
    fat-soluble, 227, 227*t*
    loss of, through cooking, 223
    and performance, 229
    synthetic versus natural, 228
    water-soluble, 227, 228*t*
Vulva, 281

Waist/hip ratio (WHR), 242, 243
Walnuts, cholesterol lowering effect of, 166
Warm-ups for exercise, 49–50
Water
    loss of, during exercise, 65
    and nutrition, 230–232
Water Diet (Stillman), 252*t*
Water-soluble vitamins, 227, 228*t*
Weight (body)
    desirable, 264–265, 337
    and earning power, 242
Weight-bearing exercises
    aerobic, 100
    kCal expenditure during, 245
Weight cycling, 253–254
Weight loss, 163, 255
Weight training, 102, 105–106, 109
Weight Training: Scientific Approach (Stone and O'Bryant), 109
Weight Training-Steps to Success (Baechle and Groves), 109
Weight Watchers Quick Success Program, 251*t*

Wellness
    assessment of, 305–307
    and body composition, 241–243
    definition of, 4–6
    dimensions of, 4–6
    effect of stress on, 203–204
    factors of, 6*f*
    and flexibility, 73–74
    health habits in, 8–11
    and muscular training, 99–102
    safety tips for, 18
    self-responsibility for, 6
Wind chill index, 66*t*
Women
    and alcohol, 276
    back extension test standards for, 314*t*
    BMI and weight classification for, 258*t*
    bone loss in, 186
    and cardiovascular disease, 158
    deaths from AIDS, 284*t*
    long-distance running for, 12
    muscle endurance standards for, 318*t*
    relative cardiorespiratory fitness levels for, 322*t*–333*t*
    shoulder flexion test standards for, 315*t*
    sit-and-reach test standards for, 314*t*
    skinfold measurements for, 263*t*
    smoking and lung cancer in, 199*f*
    standards for partial curl-up test, 319*t*
    strength-to-body-weight ratio for, 317*t*
    weight training for, 102

Yoga plow, risks with, 86*f*